COPYRIGHT PAGE

For information, or to order write:
Jennifer Hart
Hart 2 Heart Innovations
PO Box 580
Ashland, OR 97520
E-mail: jennifer@hart2heart.com
www.hart2heart.com
www.MarleyRides.com

Cover design by Jennifer Hart and Jeff Altemus

Marley Rides by Jennifer Hart
ISBN: 0-9777632-2-6
Printed in the United States of America

10 9 8 7 6 5 4 3 2

"The great hope for society is individual character."

William Ellery Channing

Marley Rides is dedicated to
Catie, Rhys, Julia, and Constant.
For their unconditional love and encouragement—
a reminder to live another day.

Marley Up!

TABLE OF CONTENTS

ACKNOWLEDGEMENTS

Without the following people, this story would not be worth writing about. Thank you for your part in our lives and for the creation of Marley Rides.

Marley Pratt
Catie Pratt
Drew Pratt
Cindy Warzyn
Laura Blount
Vanessa Blount
Rhys Rounds
Selene Foster
Jeff Altemus
Jay Newman
Constant Hine
Sunny Kieley
Andrea Freewater
John & Sharon Javna
Angela Kern
Kim Strubel
Reagan Burrell
Lucas Morgan
Luke Thomas
Debbie Thornton
Dermaris McNarmara
Kate, Katie, Tim, Jim, & Pat
Nicky Hardenbergh
Garrick Cole
Joseph & Julia Gunnels
Winston, Peter, & Rawley
Tim & KC Little
Martha Little
Claudia Bauer
John Dollison
Gordon & Maggie Javna
Debra Gates
Eric Stahlman
Dee & Kellar
Adam & Dena
Jennifer Strange
Adam Silver
Sean Grace
Dal Carver
Denise Wingler
Dustin & Shaney
Thom Little
Julia Papps
Allen Orso
Dan Kock
Paul Stanley
Annie McIntyre
Sage, Zipper, Salsa, & Gracie
Steve Scholl
Lorraine Katena
Kim Faerber
Brian Moreland
Susan Leavitt
Elizabeth & Rex Morgan
Colestin Rural Fire Dept.
Cynthia & Wes Norton
Jennifer & Alex Dykema
Sooling Jay Rounds
Nan Inglis
Catherine Riesgo

***"I may be going to hell in a bucket,
but at least I'm enjoying the ride."***

—The Grateful Dead

PROLOGUE

ONCE THERE WAS A BOY
by Selene Foster

Once, in the beginning, when I had just moved to Ashland, Marley and I had a talk outside during a party, sitting on the top of the monkey bars in the back yard. He knew he had cancer and he wanted money and things to do. He didn't want answers from me, or even suggestions; he wanted to be heard. A year later, I sat with his sister Catie around a campfire at a family reunion. We had learned Marley's cancer had metastasized, and there was very little anyone could do. I had no solutions. Catie had nothing to be comforted by. She sobbed in the firelight and it made me feel better. In the face of indecision, indirection, the lack of answers, one must do the only thing one can do: the obvious.

Once I sat on the top of a high hill with Marley and talked about how beautiful the land was. Once he told me how many times he had given roses to girls at school and had them given back. Once he held my hand through my father's funeral. It was never his words that made me love him, although he once told me I don't take enough risks—and that has changed me forever. It was his willingness to live without answers, or even attempts at answers, that changed me.

He was an ass half the time, but he knew that what I needed was impartial and unobstructed love, and that this could be imparted with the smallest of gestures. He would reach out the instant before I gave up trying to help him. The night before he died, he made the smallest of movements to kiss my cheek, just enough to make it okay for me.

There is no making sense of who he was. There is no explaining the impulse we all had: To do anything for him. Our daily experience of living with the knowledge that he would die did not arrest our own needs. His indignation was fierce. He demanded attention. He made friends with the dirty, smelly guy on the corner. He saved us all from certain normalcy.

INTRODUCTION

Passing the Torch

This tale chronicles the adventures of Marley's 18-year visit to Earth. It begins with the letters I wrote to my son before he was born. The rest of this book is based on e-mails written to "Marley's Network"—those who joined this family before you. Also included are new letters written to you as my narrative and stories written by friends and family. I call these submissions "The Butterfly Effect" as an example that all we do, as individuals, influences everything else.

I feel it is of vital importance to recount what our family learned about communication, cancer, doctors, fear, and the cowboy way of living and dying—information you may need now or when you encounter sickness and death.

Everyone dies, even extraordinary people. Yet very few families seem to share their stories, thereby leaving the rest of us without their valuable knowledge. I offer to you here the stories provided by Marley's life and death.

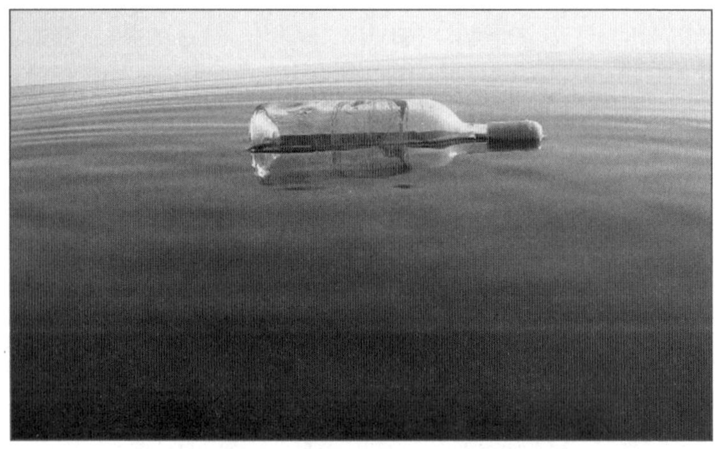

"Message in a Bottle"
An ongoing art project by Jay Little

Photo: Jay Little

Chapter One:
The Fine Art of Parenting

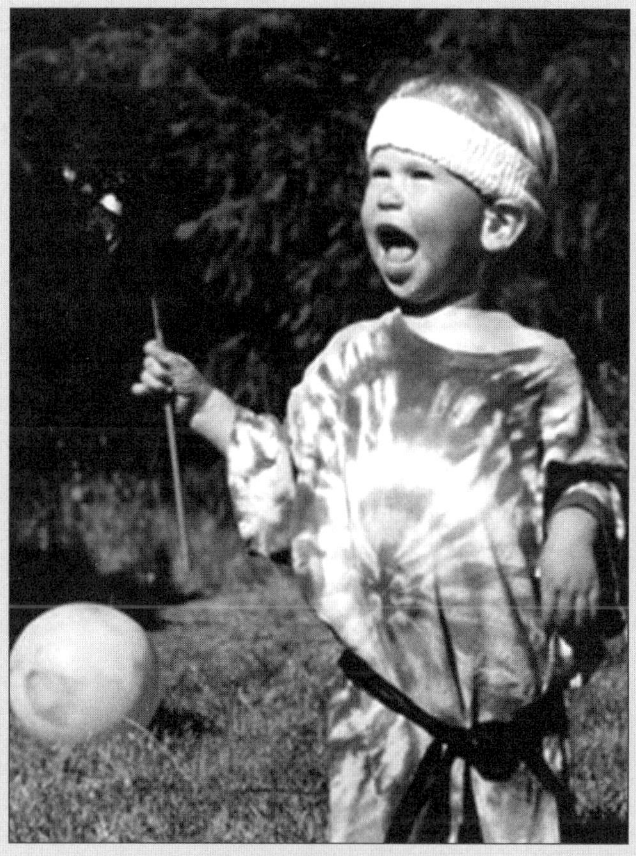

Meet Marley

Photo: Jennifer

DREAMSCAPE

Winds of Change

I was standing in a field of three foot high blue grass. A gentle breeze was making the tall, slender blades flow in wave-like patterns. Never in my wildest dreams had I seen grass that color of neon blue. The sound and sight of my surroundings took my breath away. I stood below the crystal clear pale blue sky, filled with a total sense of calm.

In an instant, clouds started forming in the distance, and before I knew what was happening, they began to rush toward me. The wind started blowing harder, creating a clearly defined path in the grass. The grass bent sideways like opposing waves, parting from the horizon to my feet. In the distance I saw a brilliant ball of light rolling down the path. It was coming at me with an incredible speed, but I couldn't move. I was frozen not only by the beauty of this ball of light, but by the growing intensity of my feelings. The closer it came, the more I was filled with a joy a thousand times more powerful than anything I knew.

I stretched my arms open wide as if to embrace the oncoming sphere, though it was far larger than I. When it was just a few feet away, I thought I was going to pop witnessing its indescribable beauty. I was overwhelmed with the most unusual feeling of being totally loved. As it engulfed me, it knocked me backward ever so gently, in a slow motion fall. I thought I had died and gone to heaven. I was in a state of complete and unadulterated bliss. I was Home! And then it was dark.

A tear rolled from my right eye and landed in my ear. I awoke to find myself looking up at the rear dome light on the ceiling of my Suburban. I wiped the tear away and rolled my head to the left to see Rhys sleeping soundly next to me under a pile of down blankets. The dream came back to me and I wrapped my arms around myself and cried from the feeling of joy lost.

Why I was sleeping in the truck with Rhys? I sat up in a panic and looked out the window. My rig was parked in Drew's front yard. Drew was the father of my two children, Marley and Catie.

He and his wife Cindy had built the two-story white house I was blankly staring at. The dream was forgotten as reality hit me hard. Marley! My heart started beating fast, and it felt like I had been punched hard in the solar plexus.

Was this really real or was I in another dream? How could I go from feeling so undeniably full to so incredibly empty so fast? Marley? Why wasn't I with Marley? And then I remembered the night before. I was not by his side because my beautiful son had died six hours earlier. I slumped forward, sitting in my nest of blankets and put my head in my hands. Oh God! Was it really true?

I quietly slipped on my shorts and T-shirt. I didn't want to wake Rhys, but I needed to go be with Marley. I gently kicked the back door open and crawled out of the Suburban. It was 5 A.M. on a cool, clear summer morning. A slight breeze was blowing through the tall green grass of the hayfields surrounding the house. The silence was deafening. It was too early for the birds. The three cow dogs weren't even awake yet. In my bare feet, I quietly walked up the steps of the front porch and snuck in the front door. No one was stirring anywhere in the house.

I walked through the living room and past the kitchen. In the hall, a candle was still burning outside of Marley's bedroom. I slowly opened the door and saw his body. He was lying face up, looking as if he were just resting. I froze. I held my breath and watched his chest for any movement. The lace curtains, gently flapping in the breeze, were the only things moving. I wrapped my arms around myself for support and just stood there. My boy was dead.

Then the feeling of the dream came back and I started to cry, feeling the joy that must have been his when he died. He was free! He was now free to ride the world's largest ATV through the thickest mud ever. He could ride his horse again and soar over the highest jumps on his bike. He was free to ride anything he wanted for as long as he wanted without any pain or worries.

I wiped my tears away and looked around. I saw Drew through the lace-covered windows, wandering, as if lost, in the field just outside Marley's room. Drew's guitar was propped against the wall next to Marley's bed. Laying on the floor next to it was the book he kept his sheet music in. I had made that book for Drew eighteen years before, and it still had the same black-and-white photo of Marley on the cover. I knew he must have been quietly singing to Marley in the pre-dawn hours. My heart melted for Drew's pain—our firstborn was gone.

It was my turn to sit with Marley. I went to the closet and retrieved my sketch pad and pencil. I spent the next hour looking at Marley—really looking at Marley—the way I do only when drawing things. I thought I knew every molecule of Marley—every curve, scar, and line—but I was to learn how every one of his eyebrow hairs touched the next, and I felt the curves of his lips through the tip of my pencil. During that precious time alone with my son's face, I was in a state of grace. His eyes were slightly open, and within them, I glimpsed another world.

I knew I was recording this special day in a way no photograph could capture. Because I was looking at him so intensely, I was able to notice the minute movements of his torso. Even six hours after death, the muscles were still relaxing, gases traveling up while gravity was pulling his blood down. They were the micromovements of watching bamboo grow—but much slower, and more subtle than watching the moon slide over the crest of a mountain.

Drew started prowling closer. I knew he wanted more time with Marley's body. I tapped on the window to tell him I was ready. I stood next to the bed looking down at my 18-year-old son, lying naked under his favorite John Deere blanket, wearing the colorful necklace his Uncle Jay had made for him. His long arms were folded across his chest. He looked so peaceful.

Drew entered the room, looking hollow. I wished I could give him my dream to hold on to. He sat down and just stared at Marley's body. As I passed him to leave, I put my hand on his shoulder and remembered first meeting him and all the training we had done in preparation for this moment.

A GLINT IN MAMA'S EYE

Desert Songs

In 1981, Drew and I met in Marin County, California, while working together at Rites of Passage, Inc. Drew and I lived and worked together for four years, guiding monthly groups of youths and adults to the desert wilderness to mark various life transitions. These rite-of-passage experiences included a three-day solo while fasting. Watching hundreds of people face their fears was awesome work. We loved teaching people how to survive alone in the wilderness and witnessing what happened when people relied on their intuition, trusting the lessons that the natural world offered.

Drew and I learned how to let people face the consequences of their own choices. We also learned how important it is to listen to the guide within ourselves. Even though we loved what we did and had no intelligent reason to stop, we knew in our guts that it was time to focus on something new. Just what exactly, we didn't know. We just had to trust. So in the spring of 1984, we prepared to resigned.

> ***"We are driven toward a higher perfection as surely as the sun pulls the life in the seed toward its light."***
>
> **—Gloria Karpinski**

One of our last trips was leading a group of high school seniors that were marking their passage from children to adults. It was a church group that wanted to do something important together, something dangerous and memorable as they prepared to go out into the world. It was evening when we arrived in a magical desert canyon and set up base camp. The following morning, each teenager picked a direction to explore in order to find their solo spot. They paired up with whoever was going in their direction while Drew and I stayed in base camp.

Hours after the six pairs of kids had left base camp and the hot desert sun warmed the surface of the earth, hordes of baby rattlesnakes started venturing out of their dens. They were everywhere! We knew this was very special—never before had we experienced this—tarantula migrations, yes, but not this. We could only hope the kids would remember what they had been taught: to walk in balance, and to be hyper-aware of the world around them. That evening we all agreed to continue the trip as planned, though many of them had encountered the snakes as well. The following morning, we said good-bye to the kids as they left us to start their three-day solos. We had taught them all we could. It was time to let them discover their inner teachers.

As dawn broke the next morning, Drew and I made love. Snuggling afterwards, we noticed a six-inch baby rattlesnake curled up very close to our sleeping bags, under a nearby bush. We weren't afraid—we knew enough about snakes to be able to lie there together and observe its miniature beauty. That was the morning Marley was conceived.

Watching the Grass Grow

Before the tests could be accurate, I knew I was pregnant. The timing was perfect to start spending more time at home. Thankfully, we had the means to survive without needing jobs. As an adult orphan, I had inherited some money, which allowed me to focus on the grass growing, flies buzzing, clouds changing, and my ever-growing belly. Drew was a luthier (a maker of stringed instruments), and worked at home.

I spent those nine months focusing on the changes within, meditating, and writing to our unborn baby, who we called "Cosmo." It was a very sweet, calm time for Drew and me. It was an unforgettable rite of passage for one of the most monumental transitions of our lives—becoming parents.

"Unless one says good-bye to what one loves, and unless one travels to completely new territories, one can expect merely a long wearing away of oneself and an eventual extinction."

—Jean Dubuffet

Written by me, two weeks before Marley
(AKA "Cosmo") was born
January 17, 1985

PARENTAL INTENTIONS

Dear Cosmo,

It is my intention to love you unconditionally throughout this life. There will inevitably be times of closeness and separateness, but always I will love you as I love myself.

It is my intention to be aware of your individual needs in order to manifest your total Self. This awareness will help me to be able to guide you toward the path you have chosen so *you* can acquire the knowledge you desire. I will not try to make you see the world through my purpose.

As your parent, it is my intention never to lie to you. I will do my best to be there for you when you need me to support you in the most helpful way.

It is my intention to be a good mother deserving of your choice, as one who will be able to provide you with many of the tools you will need to live a full and meaningful life.

I simply wish to love you and to be able to receive love from you.

Thank you, my little one, for choosing us; it has changed me considerably already.

Peace unto you, child,
Jennifer

"The future belongs to those who believe in the beauty of their dreams."

—Eleanor Roosevelt

IGNORANCE IS BLISS

Cosmic Education

The way I figure it, babies begin as cosmic beings, ready for rebirth, that hover around connecting couples. They are busy scanning potential human parents that will provide them with the circumstances for their continued growth as a soul. I've felt them during times of lovemaking, some gently knocking on my door asking if I'm ready and willing, politely waiting for the answer, and some with the gentleness of a bulldozer, not caring what I had to say about anything. Marley was of the bulldozer variety.

> ***"Grown-ups never understand anything for themselves, and it is tiresome for children to be always and forever explaining things to them."***
>
> **—Antoine de Saint-Exupery, *The Little Prince***

When I got pregnant, it felt like this child had chosen Drew and me whether we were ready or not. We didn't feel prepared to enter the world of parenting but, Marley was right, we were ready. I spent those nine months of pregnancy devouring books about birthing and parenting. Marley was overdue, I was tired of being pregnant, and I was getting impatient. I was completely oblivious of what I would face. Ignorance can be bliss—without it, far fewer children would be born!

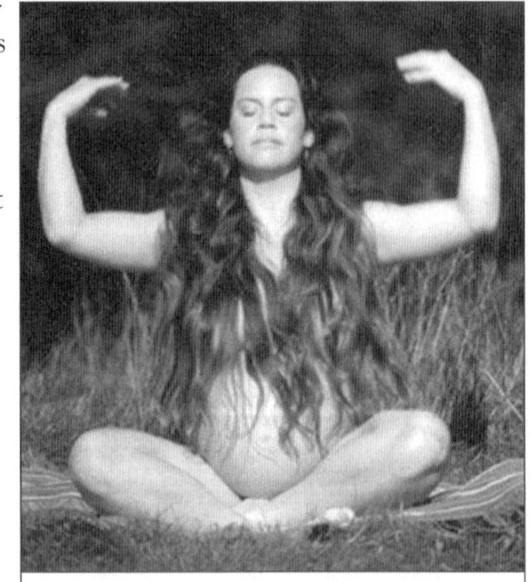

Yours truly, nine months pregnant.
Photo: Drew Pratt

THE BIRTH OF A STAR

Home Sweet Home

On February 6th, 1985, Marley Jacob Pratt was born at 11:15 P.M. Where Marley was to be born was never questioned. Home is where the heart is; besides, I had never been in a hospital. I had watched both of my parents die at home, and I had watched two of my nephews being birthed at home. To us, it didn't make sense to go to a hospital to do what people have been doing at home for centuries.

At two in the afternoon, a member of our birthing team (two midwives and a doctor) came to check on my dilation. She asked us if we had everything ready. "Yes, Ma'am! Triple checked and ready for action!" She examined me, rolled her eyes upward, said we had plenty of time, and left. Ugggh! We were bored of being excited, so we took a nap.

When we woke up, the wind was starting to howl; a storm was brewing. Our house was built halfway up a steep ravine, among towering ponderosa and redwood trees. Being in that house during a storm was something both Drew and I always liked. The view from our downstairs bedroom was of massive tree trunks, just feet from the windows, slowly swaying, which gave the eerie impression that the whole house was moving.

The Cosmo Cometh

We waited until the last minute to call the midwives again. We didn't want them to drive so far just to wave a hand and say, "You've got plenty of time!" Unfortunately, we didn't consider how the storm would slow them down.

The final labor stages lasted only a few minutes, and the doctor arrived just seconds before Marley burst forth. From my perspective, it seemed like Marley thought it would be really cool to see if he could fly to the opposite wall. After our slimy newborn was resting on my chest, the doctor made some comment about adding a catcher's mitt to his medical kit. This was the method of living that Marley would adhere to for the rest of his days; he would take his sweet time until he knew he was sure of the situation, and then he'd forget the brakes and go full tilt boogy.

Transitions

As soon as Marley arrived, it occurred to me that nine and a half months wasn't enough time to prepare. Caring for a colicky newborn first child is, in my opinion, the most exhausting, selfless act a person can do (although caring for the dying is a very close second).

From the beginning, Marley had a voracious appetite that kept me busier than I had ever been in my life. He never did break the habit of gulping air when he drank—whether it was milk from my breast or Mountain Dew from a can. By the time he was eighteen, he had perfected belching and farting as an art form.

My favorite memory of Marley's first week: Him lying on my chest while soaking in our big claw foot bathtub, watching the trees sway in the February winds. It had been a long night and the bath was our relief; a warm, watery sanctuary that was salve for the war wounds of no sleep, clothes soaked with breast milk, and the frustration of not understanding my newborn's language.

Marley was relaxed and happy for the first time in hours. So relaxed, in fact, he finally released all of the milky food and gaseous glory that had been tormenting him. Unfortunately, it did not come in the form of a benign belch—this was the stuff nightmares are made of and plants thrive on. Once past the brief state of shock, I called for Drew's assistance. He entered the bathroom, made a face like one of those old ladies made from a dried apple, and said, "Jesus H. Christ! What happened?" I was surrounded by a thick film of yellow-orange oily curds—Marley had taken a crap. All we could do was laugh and start the bath over again. From the beginning, this child was my instructor in patience, humor, unconditional loving, and perseverance.

"A weed is no more than a flower in disguise."

—James Russell Lowell

MAKING THE MOVE

Retreating Home

When Marley was six months old, we moved to Ashland, Oregon. Within two days of our first visit to this town, we bought five acres of wild land, complete with a two-room rustic cabin, running water, but no electricity.

The morning after we arrived at our little cabin, Drew unloaded the moving van while I took a break to change Marley's wet diaper. It was a chilly June morning, so I was kneeling in front of the wood stove with Marley on the floor. In a whoosh of energy, a hot coal leapt out of the stove and landed right in Marley's belly button. I grabbed it within a quarter second and was lifting my screaming baby as I heard a car door slam and Drew exclaim, "You're the last person I expected to see!" Seconds later, my sister Constant found me amid stacks of boxes, soothing Marley.

One year earlier, Constant had begun a spiritual sabbatical to end old patterns. This included not associating with family. We were very close friends, as well as sisters, so this was difficult. She even missed the birth of her nephew. I wasn't aware that her retreat had ended—or that she had moved to Ashland just two days before we did.

Both of us had followed our intuition, guided by our meditations, and had landed in the same town just days apart. Constant had come to tell me that our 21-year-old nephew, Sean, had died in an auto accident. We hugged and cried and then hugged some more and laughed at the bizarre circumstances.

Both of my parents had already died, but this was the first accidental death I had experienced. I was not prepared for the shock of disbelief. I was stunned. I swayed in my rocking chair, holding my own boy-child as close as possible, unable to comprehend what my brother Ric, his wife Mollie, and their other son Charlie were feeling. All I could feel was the dark void of the space that Sean once consumed. I felt hollow.

For months, I felt guilty that I had a baby to cuddle and love while Ric and Mollie were suffering the loss of their youngest. As cruel as it felt, I knew this kind of pain was nature's way. It was no use shaking my clenched fists angrily at the heavens for stealing Sean so quickly and so young. I knew there was absolutely nothing I could do to mend the hearts of those he left behind.

"Whom the gods love dies young."

—Menander

Big Boy Toys

My way of healing was to share my memories of Sean with my towheaded son. I would poke Marley's belly button with my finger as I told him about Sean's love for fast cars, motorcycles, and snowmobiles. As Marley grew, I wondered how those stories influenced him.

From the minute Marley could manipulate his hands, his choice of toy had wheels on it. If it went fast, especially if it went fast loudly, it was sure to please the boy. Sometimes I thought Marley picked the wrong parent. My brothers, Tip and Ric, lived to win races and crash cars. I simply didn't inherit that go-fast gene. Marley had only met my brothers once, but he felt a kinship for their ways—their need for speed, their love of hunting, and their bountiful acquisition of all large toys.

Marley's dad liked snow skiing, surfing, and other water sports, but Drew was never into racing motorcycles or snowmobiles, demolition derbies, hunting, or monster trucks. Marley's desire for these things certainly didn't come from me or anyone Drew and I were hanging around with—a bunch of tree-hugging dirt worshippers.

By the time he was two years old, I knew moving to the country was one of the smartest things Drew and I had ever done. Marley was on a path of his own, one that had to be honored. I am thankful I had Ric and Tip as reference points for this diehard mentality, and always hoped the spirit of Sean would help keep Marley safe.

Written by me when Marley was almost three years old
December 12, 1987

NO WORRIES!

Dearest Marley,

My little one, do you have a fever still? You're so sick and cuddly. It's a shame when you are zapped of energy but I secretly adore the way you love me when you're feelin' bad. You cuddle so close and need me so much, it feels like we want to crawl so near that we swallow each other's love and become one. Thank you for letting me love you so completely. You are the only one I've known in my life brave enough to let me love you fully, the way I've dreamed of one soul melding with another. You actually allow me in.

I don't know, sometimes I feel I'm normal enough, but other times, I question my parenting skills and my ability to pretend to act like other people do. You never question me. I don't question you. You're still not talking. Everyone says it's because you don't have to. They say it's because I know what you're saying non-verbally and I don't MAKE you say it. Hogwash!

You're still nursing at dawn and at nap time, and I'm not gonna do diddly squat about it. You like the grounding and I like being close to you. So there! Drew seems to be fine with everything, so I'm not too worried. God, I hope you're "normal" when you're grown. I'm bucking the system, and I hope my instinctive courage pays off with a well adjusted, flexible, loving, self-assured, independent man.

I'll pray for you. Will you pray for me? We need all the help we can get.

I love you, child,
Mom

THERE ARE NO ACCIDENTS

No Fear

Being cautious was not one of Marley's priorities. I don't think the concept existed in his reality. He seemed to have the impression that he could take care of any situation he got himself into. He could—most of the time—but it sure scared those of us responsible for him.

For instance, when he was almost two years old, he pulled a stunt I'll never forget. Drew and I were on the barn roof, nailing down the plywood. We looked over the edge of the roof to check on Marley, playing in his sand pile, but he was nowhere to be seen. Drew and I called for him just as he popped his little bleach-blond head up over the edge of the roof, making one of his classic "here I am" sounds. We froze and held our breath in fear: He was at the very top of a 22-foot ladder! Trying to remain calm, we slid down the roof towards him before he could make a move. He didn't think there was anything wrong—he was simply investigating what we were doing up on the roof! I could feel my grey hairs growing.

Marley was adventurous and competent...well, 95 percent of the time. He had gained our trust over the years and was given a long leash to explore our wild world. He was self-sufficient and incredibly creative. He lost a lot of tools and buried a lot of toys, but he entertained himself well and generally stayed out of trouble. I'm focusing on the five percent of mishaps, because they're notable times, and I learned what made Marley tick and how he handled adversity.

His first minor accident happened when he was two. Running while carrying a stick, he tripped and jammed one end of the stick up into the roof of his mouth. It was a clean U-shaped cut, but it bled profusely. As I picked him up to carry him to the house, I felt the warmth of his blood coat my back in wetness. The only thing I could think to do was slide a popsicle up into the hole left by the stick. This stopped the bleeding, numbed the pain, and held the flap of skin in its proper place while the blood clotted. He was brave, very brave, faithfully following my instructions on how to stay calm.

His second accident happened when he fell off our slide while speed-sliding, dislocating his foot. This only slowed him down for a few frustrating days. He had an unusually high pain tolerance and healed remarkably fast. He mended with a speed that made us wonder what planet he hailed from.

Under Pressure

I spanked Marley twice in his life. Both times for the same crime: playing with fire. It's ironic that firefighting was the profession he later chose. His first experience was at three years old. It was in the wee hours of dawn, before Drew and I woke. He decided to while away the early morning hours building a small fire with twigs. The only problem was he chose to do this four feet away from the 500-gallon propane tank.

Drew and I woke up identifying the smell of wood smoke wafting in through the open windows. Fire is something we feared, living in the dry woods of southern Oregon. We levitated from our dreamy states and were dressed and ready for action in seconds flat.

His little fire had started to spread, igniting the very dry grass nearby. Marley knew the fire was out of control and was already at the scene, armed with the garden hose. To Marley's dismay, the hose was three feet shy of reaching the fire and our limited water pressure didn't help. (Urinating on the fire would have been more effective.) In the end, all was well—no explosions or forest fires.

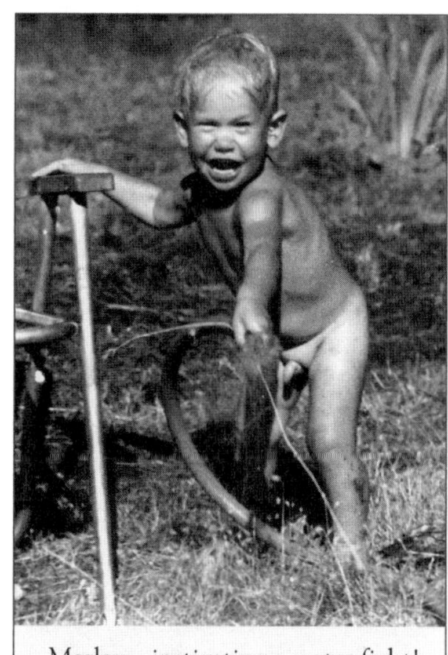

Marley—instigating a water fight!

The Butterfly Effect

RICH MEMORIES OF MARLEY
by Llyn Peabody

I loved the summers I lived with Jennifer and Drew, helping them parent Marley. Who was actually parenting whom, I'll never know. In my mind's eye, I see his wide smile that seemed a size or two too large for his grinning face. He was always such a special and unusual being. I felt special just by being associated with him.

I loved watching Marley tackle learning to walk on the rough, uneven surface of the land they called Light Haven. And how, even before he was four years old, he could out-hike most city-adults. He navigated the land around Light Haven with an ease and confidence that belied his years. I have happy memories of water fights around and *IN* the house, and of Marley's mischievous delight in instigating these wild times. Even as a little kid, he was so good at reminding all of us "grown-ups" to have fun and not take life too seriously!

As he grew older, Marley gave me the gift of feeling loved by a teenager. I have always felt shy to reach out physically or emotionally to teenagers, figuring that they would reject my overtures. Marley took care of that by being the initiator. He brought me into his world—openly, lovingly, and with great confidence. Because of him, I've had more courage to connect with other teens in my life.

He was always a go-getter. Always pushing the boundaries. Always doing things his own way. And yet, he had this dear, dear sweetness that seemed otherworldly—dare I say, angelic? I guess we only got to borrow him for a short time. Perhaps he was on loan to us to remind us of the preciousness and brevity of our time here on Earth—to remind us to be clear in our priorities, because none of us ever know how much time we've got.

Chapter Two:
Marley Up!

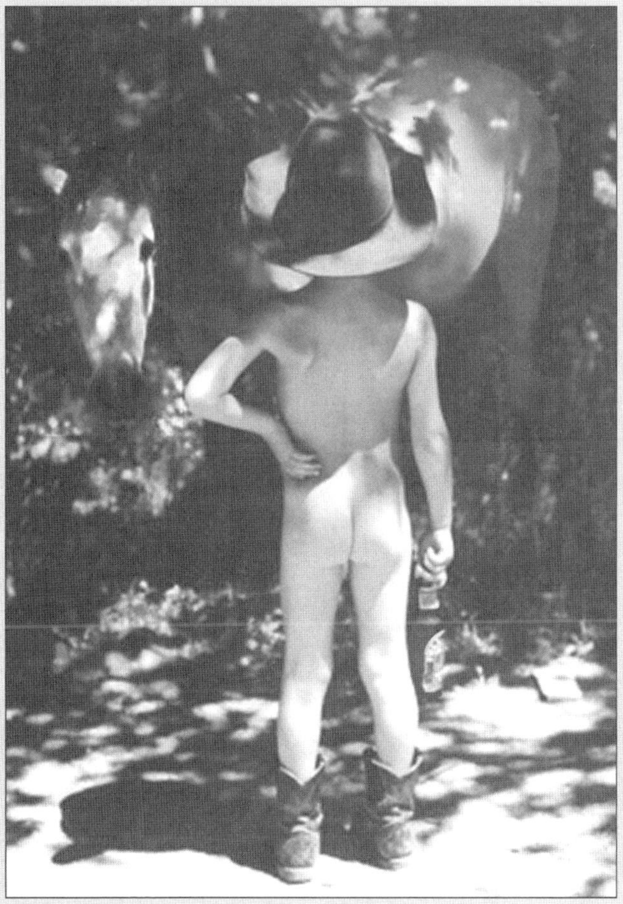

Marley, age five, frustrated with his horse, Nike.

Photo: Jennifer

Letter sent to my family
May 16, 1989

SPEECH! SPEECH!

Dear Family,

Here's some news for you! Another family member is on its way. A girl, this time, we hope. Yes, a baby…a Christmas baby (actually she's due December 7th).

The reason I'm writing is to let you know what's going on with our firstborn. Marley's now four years old and is a beautiful, bright boy. He's into horseback riding in a big way. He and Drew have been taking daily hour-and-a-half long rides. He goes to preschool and gymnastics class and even has a girlfriend (our neighbor, Brianna). Marley is a high-energy kid, filled with loads of common sense and a great imagination. He's not like other kids in a unique way...he doesn't speak the English language.

He communicates with a variety of sounds, great expressions, and a fairly large "vocabulary" of hand signs (American sign language). He fully understands everything, it just doesn't come back out with verbal words. Strange! Anyway, we've been to four doctors, a psychic, and several specialists. We've had his hearing tested twice and his oral motor capabilities tested; apparently there's nothing wrong with his hearing or the shape of his mouth, or the way he uses his tongue. He can make sounds, but he cannot put them together to form words (other than "mama," "dada," "pop," "yeah," "help," and "boom"). He never did the baby chatter that you commonly hear one-year-old kids do, although he makes lots of beautiful sounds when he sings.

The term Western medicine is using to describe this handicap is *Developmental Apraxia*. Which basically means the connection in the brain to the speech center is "turned off," thus he cannot get the information from his master computer to tell his tongue and lips how to work to form consonant sounds or to put more than one group of sounds together. The word "help" is a big one (take a minute to sound it out and break down the different movements of your tongue and lips.) It takes Marley major concentration to form this word.

There seems to be no apparent cause. The cure? They say there is a chance for him to learn to speak with therapy (taking anywhere from 3 to 10 years). It may or may not ever sound "normal," although technology has devised many ways of helping these folks communicate with computer aid.

Alternative medicine has a slightly different twist. We were told "Mars Bar" has a lot of psychic energy, and he uses this to communicate with. They said, for reasons with an unidentified purpose, he has chosen not to use the "normal" ways of verbally communicating. In other words he has "turned off" this ability, but is also able to "turn it on" when he feels it is necessary to communicate with words.

I think they both said about the same thing, except the nontraditional view sees Marley in control of when speech will occur. This has been my sense for a long time; that it's not just a rebellion, "I won't talk," but "I can't talk now."

So what do we do? We checked out a special school for the language impaired. None of us liked it but the concept was okay. At least the staff all used sign language. The idea of Marley finally being understood by other people was extraordinary to us. But they run the program with such limited brain power and imagination that we decided to reject it. We're looking into hiring a private therapist.

I would like to ask all of you to consider learning sign language. It's a wonderful second language to have under your belt, and it may be the only way you and Marley will be able to communicate. Until now, I don't think our family has ever encountered a handicap other than dyslexia. It's time to think about what you're willing to do in order to communicate with your nephew, cousin, or grandson. Learning a different language can take some time, so don't wait until the last minute if you choose to give it a try.

We appreciate your love and support and thank you for considering working with us on this project. For those of you who haven't yet met Mars, I think you will find him a loveable, delightful, funny little boy who wants to play ALL THE TIME! I hope you will meet him soon—his little sibling-to-be, too!

With joy and much love,
Jennifer

"The problem is not that there are problems. The problem is expecting otherwise and thinking that having problems is a problem."

—Theodore Rubin

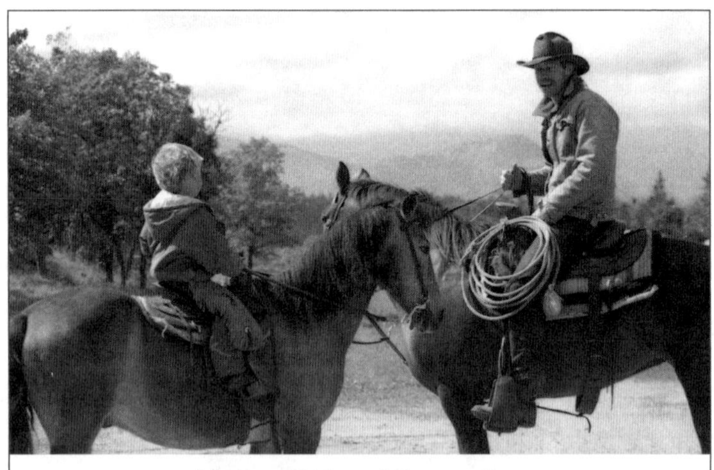

Marley on Nike and Drew on Star

The Butterfly Effect

GRADE SCHOOL SPEECH
by Selene Foster (age 11)

If you see an elf running around with a sonic wave device hanging on his ear, don't call the Marines, it's Marley, my cousin, the subject of my speech. Actually, I think of him more as the little brother I never had. To explain my opening line I'll have to say that Marley is special. The sonic wave device is really just a piece of skin on his ear that's been there all his four-year-old life. The doctors say that it doesn't do anything, but I'm not sure they're right.

First of all, I'll tell you a little bit about Marley. He has blond hair, blue eyes, he is sweet, sensitive, outgoing, and very intelligent, despite his handicap. That's another thing I need to tell you about, his handicap. But, I really wouldn't call it that because it doesn't seem to slow him down any or bother him much, it just gets frustrating sometimes and he does have temper tantrums because of that frustration. Specialists say that there is a little part of his brain that doesn't work. This means that he'll probably never be able to talk. This also means that he'll probably never be able to go to a regular school or lead a normal life. However, I don't believe it. He says some words, so I think he just doesn't want to talk. At least I did think that, but now I realize that he really does have a problem. He taught me that. He knows he is different. I overheard him telling his mom that he really wants to go to a speech therapist.

He and I have a special relationship and it grows every time I see him. Right now I am looking forward to the next time I can visit. I always am. My aunt tells me Marley always asks her when I will come for a visit and that he continually asks how I am. This makes me one of the happiest people alive. When I do come to visit, he immediately latches on to me, and insists that he tell me everything new that has happened. Then he shows me all the new animals he has gotten. I love it.

When I say he "tells me," I mean he signs. Signing has been a big part of his learning, and I am now in the process of learning how to sign so that I can understand him more easily. He is so good at signing that he now surpasses his mom.

I have a horse that recently died. After I told my aunt on the phone, she told Marley. She said he cried for twenty minutes and was worried about me. When I hear things like that, it brings me to tears and I want to tell him how much I love him.

I have many other stories. Just the other day, he went up to my aunt Jennifer, and "said" that the door needed to be closed, (usually he would have just closed the door himself). Jennifer told him he could go ahead and close it, but he didn't. Instead he signed to her that she needed to do it so that his ten piglets wouldn't get out. After Jennifer told my mom this story my mom asked when they had gotten the piglets. Jennifer said they hadn't, but apparently Marley thought so! He is always surprising someone with something.

Another thing Marley is famous for are girls. I know that you might think that he would be shy, and sometimes he is. But, when it comes to girls, he's a tiger. At the pool, at the arcade, it doesn't matter where, if Marley's around, you've got to watch out. Many a time he has gone up to a girl, grabbed her hand, kissed her on the cheek, and dragged her around until it was time to leave.

There is so much else I could say about him, but I don't know how to put it into words, so I'll end by telling you what he has taught me. He has taught me patience, courage, how to accept things as they are, how to get the most out of everything, and most of all—how to love. I hope that one day he will be able to read this and fully appreciate and realize how much I really do love him.

Thank you for taking the time to listen to me speak.
Good night.

COWBOY TROUBLES

Horsing Around

One thing I am truly amazed at is how few times Marley really hurt himself. He was taken to the emergency room only once until he tangled with cancer at 15 years old. That's mind-boggling, considering how active and daring he was.

When Marley was five years old, he tried to load his pony in the horse trailer alone. Our trailer was the old fashioned kind, sporting a ramp rather than the swinging door that was later proven safer. The ramp was fivefeet square, made of steel and thick planks of wood, designed to support 1,000 pounds of bucking horseflesh. Marley must have thought he was much stronger and taller than he was, because his plan included lowering this heavy ramp.

From what would be a block away in city terms, Drew and I heard Marley's bloodcurdling scream. We ran up the gravel drive to find his leg pinned between the ramp and the dirt road, with a three-inch bolt embedded in his calf. After patching the hole and stabilizing his broken leg, we calmly endured the 25-minute drive to Ashland's hospital. I knew there was something strange about this kid because he, too, was remaining calm, like this was another adventure—a field trip to the ER!

It was then that I learned his pain threshold was abnormally high. A few days later, he was good to go, ready to show off his fancy, painted cast. Why slow down when you can have fun? Having a cast didn't stop him from riding horses, running, climbing, wrestling, or getting into mischief. I had to fight the urge to protect this little kid who talked without saying any words—but there wasn't much I could do to stop him.

"When a great ship is in harbor and moored,
it is safe, there can be no doubt.
But that is not what great ships are built for."

—Clarissa Pinkola Estes

August 3, 1990

UNCONDITIONAL LOVE

Dear Marley,

I just want to tell you how much I love you! You are five and a half years old. What an age! Sometimes you drive me crazy, but through it all you are my best friend. We are with each other all day long, every day. We've been busy this summer going to summer camp at the YMCA and to speech therapy in Medford. Even when I'm a real crankcase, you're always there for me in the end. I don't know how you put up with me and still try so hard to please me.

Your sister, Catie, is eight months old and she loves you so much. You're a great big brother. Thank you for letting me watch how you look at her when she sleeps. Such adoring, I've never witnessed, only felt. For a rough-and-tumble guy, you sure know how to be gentle and sweet. I am amazed by the way you, the one who takes such pleasure in pulverizing rocks, are so incredibly tender with your baby sister, handling her with the perfect combination of strength and care.

Your ever lovin' Mom

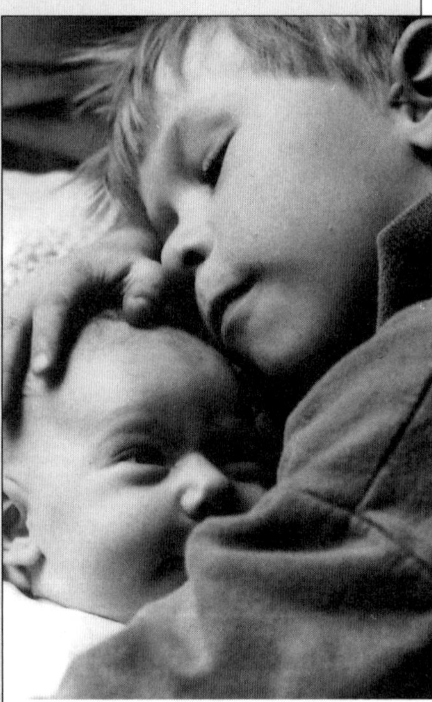

Mars with his baby sister, Catie (Note the polyp or "sonic wave device" on his ear. At his request, it was removed when he was seven.)

PASSING THE TEST

It's Elementary

Before Marley could enter the public school system, he needed to be assessed for eligibility for special education services. When he was five and a half years old, Janet, the Speech Language Pathologist for our district, was asked to do an evaluation. She visited him at his preschool summer camp and, as a part of his assessment, wrote:

> "During the informal speech/language observation, Marley displayed age-appropriate play skills. He participated with other children, but only communicated with gestures and noises. He appeared to have no interest in verbalizing. He displayed the functions of asking, showing, telling, and requesting at a pre-linguistic level. It was apparent Marley used direct eye contact while communicating and was understanding questions asked of him and directions given."

He had been given two labels, *Apraxia* and *Aphasia*, but both were deemed inaccurate. Because no one could come up with a better label to afford him the services we knew he needed, we found a loophole: percentages. The final report stated that Marley demonstrated severely limited oral expressive language development, scoring a 67 percent delay. That percentile was good enough for the state's requirements. Marley could go to school! The following year, when he entered kindergarten, Janet began her role as Marley's speech therapist for the next eight years.

During an interview with Janet ten years later, she was asked if she remembered the first time she met Marley. A warm smile spread across her face as she said, "Oh yes! I went to observe him when he was five years old. He had been told I was coming, and I was expecting him to be shy and withholding. But as soon as I entered the room, he ran up to me smiling, gave my legs a hug, and took my hand. I was instantly his friend and he wanted to show me everything." For the rest of his days, Marley adored Janet, and honored her for his ability to speak.

Letter written to my clan
New Year's Day, 1991

HOLIDAY UPDATE

Dear Ones,

It was a wonderful Christmas! We spent this holiday wrapped in warmth and love in our ever-expanding home, nestled in the mountains. Santa was very generous and Marley was a great receiver, taking his time, exploring each gift with interest and thanks. A remote controlled cement mixer actually brought tears of joy to my boy! Because of my children, for the first time as an adult, I'm actually looking forward to next Christmas.

For two weeks, the temperatures have hovered around twenty degrees. Oregon is simply not prepared for these temperatures. The electricity, gas, and water went out for much of Ashland during this Arctic freeze, and many have been residing in the gymnasiums of our local schools. Fortunately we weren't so badly hit because we use wood for heat, propane for most utilities, and a generator that provides electricity to pump our well water and to charge the 12-volt system used for lights. Unfortunately, our water pipes *did* freeze. So we are carrying water from town in many 5-gallon containers to supply water for thirsty animals and our household needs.

Before the freeze hit, Drew had nearly completed a new extension; an office and a bathroom with a compost toilet. Yes, folks! No more midnight runs to the outhouse in the snow. We're moving up in the world. Another lifesaving addition this year has been a large covered front porch. Now there's a place to stack firewood, kick off mud covered boots, and a place to be outside while the skies cry. A true blessing.

I have found a beloved friend who is a godsend in my life.

Friends of this quality and depth don't come along every day! Cindy lives in Ashland with her husband and two daughters. Vanessa is a year younger than Marley, but they are both in the same preschool class, which is how we met. Laura is just ten months older than Catie, and both pairs of kids adore each other. Laura and Marley even share the same birthday!

Drew is now a farrier, shoeing horses, a perfect career choice for his rare personality type. It's dangerous and exciting, it's hard work and rewarding, and it's ever-changing and flexible. A demanding job not many can withstand but, then again, we're talking about Drew (Doo da loo, as Marley calls him). When Drew's not shoeing horses, he's adding on to the house, redesigning the existing system, taking long horseback rides in the mountains with Marley, or curled up reading a never ending supply of western novels. A true cowboy. His fantasy is a 100-acre ranch with lots of horses and cattle to roundup.

Marley will be six years old in February. He has grown tall and beautiful. His words, limited to five last January, have rapidly multiplied. He now uses full sentences, one right after another. (Currently his speech is at about a three-year-old level.) He still uses sign language and/or sounds for words he doesn't know or cannot manage. Imagine, it's the first time I can listen to my son without having to always be within eyesight!

Last January, just after Catie was born, Marley had PE tubes placed in his eardrums due to repeated ear aches. This procedure equalized the pressure and allowed for adequate drainage. It was a 20-minute out-patient surgery done in the local hospital. We're not sure whether it was the surgery or Catie's birth that influenced his desire and/or ability to speak, but regardless, we're thrilled about the shift.

Marley is an amazingly bright and loving boy whose zest for living and learning seems to far outweigh the pain he has had to live with. Not only has he dealt with intensely painful earaches and the frustration of not being able to communicate with others without my help, he has also had an acute and chronic stomach disease.

After ten doctors, thousands of dollars, and two and a half years of pain, we took Marley to Stanford Medical Center for two days of tests, climaxing with two surgical procedures; a *bronchoscopy* (a camera tube snaked down his throat) and a *colonoscopy* (the same but from the other end). He made us very nervous when he stayed under the anesthesia much longer than expected. But in the end, a diagnosis was made: He had a bacteria called *Urcenia* and a parasite called *Blastycis Hominus*. Both are extremely microscopic and rarely seen, apparently the reason our local doctors and lab technicians were unable to explain the cause of pain.

Now, after two weeks of being on two different antibiotics, Marley has only had five bad days. I'm skeptical about the cure, due to the fact he's been on so many antibiotics for his ear troubles. I wonder sometimes if the cure for the ears wasn't possibly the cause of the stomach disorder. At least we are relieved to know there's really something in there and it's not all in his head.

It's been very hard to see my boy in such pain and not be able to find a solution. This stomach problem has been the cause of Marley's hyperactive behavior (he says he had bees in his belly and moving fast was his solution). It's been really nice to have my boy back now that he's feeling better. Keep your fingers crossed!

Catie just had her first birthday. She's a pretty little "knee leech" that loves to dance. She's always happy and loves wrestling with her brother, whom she adores. Marley is the best big brother in the world—it's so cool the way he loves her. We just got an Olympic-sized trampoline, and Catie squeals with delight as Marley endlessly bounces her on it.

The animals still fill our lives. We presently have three horses, one dog called Sage who faithfully sticks close to the kids at all times, and two cats. Pretty Kitty helps pay the bills, producing continual crops of Himalayan kittens, which we sell for $20 each. We also have a bunch of laying hens, one mean rooster that we're all scared of, and a very funny guinea pig that roams free but is faithful to the homestead.

We hope you come to visit soon. You're always welcome. You'll probably want a four-wheel drive vehicle to get down our driveway. When you do come, remember to watch out for Marley's trucks frozen in the puddles, and don't worry about Sage; she barks but she doesn't bite. Our guest house is small but has a really comfy featherbed and a shower. (Well, that won't do you much good 'til the pipes thaw.) Hell, forget about visiting until springtime—we just decided to pack up and go to Baja for awhile! Yahoo!

We love you,
Jennifer

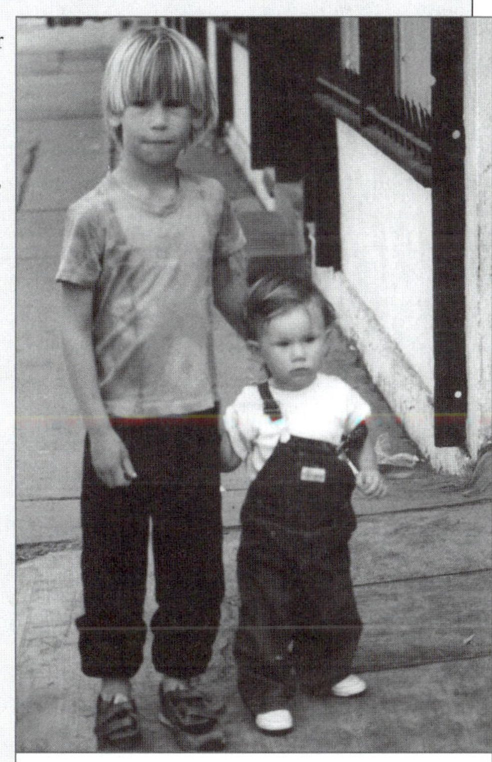

Marley and Catie in San Felipe, Baja

PLEASURES AND PITFALLS

Responsibility

From parenting, I learned the ability to respond—even when I didn't want to. I had felt the joys of love from parents, siblings, friends, and mates, but no one could have prepared me for the utter bliss of smelling a newborn, the incomprehensible butter softness of new skin, and the intimacy that's not only allowed, but required. The most amazing thing was understanding, on a cellular level, that this little human will die...DIE...if it's not cared for, and it will pay the price later for negligence now.

I never wanted kids. That was supposed to be my sisters' job. They were supposed to have the kids, and I was to be the best auntie known to humankind. I believed I didn't need kids to know what responsibility was, because I was an adult orphan responsible for myself in a way none of my peers or even siblings were. (That's a complicated story, I'll explain later, I promise.)

When the going got tough, most folks my age had at least one parent to fall back on. Yet, for me, the rite of passage from individual to parent was the very lesson I needed. I was, for the first time, responsible for someone else, and I knew what commitment meant: 'til death do us part, for better or for worse, for richer or for poorer, in sickness and in health.

Commitment Sample, Part I

Many of us throw around the term "commitment" with relative ease. I really had no concept of what it meant until I had a baby. At 17 years old, I married a man I had loved since I was 13. Yet after nine years of loving him, we divorced because I wanted to feel free. Vows...whatever! Things change.

My role models were confusing. On one hand, I had my parents (here comes that complicated story I promised you). My mother, Virginia, was married to Phil, and they had four kids; Tip, Ric, Julia, and Constant. My father, Alden, was married to Liz, and they had four children; Andrea, Meredith, Martha, and Tim. (Both sets of kids were approximately the same ages.)

Phil and Virginia had built a new house on the hill above the one they lived in, and Alden and Liz bought their old house. We're talkin' a rural small town—Wayzata, Minnesota, in 1958. To make a long story short, Mom and Dad fell in love and so did Phil and Liz. Both couples divorced and, days later, married their new loves. Phil and Dad packed their belongings, and each moved into the house of his new wife and legally adopted her four kids. Constant, for example, went to kindergarten that morning with one last name and returned home that afternoon to a new last name and a different dad. Meanwhile, just to make things a little more complicated—Mom was nine months pregnant. Eleven days after Mom and Dad were married…ta da…I was born! Nine months after that, Jay was born to Phil and Liz.

Poor Phil had to move back into the house he had just moved out of, so he and Liz built another one on the other side of the hill. The two families lived next to each other for eight years until Phil and Liz and their five kids moved to California. Mom, Dad, Constant, and I moved to Miami. Tip and Ric, adults with independent lives, stayed in Wayzata, and Julia remained at college.

Commitment Sample, Part II

On the other hand, I had Gladyce and Phil (another Phil) as the example of an old-fashioned, farm-style, 'til death do us part kind of marriage. Mom and Dad went on their honeymoon two weeks after I was born, and left me in the highly capable hands of Gladyce, who helped both Liz and Mom with domestic chores. Gladyce and Phil lived on a dairy farm that I considered my second home, as Mom and Dad traveled a lot. Gladyce and Phil are now both in their 90's and have been married longer than most people live.

I'm thankful I had examples of two very different life styles available to me. I felt what two very different brands of motherly love felt like. When it was my turn to mother, my technique fell somewhere between Mom's pioneering style of the future and Gladyce's old-fashioned style.

History Repeating Itself

My parents weren't the only couple with a complicated love scenario. I had to ask myself why we sometimes create situations that mirror circumstance of the past, as this soap opera story became even more absurd. (Some things are just too weird to ignore.)

Marley and Vanessa were in preschool together—that's how I met Cindy. She had a babe in arms (Laura) and I had a babe in the oven (Catie). We became inseparable friends for the next three years. Cindy, her husband Marlo, and their two kids would hang out with us for BBQ's, waterskiing, etc. Everybody got along, especially the four kids.

Marley and Vanessa adored each other. One night when we were at Marlo and Cindy's, the kids announced that they were going to get married. A few weeks later, Drew and Cindy realized they had fallen in love with each other.

After ten stormy, emotional months, both marriages were dissolved. Drew moved up on the hill above our property and started courting Cindy. Had Marlo and I connected, it would have been exactly the same type of switch that my parents had made thirty years earlier.

In the end, Drew and Cindy got married, so Laura and Vanessa became Marley and Catie's stepsisters, which suited them just fine. Marlo and Cindy set up the same schedule for the kids that Drew and I had—two weeks on, two weeks off. And everyone lived happily ever after. Tra la la!

Even though I never wanted to have children, I know that becoming a mother was the most important gift the spirits ever gave me. It is my children that taught me about commitment and about being alive—about really living! I always hoped to repay their gifts by being a great parent, helping them to love, live, and die well.

"Our children change us…
whether they live or not."

—Lois McMaster Bujold

GROWING PAINS

Square Hole, Round Peg

Marley spent two years in kindergarten and was seven years old by the time he was ready to start first grade. I had fought hard to get him into a school that would adapt to his special needs, rather than trying to make him fit their curriculum. His elementary school was amazing. During the years he was in kindergarten, this school helped students learn sign language and began to implement an old-school concept: blended classes.

Marley's first blended class consisted of both first and second graders. A wondrously creative woman named Pat was his teacher for both years. It was a brilliant plan that let the kids learn at their own pace. The kids also had time to learn how to communicate with Marley while he slowly learned to speak our language.

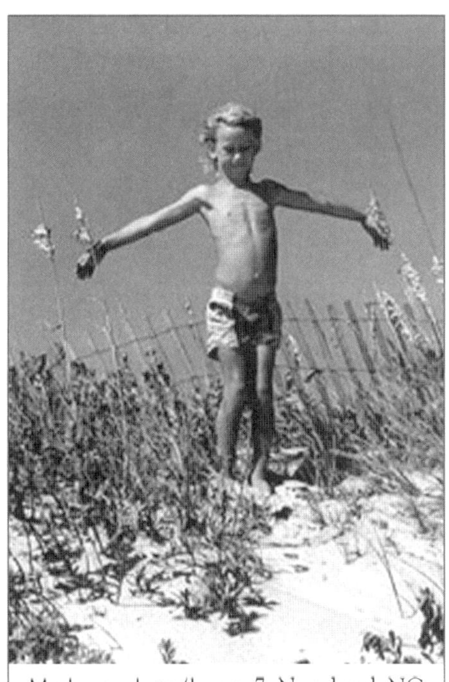
Marley ready to fly, age 7, Nags head, NC

For the next two years, Tim was Marley's teacher for a third and fourth grade blend. Most of his classmates had graduated with Marley from Pat's class to Tim's class. Being with the same bunch of kids was his saving grace. They had already learned to accept Marley for who he was and had the patience to help teach him social skills without stomping on his self-esteem in the process.

It became apparent that Marley simply didn't understand the

abstract nature of symbols. Seeing letters and trying to match a sound that related was incredibly confusing and frustrating for him. Whenever the class focused on English, Marley would go with Janet, who helped him with his speech. It was the same with numbers. When the class studied math, Marley would go to Nancy, his special-ed teacher, for one-on-one help.

An example of how Marley's brain worked: If Nancy was teaching math skills and asked him what two plus two was, he wouldn't know. But if she asked him how many tires a truck needed, he'd ask, "What kind a tfwuck? A semi or one like my dad's? My dad's tfwuck needs foua tiyas." And he'd launch into a story about the time his dad almost rolled his truck off a cliff. He was so animated, it was difficult not to fall completely in love with him.

"I never let schooling interfere with my education."

—-Mark Twain

Throughout his elementary education, Nancy was a master at inventing ways to teach Marley. She incorporated "life skills" into Marley's special curriculum. For many years, Marley had two jobs; one in a nearby plant nursery and the other in the school cafeteria. He especially loved working in the kitchen because he got second helpings for his effort.

Going Psycho

When Marley was in the third grade, it was time for him to be retested for continued special education. It took Don, the school district's psychotherapist, several months and a wide variety of tests to determine if Marley was officially handicapped. It was the responsibility of this one man to give Marley an effective label that would allow Marley special services until he graduated from high school. When his report was complete, a meeting was called. Tim, Pat, Nancy, Janet, the principal, Drew, Cindy, and I all gathered to read the report aloud.

Don's nine-page Psycho-Educational Report was either going to make or break Marley's future in education.

> "Initial Contact: Ordinarily during the initial period, there is some tension as the examiner and the child 'adjust' to each other and to the evaluative situation. In this case, Marley accompanied me quite willingly and did not show any undue signs of distress or tension. Marley was a delightful but low-functioning student who warmed up rather quickly to me. It takes a while to understand Marley's verbal output, but after one becomes used to his language it is much less of a problem."

Before Don explained the details of all the tests, he did a "Summary of Report" that really worried us.

> "Current testing indicates Marley is classified as being in the Borderline and Intellectually Deficient (mildly mentally retarded) range. There were, however, some definite indicators that exceeded these global scores. Clearly Marley presents a difficult diagnostic problem. He has many of the traditional signs of mental retardation and yet there are sufficient strengths that would, in my opinion, make a determination of mental retardation erroneous."

We all moaned, fearing that Don's confusion would mean Marley might face a bleak future without special aid. But in the end, Don's final summary gave us what we needed.

> "From my numerous interactions with Marley, I will state that he does not appear to me to behave like a 'typical' retarded child. He has some areas of strength that approach the average range. I have to say, as well, that when it comes to the very abstract nature of 'learning,' that his scores are quite like that of a mildly retarded student. He is much what I think of as a boy who is '*retarded between 9 A.M. and 3 P.M.*'—i.e., primarily for the purposes of learning academics. His breadth of knowledge in interest in things outside of 'book learning' are much stronger, and I think it would be a disservice to Marley to label him mentally retarded, though he is, functionally, when it comes to school-

> ing in academics."

That was that! We all cheered. We had Don's label, (which he purposely put in quotes) to put on Marley's documents. Once signed by all of us, Don's assessment would not be challenged.

Sticking Together

By the time Marley was ready for fifth grade, for some mysterious reason Tim and Pat resigned their posts and joined forces to team-teach fifth and sixth grades. Pat primarily worked with the younger students while Tim focused on the older ones. This meant that for his last two years years of elementary school, Marley would be able to float between two classrooms with the same two teachers and the same students he had had since the first grade.

Marley began to thrive in school when he was 11 years old. The following progress report describes Marley's abilities during the last two years of his elementary education:

> "Marley seems much more comfortable about approaching academic topics. Because he is now adding and subtracting, he can play many of the math games with other students in Pat's room.
>
> Marley is very adept at traveling between the rooms. He works in Pat's class for some of the academics but feels more socially connected to the students in Tim's. He is very independent but also interacts well with other students.
>
> Marley is an incredibly dependable student. He is the person both classes rely on when something needs to be done just so and right away. More than any other student, he knows his way around the school and knows where things are and how they work."

I was amazed Marley did such a great job of hanging in there with school. Sometimes it felt like a survival test, and I held my breath throughout most of those early years. But when the going got tough, he'd either find a way around the trouble or he'd cowboy up and keep trying.

THE GOOD, THE BAD, AND THE UGLY

Stuck in the Middle

When Marley was 13 years old he entered middle school. Most of his peers were one to two years younger than him, and were far superior academically. The combination could have been devastating, but he was placed in a "cross-grade" program that was similar to his earlier education. There were six teachers that worked as a team for both seventh and eighth grades. All classes were in one hall, which made it much easier for Marley to navigate in unfamiliar territory with new rules.

Marley loved his first year at the middle school. The special services were fairly limited at this school, so when the regular class focus was beyond his comprehension, he got to socialize one-on-one with the teachers and counselors. Two of his favorite people were the nurse, Beth, and a new counselor named Abdi. They ended up being Marley's saving graces at the middle school. They were always there for him *and* they loved listening to stories about Marley's wild adventures (some of which, I'm kind of sure, were true!)

The second year wasn't as much fun for him. Nothing inspired him. I think it started to dawn on him that life wasn't going to be easy without a few of the basic concepts he was missing. He tried to rely on his loving charm, but that wasn't working with many of the girls. He was a romantic and would bring girls roses. Many of them loved his attention, but didn't want to accept his favor for fear that their social status would be lowered by associating with the "odd kid."

Marley looked and moved like a normal 14-year-old, but he talked in a strange way and he couldn't read or write. He covered up how much he didn't understand so well that we didn't always know how much help he needed. For instance, sometimes after bathing, his hair still looked greasy. It took us years to figure out it was because he couldn't tell which bottle was the shampoo and which was the conditioner. It was a 50/50 chance he would wash his hair with the conditioner. He started looking much better after we taught him to recognize the word "shampoo."

One of his teachers pointed out, "He has difficulty using the correct verb tense and seldom uses the past tense." This, combined with not fully understanding the concept of numbers, made for some fascinating storytelling.

One example is when Marley told a teacher about an accident that Drew had as a youth. Marley made it seem like it happened yesterday, and the cliff Drew drove off wasn't 600 feet, it was really only 6 feet. But to a listener, it all sounded possible. Fantastic but possible. Marley's teacher was very concerned, and asked me how Drew was getting along after the accident. Huh? I listened to the re-telling of the story and understood the confusion. Another example is when Marley said, "That car could haul ass, it could rev up to 600,000 rpm in second gear!" I knew to translate that to 6,000 rpm. But when Marley referred to the cost of things, misunderstandings could get a little pricey.

For the first time, Marley was surrounded by peers who were unfamiliar with how he looked at life upside down. I think he was often misunderstood, made fun of, and accused of lying. Most of the time he just didn't want to deal with trying and failing to make new friends. He was miserable. On most mornings that year, I would have to drag him out of bed, as he loudly complained about how stupid school was.

Catie loved school and would be furious at Marley for threatening to make her late. When she would start screaming at Marley to hurry up, his reaction was to move slower and then she'd start yelling at me! I hated those mornings. I hated fighting or having to be the stern, consequence-wielding parent. There were some mornings when he refused to get ready. After a verbal battle, I'd make Marley dress in the car after threatening to take all of his bikes to Goodwill. Many of the mornings during the first part of that year were a drag. We all suffered through Marley's suffering. Little did I know what was to come.

"If you're going through hell, keep going."

—Winston Churchill

Chapter Three:
A Crash Course in Medicine

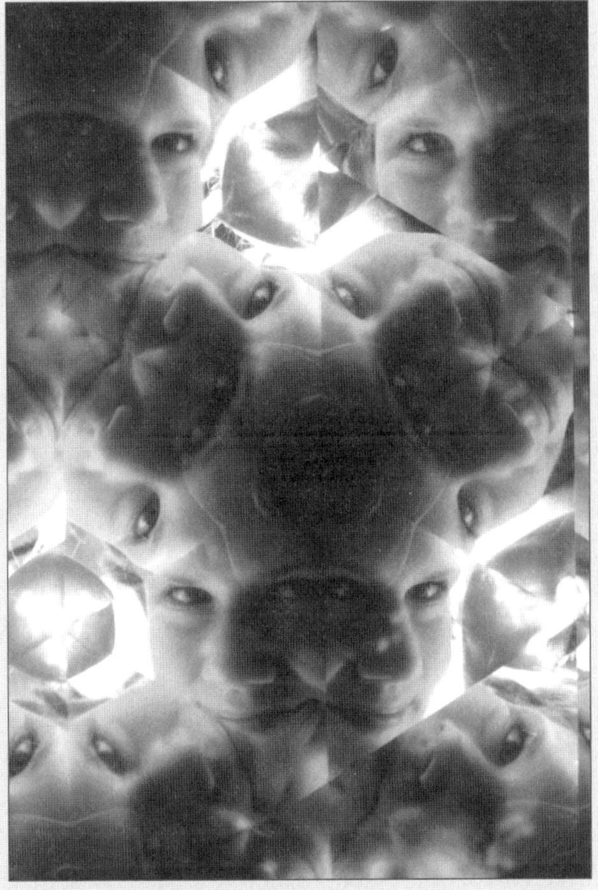

"Which end is up?" (Catie through a kaleidoscope.)

Photo: Jay Newman

HIGH PRESSURE PARENTING

A Change of Plans

Most of us tend to live in a world full of assumptions. We might make plans for tomorrow and assume our alarm will go off, the car will start, and the destination will be there in the morning. The reality is, a thousand and one things could happen to change those plans, but that doesn't occur to us most of the time.

When I first became a parent, I didn't know about all the things that could go wrong. I knew my kids would get sick, and I thought my job was to nurse them back to health. By the time Marley was 15 years old, he had taught me that sometimes kids can be sick and doctors don't always know what's wrong and there isn't always a cure.

On "switch" day, I went to the middle school to pick Marley up and his stepsister, Laura, told me to meet Drew and Marley at the doctor's office. I didn't think much of it. I picked Catie up and headed for Marley. When I got to the doctor's, Drew said they thought Marley might have pneumonia. I just figured I was going to start my two-week shift with the kids being a nursemaid.

It was Friday afternoon, and it was dark by the time the doctor had done an exam and told us we needed X-rays at our small local hospital. Drew left Marley and Catie in my care. Because it was after hours, we couldn't *just* get X-rays, we had to go through the whole emergency room procedure. After waiting forever and getting yet another physical exam, the X-rays were taken and the official diagnosis was delivered. It was all there in black and white. Marley had pneumonia. I thought, "No big deal. I can handle this." We were given antibiotics and discharged. On our way out, we were handed a computer printout, defining pneumonia.

> "Pneumonia is an inflammation of the lung(s). It is an infection caused by inhaling one of three types of irritants: viral, bacterial, or fungal. This disease is treated with antibiotics, plenty of fluids, and bed rest."

We dutifully went home and propped him in a recliner in the living room with plenty of fluids. On Sunday, I started to worry. His symptoms had changed for the worse. The antibiotics weren't doing the trick. I watched Marley's eyes roll white with an intense "I'm-going-to-suffocate" fear because his lungs simply couldn't take in enough air. It was very scary when I realized he might be in serious trouble. I called Drew.

Leaping into the Unknown

It was leap day, February 29th, 2000. Our friend Dee was in labor with her firstborn, and I was supposed to notify everyone when baby Kellar was born. I called the first person on the phone list and passed the responsibility on. I had to get my boy to the hospital. It was late, and Catie was asleep. Our friend Liz agreed to stay with her and keep the wood stove stoked. Drew and Cindy were going to meet me at the ER in Medford, 40 minutes north. We had decided that if Marley needed emergency care, we were going to a larger hospital with better equipment and more experienced doctors. (From then on, Medford symbolized bad experiences, so henceforth, I refer to it as "Dreadford.")

The infection in Marley's lung landed him in the Intensive Care Unit (ICU) for almost two weeks. Marley's case of pneumonia escalated so quickly we had a hard time keeping up with what the doctors were saying. It was one emergency situation after another. It felt like a nightmare that I couldn't wake up from.

During those 12 days in the hospital, I felt lost and queasy most of the time. At first I thought it was a normal nervous response, but then I noticed that whenever I walked outside, the feeling disappeared. I figured it must have been a combination of fluorescent lighting, heavy-duty cleaning fluids, and using the elevators. Regardless of the discomfort I felt, I knew I couldn't leave my son alone.

After many gruesome procedures, Marley started recovering and we were able to bring him home.

I wasn't prepared for how strong we would all have to be. I wasn't prepared for having to be in a relationship with Drew and Cindy again. I felt dizzy and scared like I was on the roller coaster from hell.

FLUID FACTS

Catie's Report

During the visits with her brother in ICU, Catie spent her time drawing diagrams of all the tubes and machines attached to Marley. She, like her three parents, needed to be able to wrap her brain around a situation to make it less scary and unfamiliar.

With Marley as our teacher, we learned a new fact about pneumonia. Catie used the information to write a school report, adding another cause omitted on the hospital's original handout.

Pneumonia
by Catie Pratt (age 10)

Pneumonia is when you have fluid in the lung caused by an infection. Pneumonia is usually caused by one of four things.

The first is bacteria, which is an organism that is so small you can only see it under a microscope. It can also be caused by a virus, which is even smaller than bacteria. Common diseases that a virus can cause are: the common cold, flu, strep throat, smallpox, and mumps. Another cause is a fungal infection. Fungi can also cause Ringworm, Candida, or Athlete's Foot. The last possible cause is aspirating foreign material like chemicals, a peanut, or, in my brother's case, a piece of chicken.

Before the development of antibiotic drugs in the 1940's, pneumonia killed about a third of its victims. Today, with the proper medical treatments, 95 percent recover. But pneumonia is still a leading cause of death.

RECEIVING THE NEWS

Marley's Western Rest Home

Marley's horrific health drama had faded away with the cold winter months. We were all recovering, delighted that spring was fast approaching—a time for new beginnings. Just when we thought the stormy weather was over, Marley's energy started to dwindle. He no longer wanted to play, complaining that his back hurt and he was again having trouble taking big breaths. We took him back to the doctor for another round of tests. When the doctor summoned us for a meeting, we knew bad news was brewing.

"What if you slept,
and what if in your sleep you dreamed,
and what if in your dream you went to heaven
and there you plucked a strange and beautiful flower,
and what if when you awoke you had
the flower in your hand? Oh, what then?"

—Samuel Taylor Coleridge

There's something simply rude about the design of most medical examining rooms. The one we were sitting in was a square 12-foot box, painted a horrible shade of green. It was barren of any wall art or window covering. The contents of this room consisted of a gray metal desk, a chair, a stool, a trash can, and an examining table covered with slick, white paper.

We were patiently waiting for the doctor to tell us the results of the most recent tests. I sat at the desk, tapping my fingers on the arm of the chair. Marley was spinning on the stool a few feet away. After a few excruciatingly silent minutes, Marley rolled the stool next to me, leaving a small trail of dried mud clods from his boots behind him. Marley leaned forward and said he had an idea. He wanted to start a new business. My mouth dropped open as I stared at him. He rarely talked of future plans except for how high he planned to jump his bike or what kind of all-terrain vehicle (ATV) he wanted. Until this moment, his dreams were always simple and very immediate.

Marley was serious about his plan, which he called his "Western Rest Home." The plan was to give crippled cowboys and elderly ranchers a comfortable place to spend their last days, doing the things that had made their lives worth living. He described his idea in detail—from the width of the wraparound porch to the dimensions of the greenhouse.

He described the layout of the bedrooms, which would come equipped with refrigerators for whiskey and beer. The beds could be hospital beds, but they would have colorful flannel sheets instead of thin white ones. To add color and comfort, the blankets would be down or woven wool. Native American style tapestries and "really cool art" would hang on the walls throughout this enormous log structure.

The guests could relax on the front porch and smoke their fat cigars and shoot at targets. If they wanted to go hunting, an ATV with a flatbed trailer would take them into the woods. He even designed the flatbed to have hooks to secure their wheelchairs to. If they wanted to go horseback riding, he had an idea of how to design the saddles to accommodate IV hookups. For the gardeners, the large greenhouse would have plant beds at the right height and angle to be wheelchair accessible.

He thought of every detail. He described what the staff would wear and what they would look like; all young, strong, and beautiful. He made my mouth water as he went over the daily menus and explained how, in case the old rancher women wanted to help cook, the kitchen would be modified for their convenience. Every room would have a view of the Cascade Mountains or the gardens in the courtyard. The hayfield would be visible from the porch so that during the hay season the old ranchers could feel like they were a part of the process, even if they couldn't help.

His eyes sparkled as he told me every last detail. I could smell the scents, imagined seeing spittoons being cleaned daily, and could hear the extraordinary stories of these old folks. I wanted to hear more, but…the door opened. I had been so wrapped up in Marley's story that I had completely forgotten why we were there.

Foul Weather Ahead

The girls played outside the doctor's office, while Drew and Cindy waited in the lobby and I waited with Marley in the examining room. I had been thoroughly entertained by Marley's plan to create his Western Rest Home until the doctor walked in with Drew and Cindy on his heels.

Unbelievable words spilled from the doctor's mouth. He kept going over the same details, coming up with the same conclusion. He explained there was a fifth cause for pneumonia. He said that Marley didn't inhale a piece of chicken taco into his lungs as we first suspected; it was caused by a tumor growing in his left lung. For a few seconds I felt like I was lifting out of my body; I could see everyone in the room, but my ears were ringing and I didn't feel connected at all…to anything. Marley had lung cancer.

When there was nothing more the doctor could say, we walked out of the prison-like cubicle. I'm sure I looked calm, fortified with that supernatural kind of strength mothers can muster when their family is under fire. Internally, it felt as though I was staggering, as if I'd been told that a hurricane was speeding straight toward us and all exits were blocked. In the back of my frozen brain I could find only one thought, "Leave it to Marley to come up with something like this."

We left the doctor's office to join the rest of the family outside. It was a beautiful, sun-filled April morning and Cindy's two daughters, Laura and Vanessa, had been playing tag with Catie in the sea of fresh cut green grass. In the middle of this manicured lawn was one stone bench. That's where we gathered to relay the news to the girls. Drew and Catie sat on the bench as Marley, Cindy, Vanessa, Laura, and I formed a circle before them on the grass.

Drew slumped slightly forward and sighed. His head was bowed low as he took off his cap, squeezed it in his free hand, and slapped it against his thigh as if to brush off the dust after a long horseback ride. It didn't take too many words before the tears began to drop onto his jeans. His voice quivered only slightly as the three girls listened intently. Catie instinctively moved in to nuzzle closer to her dad. She knew something was terribly wrong as she watched Drew.

Batten Down the Hatches

Drew took a deep breath and said, "Well, it turns out that Marley didn't aspirate on that piece of chicken at school after all. Instead, he got pneumonia because there's a tumor in his lung. Marley has lung cancer. He's got a kind of cancer they call "squamous," and they did all those tests to make absolutely sure. I guess they've never seen this kind of cancer in a kid."

Vanessa, the oldest of the girls, was shaken but curious and asked, "Are they *really* sure?"

It was a good question, but there was only one short answer, "Yup."

Laura calmly asked, "What happens now? What are we going to do?" I had known Laura since she was a wee babe and always marveled that nothing seemed to rock her off balance.

Cindy sighed and explained, "Well, the two doctors we have now said from here on, this is out of their league. I guess now we need to find a new doctor while we learn as much about this as possible on our own."

Catie was crying. She looked up at her dad and quietly asked, "Is Marley going to be okay?"

Drew put his arm around Catie and almost whispered, "We sure hope so. There's a lot we don't know yet."

Marley was quietly sitting on the grass, leaning back on his outstretched arms, chewing on a long blade of grass. Our stomachs were in knots and an uncomfortable silence swept over us. When there were no more answers, we wandered over to Drew's truck, not really wanting to separate.

It was switch day. I'd had the kids for two busy weeks of juggling work, school, and a sick boy. All of a sudden, the kids drove away with Drew and Cindy, and I found myself standing in the parking lot alone. I was numb. I couldn't believe this was really happening.

I had to drive 20 minutes back to Ashland to go to work. I

thought about going home to recover, but it dawned on me that life wasn't going to stop because my son was sick. The tasks required both at work and at home couldn't be ignored just because I was scared.

Shocked by the proportions of the storm we were facing, I drove back to the office to the folks I worked with—they were the closest thing to family I had locally. As awful as this situation was, after I finished telling the news to my clan at work, I knew someone could and would make me laugh. Sure enough, Jay, the jester of the crew, broke the tension and sadness that was filling the office. He did a perfect imitation of my desire to deny the diagnosis with the following quote from one of Marley's favorite movies:

"It's NOT a 'tuma.'"

—John Kimble (Arnold Schwarzenegger)
Kindergarten Cop

Communicating with the Clan

The last thing I felt like doing was talking to my family on the phone for the next few hours. Just the process of contacting my five sisters and three brothers would have taken forever. I realized I needed to create a new way of communicating this news to other family members and friends. Too many people knew and loved Marley, and they all needed to be kept in the loop. I stayed late at the office to use the computer and started drafting a letter. I started at the beginning and tried to explain everything. I sent the e-mail update to everyone who knew Marley.

From that day forward, Marley's Network was officially formed. I had no idea how incredibly important this communication technique would become. Every time information needed to be updated, I just sent another e-mail. I also didn't expect how comforting it would be to write about what we were experiencing. At the time, it simply seemed like a logical solution. The process of communicating kept me focused, connected, and relatively clearheaded for the duration of Marley's journey.

Wednesday, April 12, 2000
Subject: "MARLEY NETWORK UPDATE – #1"

Dear Ones,

This is the first of many e-mails designed to invite all the people in my life to join forces. I'm up against the most important event in my life, and I have a very strong feeling that it's critically important we go through this together. It's an unusual story, and it's going to affect many of us for the rest of our lives. Sit down and prepare yourselves.

My son Marley is very sick and is facing choices few of us will ever know. As his mother and advocate, I call on all of you to form a well-oiled machine that's prepared to handle *anything* we're faced with.

I do my best to manage Bathroom Readers' Press, a publishing company that is currently for sale. I work with an exceptional team of people. I'm good at what I do; communicate, organize, and delegate. It occurred to me that I need to use my professional skills in my personal life so I can have the time and energy to care for my son and daughter, continue to run a business, and still have time and energy to care for myself. To pull this off, I need your help. If we unite and stay informed, we can make a difference to a unique and worthy young warrior.

I want to describe the players and recap the recent history of events. Soon I will send a list of possible needs and "job descriptions" for those of you who'd like to help but don't know how. It's time to get organized.

The Star: Marley Jacob Pratt (15 years old), born Feb. 6, 1985.

The Lead Characters: Drew (father), Cindy (stepmother), Catie (sister, 10 years old), Vanessa (stepsister, 14 years old), Laura (stepsister, 11 years old), and me (Marley's mother).

The Supporting Cast: You.

The Plot: Marley is a unique and well-loved individual whose special spirit has wiggled into the hearts of many. Trying to define Marley is like trying to make sense of chaos. He's had a radical history of undiagnosed irregularities throughout his short stay on Earth. In spite of his life hurdles, he's a tall, strong teenager who has a remarkable sense of self and the rare ability to express love.

On Leap Day, Marley went to the emergency room with pneumonia, which escalated beyond the expected. The first two weeks in March consisted of one procedure after another, and he has the war wounds to prove it! At first, the emergency room doctors tried to suck the fluid from his lung with a long syringe (didn't work). Next, a lung specialist put three half-inch drain tubes into his side because the fluid had escaped into the *pleural cavity* around the lung (didn't work). A surgeon was called in to do a *thoracotomy*, an incision from his nipple to the top of his shoulder blade, designed to clear out all the *empaema* (thick fluid) from the cavity around his lung. At the same time, the surgeon elected to do a procedure called a *bronchoscopy* (several tubes up a nostril lead-

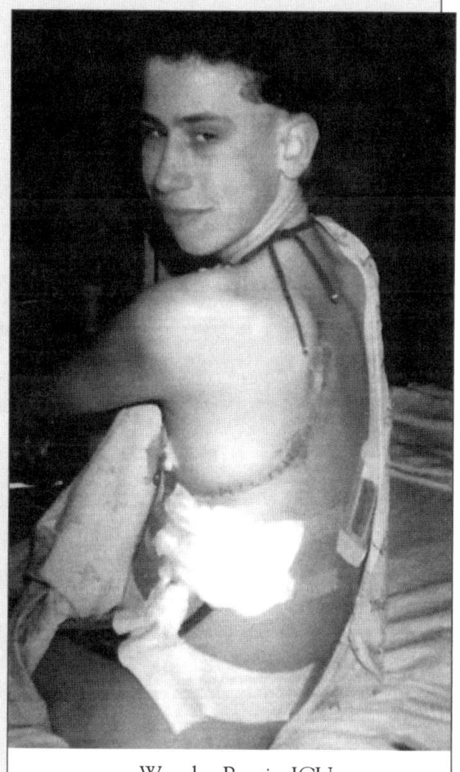

Wonder Boy in ICU

ing down into his lung). A "foreign body" was identified, looking like a piece of meat. This explained why the antibiotics didn't do the trick and why the infection persisted. Marley recalled choking on a chicken taco at school. The way he eats...no wonder! It was nice to have a reason for this drama.

Two more bronchoscopies were performed to get all of whatever was in there out—piece by piece—with microscopic pinchers. These samples were also used to biopsy both his lung tissue and the "foreign body." The results came back "abnormal," indicating a tumor; but *that* couldn't be right, so it was agreed we'd let the lung heal a bit before testing it again.

During those two weeks, an incredible network of people showed their love for Marley by sending pebbles as a symbol of their healing prayers. I am still amazed at the showing of community. Marley built an incredible water fountain using the many stones and gems sent (although the container proved to be way too small!). We also did a 5 P.M. meditation daily to focus healing energy—many have continued this practice to date.

The Plot Thickens

After 12 days in the hospital, we spent one additional, truly ghastly week of Marley suffering from "spinal headaches." During surgery, a morphine IV had been inserted directly into his spine. This is called an *epidural injection* and is standard operating procedure. These incredibly painful headaches were created when the epidural needle was removed from his spine. The hole didn't properly close, and spinal fluid was slowly leaking out, causing excruciating headaches whenever he lifted his head above heart level.

This unfortunate side effect happens rarely, so no one thought it was a big deal. They suggested we wait it out—the ol' "take two aspirins and rest" medicine. Enough was enough, and we demanded attention. Seven days later, all was solved with a "blood patch." They extracted some of Marley's spinal fluid with a very long needle and injected it into the hole that was leaking. It was a fast but horrible procedure. Less than an hour later, the pain was completely gone. He leapt off the gurney, slapped his baseball cap on his head and defiantly strode out of ER, wanting nothing to do with hospitals ever again.

Drew, Cindy, and I were beside ourselves. We were outraged that the anesthesiologist hadn't told us about this cure in the beginning and instead left Marley to writhe in agony for a whole week, after two previous weeks of torture. This whole situation was intolerable. The worst part was, apparently it was a risk that we agreed to when we signed the initial paperwork, so this jerk was able to charge us an astronomical fee to perform this unusual procedure to cure a rare problem that *he* created in the first place! When he fixed the mistake in just a few minutes...well, we thought his death would have been a punishment too kind.

Meanwhile, back at the ranch...Marley made me dye anything that was white except his hospital gown—he wanted to burn that one! We had a coming-home party around a bonfire, and his wish came true. He was healing fast and was back at school in no time. He was thrilled to be reunited with his beloved bike. But alas, a few weeks ago a shift happened: his energy began to decrease and the pain in his chest started to increase.

The Climax

The lung specialist was fast to react and scheduled another round of X-rays and yet *another* bronchoscopy. Poor Marley was scared to death and threw up all the way to the hospital (a 40-minute drive), hanging out of the passenger window of Drew's truck. After an out-patient procedure, the lab results were quickly diagnosed. Our worst fear became a reality. In the superior lobe of Marley's left lung, a cancerous tumor exists. Marley has lung cancer. Gulp.

What we know, so far, is that this type of cancer is called *squamous*, a common and slow-growing cancer found in older folks. None of the general rules of this type of cancer apply because of Marley's young age. Cancer tends to be more aggressive in youth. It looks like the tumor may have already *metastasized* (spread to other areas) because apparently, some of his lymph nodes may be suspect. We need more info and a new doctor.

We have an appointment with an *oncologist* (cancer specialist) on Thursday. We're looking into finding the best teaching hospital with the most experienced and knowledgeable multidisciplinary oncology team available in the country. No one on the West coast has dealt with squamous in a 15-year-old. We're not even clear whether we're looking at pediatrics or not. (Marley is young, but with an old person's disease.) We've been told radiation and chemotherapy are the standard operating procedures. We need more information and we need it fast! Marley's life is at stake.

Epilogue

This is where you come in. We need your help because, as you know, time never seems to stand still. Our lives are full to the brim right now even without this new scenario. There's no way we can deal with this on our own.

Drew and Cindy have been working their butts off. They've just bought a ranch in the Colestin Valley and are building their dream home. They are also busy maintaining two full time careers—Drew is a farrier (horseshoer) and Cindy is an electrical contractor. My career is a dream come true and is at a critical stage. My beloved boss/friend has just sold the Bathroom Readers' Press to a San Diego corporation. My co-workers and I have been sold as a part of the package. We've been given substantial raises, but our responsibilities have increased twofold. In short, Drew, Cindy, and I are under incredible stress and need all the help we can get, not only to obtain our dreams, but to maintain our health and sanity.

Marley's little sister, Catie, needs some special attention too. She FEELS more deeply than anyone I know. When she doesn't have a safe arena to express, she tends to go into the labyrinth of Within. Unfortunately for her three parents, sometimes it's hard to be in two places at once, and some traveling may be on the horizon.

Drew and I split the custody of the children equally. Cindy and her X-husband have the same arrangement—two weeks on and two weeks off. This has been working great for many years. Both of our families live in the country and have gardens, land, and animals to tend. Neither family has a nest egg to fall back on. Thanks to my beloved boss, John, if all goes well, we'll be able to maintain and, hopefully, avoid falling into the black hole of debt. (John gave me the birthday gift of health insurance precisely one month before Marley got pneumonia.) As always, John's timing is impeccable and his gift...invaluable! Just imagine our woes if we had no insurance coverage.

Ta da!!!!! Done!!!!!
I love you all and can't thank you enough for your support,
Jennifer

***"The fearless are merely fearless.
People who act in spite of their fear
are truly brave."***

—-James A. LaFond–Lewis

LUNG CANCER 101

Know Thine Enemy

Taking a crash course in medicine felt much like dealing with the educational system. Drew, Cindy, and I had to quickly learn how to be effective advocates for Marley. We needed to understand the reasoning and methods of any procedure or prescription advised. We discovered that unless we asked questions, sometimes the professionals forgot to share critical information. The first step was to grasp how our bodies work and translate that information so even our kids could understand it.

In our bodies, we have trillions of cells, each cell containing approximately 140,000 *genes*, threads of chemicals known as *DNA*. It only takes a defect in one gene to cause cancer. One job of a gene is to organize the process of regenerating new healthy cells by replicating itself. Sounds simple enough—but when a malfunction happens, a copying error can occur. When the DNA mutates, the abnormal cells can multiply, which causes cancer.

It takes many genetic generations of mutation before cancer occurs. Once a cancer cell is born, it can take ten years of multiplying and grouping together to form a tumor that can be recognized by our current technology. This meant Marley may have been five years old when this disease took hold.

Lung Cancer

There are four types of lung cancer, each with their own set of characteristics. My father died from *small-cell carcinoma*. This is the rarest and nastiest of the four kinds, but it responds the best to chemotherapy and radiation. Marley had *squamous*, a *non-small cell carcinoma*. It usually affects people over 45 years old whose bodies have been abused by heavy smoking or carcinogenic chemicals. Generally this cancer grows slowly. In children, however, it can grow rapidly because a child's cells (healthy or not) multiply much faster than an adult's. (Ironic that my father—a long term smoker—contracted a non-smoker's cancer while Marley, with his virgin lungs, contracted squamous.)

FAITH IN DOCTORS

Who's on First?

While learning what the medical profession knows about cancer, we also found out how much they *don't* know; and their techniques of covering that up. We needed to learn their language so we could understand them. One thing we learned is that the more unsure doctors are about something, the more complex their words become.

When researching the method doctors use of "staging" cancer, we found clear confusion. This is supposed to be a way to identify the severity of the risk caused by a cancerous growth. The problem is, different kinds of cancers have specific staging systems, so it's like using three alphabets for one language. A brief explanation of this professional disorganization was found in *The Complete Cancer Survival Guide* (a must-read for anyone dealing with cancer). "The need for a standardized classification system has been addressed but not yet rectified."

I'm not implying that all doctors are bad, but once we started to experience some of the holes in the medical system, like how easy it was to lose our X-rays or how difficult it was for them to admit their mistakes, we knew it was imperative to question what we were told and to research everything. We realized it could be a matter of our son's survival to take responsibility and make sure we understood what was going on.

The benefit of educating ourselves was not being at the mercy of doctors' sometimes antiquated knowledge, conflicting opinions, and limited communication skills. The problem with educating ourselves was losing respect for that which, at first, seemed so powerfully magical.

"Those who are held wise among men,
and who search for the reason of things,
are those who bring the most sorrow on themselves."

—Euripides

UPDATING INFORMATION

High Speed

With every new day, people stopped me on the street corner or e-mailed me to say they wanted to be kept informed about Marley's health. Marley's Network was growing. Our lives had just been flipped upside down, and knowing what I was communicating to whom was a mystery.

In the beginning, when I wrote an Update Letter I had to assume the reader knew nothing of past events. This ended up working pretty well because, in reality, none of us really knew what was happening. Repeating some of the basic information helped me battle the stupor of shock and enabled me to comprehend the facts (or lack thereof).

"If you can keep your head
when all about you are losing theirs,
it's just possible you haven't grasped the situation."

—Jean Kerr

Tuesday, March 16, 2000
Subject: "THE SCOOP ON MARLEY"

Dear Family,

As most of you know, it turns out Marley didn't aspirate on food after all. Rather, he has lung cancer—squamous, by name. Apparently the tumor reached a size great enough to irritate the lung, which caused the pneumonia. When the surgeon found the tumor, it was assumed it was a foreign object until the biopsy was tested and retested. The pros couldn't believe the initial results, so they waited several weeks for the swollen tissue to calm down enough to retest for accuracy. Last week, he had his fourth bronchoscopy to grab another chunk of the lung to make absolutely sure it was indeed what they feared—lung cancer.

Cancer is rated by stages (with numbers; 1 – 4 and letters; A – D: the lower, the better.) Our local doctors think Marley's cancer is pretty far advanced, but it's hard to tell at this stage of the game. Their guess is 3A or B. It seems the tumor in the lung has already metastasized; in other words, has gone beyond the confines of the left lung. This makes it questionable as to whether or not it's even operable. The only way for them to know whether major surgery can eliminate the tumor is to do "minor" surgery to investigate. The surgical procedure would be another thoracotomy. This is problematic, since they just did this massive procedure and his muscles and nerves haven't had enough time to heal.

Our next step is to find out which hospital has the experience and technology to deal with a teenager with this kind of cancer. We don't want to have three operations if they're not all necessary. The suggested surgery and recovery will require a couple of weeks in whatever hospital is most suitable, and then follow-up therapy. We're assured the recommended radiation and/or chemotherapy can take place locally. We're swimming in conflicting professional opinions, and we're not sure what river we're in.

**Late breaking news! The doctor just called. Now they think they want to do the chemo and radiation *before* surgery. Hmmmm. Sure fills me with confidence that they know what they're talking about. Not! Must hit the books and ask intelligent questions and find a doctor with experience.

Anyway, as we know more, we'll let you know.

As my niece Selene once told me, "I love you up to God,"
Jennifer

PREPARATION

Questioning Everything

In the beginning stages of learning about cancer, the amount of research done on our behalf was extraordinary. We were learning everything from medical definitions to organizations that fund special needs. It felt useless to read most of the medical research because nothing seemed to quite describe Marley's case. The information about squamous lung cancer primarily related to older people who spent a lifetime abusing their bodies or being abused by environmental hazards.

I was swimming in statistics, questioning everything I had done that could have caused cancer to grow in my son's body. I had been handed hundreds of leads, and I was feeling completely overwhelmed by the amount of work required to follow up on just a few of them. I didn't know if I could deal. I wanted to run away. I wanted to wake up from this nightmare. I wanted to hide under the covers but knew my only course of action was to study hard, think like a detective, and be brave.

While reading reams of research, Drew and I came to the conclusion that none of the existing "rules" applied. Before us was a country-bred 15-year-old who didn't smoke anything and who ate mostly healthy food, prepared in healthy, loving homes. And yet, Marley had squamous lung cancer that from the get-go had metastasized to the lymph system. According to the books, Marley faced a wicked case of terminal high-class cancer, which meant he had about six months to live (give or take). But none of these books took into consideration that he was a headstrong teenager.

Marley's Way

Marley had an amazing way of looking at life. He seemed to fully understand what was going on, yet cared about only the facts—he didn't ask why, or what could go wrong—he just wanted answers to "what" and "when." All he cared about was the bottom line. I would have been scared shitless facing this kind of crisis, but he took it all in stride.

During the time we were scurrying around gathering information and making plans, Marley was basking in the attention. Everyone was being so nice to him! Marley hadn't been exactly easy to live with that year. He spent most of his time butting heads with everyone in authority. For Marley, the relationship that changed most beneficially was with his stepmother, Cindy, and he was glad of it. He was also excited about the possibility of traveling to a big city hospital, alone with me and Drew. From Marley's perspective, maybe having cancer wasn't so bad: Great things were happening because of it.

"When written in Chinese, the word "crisis" is composed of two characters. One represents danger and the other represents opportunity."

—John F. Kennedy

I worried about this "childlike" view and tried to play psychologist, communicating in a way I knew he'd understand. Without beating around the bush, I found opportune moments to ask digging questions like, "So do you get that this disease is trying to kill you?" He'd shrug as I continued to push the "reality" river. "The doctors worry you have…like…'til Christmas to be alive."

He'd flick a chunk of mud off his boot and matter-of-factly reply, "They don't know shit."

My knee jerk motherly response was, "Watch your mouth, boy."

Turning toward me with a straight face he'd respond with, "I can't watch it, when I can't see it!"

I'd roll my eyes, amazed that I'd walked right into his classic diversionary volley. He'd just smile and distract me by pointing out a red-tailed hawk and we'd both nod, appreciating its grace. After ten thousand such psychological inquisitions, I learned that Marley was very aware of his situation, but he chose to live in his own world, with its own rules of reality, and he had little time for anything else.

DECLARING PEACE

Forgive and Forget

My life was changing direction so fast that I was forced to use every skill I had, and needed to learn new ones as quickly as possible. Our 15-year-old had cancer, and it felt like we were on the front lines of a war. We knew what we were fighting, but we had no idea what weapons we could use, or how to wield them.

During the six years prior to Marley's diagnosis, relating with Drew and Cindy was respectful and cordial but a bit chilly. We basically stayed out of each other's way, respecting our individuality as two separate parental teams. When Laura and Catie were babies and Vanessa and Marley were in preschool together, it was as though Cindy and I shared all four kids. When Drew and I split up, my relationships with both Cindy and the girls had ended.

When Marley got pneumonia and we ended up spending 12 days in ICU together, there were some tense times. We were face to face, dealing with one gruesome procedure after another, in a very small space, under extreme emotional stress. It could've been ugly.

I bow down before the gods of grace in thanks that Drew, Cindy, and I were able to keep our past personal grievances and our present level of discomfort in perspective. Drew and Cindy respected my role as mother and I honored their roles as father and stepmother. We were thrown into leaning on each other for survival. At first it was like we were all wearing our clothes backwards—a little strained and uncomfortable—but we knew we were all in this equally and together. The only war to be fought was the one to help Marley live. We were all on the same side.

There were four children and three parents. Each clan had their clan and supporting network of friends. Leave it to Marley to unite us though extreme circumstances. I know it made all the difference in the world to Marley, having all three of his parents right there to catch him, and all three of his sisters there to discover their courage with him.

Chapter Four:
Faith in Friends

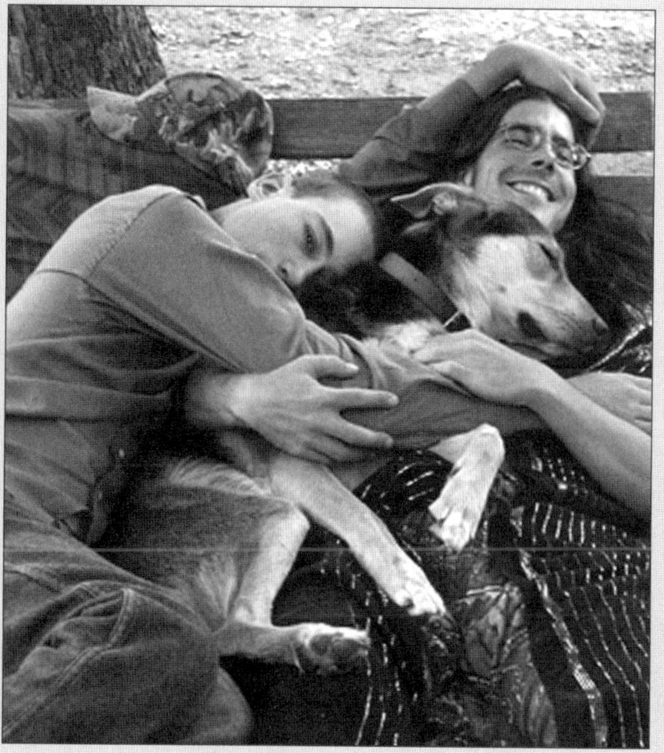

"Critters Cuddle"

Marley, Frisco, and Eric

Photo: Debbie Thornton

FRIENDS IN HIGH PLACES

Rite Aid

I was a member of a highly elective group called Evo's Porch Club [in the] A.M. (EPCAM). Every weekday morning Sunny, Cullen, Kim, Jeff, and I met at Evo's, one of Ashland's abundant coffee houses. There were seven other semi-regulars who joined us when their schedules permitted. When I arrived every morning, I never knew who the group would consist of or what the flavor of the conversation would be. But whether it was glorious or gloomy out, I could trust that EPCAM would be gathered. We found that not only were we a lifeline for each other, but our daily ritual of gathering was comforting to others as well. For instance, one woman approached us and said, "I always know everything in this strange world is okay when I see you all on the porch every morning."

Our morning ritual was as predictable as the sun rising. The EPCAM crew had wordlessly vowed to be there for each other, no matter what. We knew that if indeed the sun were to rise, at least one of us would be on Evo's porch. I didn't even like coffee. I did like knowing there was one thing in my life I could count on.

For the two weeks each month that the kids were at Drew's, I didn't have to wake early to get the kids to school. I still leapt out of bed each weekday to scurry to Evo's, regardless of how crappy or euphoric I felt because…well, because my presence was expected, and the other members of EPCAM seemed to need me as much as I needed them. This particular ritual was a physical lifeline as well as an intellectual and emotional one. If I didn't show up for two consecutive days, I'd likely get a phone call to make sure I was still alive. The same went for the other single people in

> ***Definition***
>
> **Rite**
>
> 1. Procedure in accordance with prescribed rule or custom.
>
> 2. Any formal customary observance or procedure, religious or otherwise.
>
> 3. A prescribed form or manner governing the words or actions of a ceremony of religious, social, or tribal significance.

this little tribe.

After Marley was diagnosed with cancer, there were countless mornings when I was kidless that I had to claw myself out of bed to face another day of dreading having to face another day. Sometimes in that split second when my eyes opened, life was a glorious blank slate. Then I would remember the enormous challenge before me. "Shit. This again?" I'd look at the clock and know that if I didn't get my butt down to Evo's by 8:45 A.M., Sunny was going to gripe at me for being late.

How do you spell relief? S-U-P-P-O-R-T!

According to *Webster's*, a basic definition of a family is "a group consisting of two parents and their children." F-A-M-I-L-Y: Father And Mother I Love You! In a perfect world, our biological family would be our built-in support group, but this isn't always the case. It seems, instead, that support is found from those around us—both family and friends—and is rooted in some form of ongoing ritual, formal or not. These days, gangs, religious organizations, cults, clubs, and purpose-oriented organizations all seem to fit the bill. Bottom line: Our support networks help us when the going gets tough.

"Call it a clan, call it a network,
call it a tribe, call it a family.
Whatever you call it, whoever you are,
you need one."

—Jane Howard

Aside from EPCAM and my biological family, I had the Bathroom Readers' Institute (BRI). Together we created and published annual editions of *Uncle John's Bathroom Readers*. My co-workers and I worked in close quarters and became an inseparable clan, both at work and after hours. We were a delightful combination of co-workers, siblings, best friends, and lovers. These exceptional people will forever and unconditionally be considered my non-kin clan.

A WELL-KNOWN MYSTERY

The Cowboy Way

The valley that Drew and Cindy lived in was a tight-knit community that followed "cowboy" rules; they believed in the importance of sticking together, getting back up on the horse, working hard, and making do with what they had. Many families in the Colestin Valley came from other circles of spirituality or wealth. The result was a valley full of heart-filled, influential families, with strong values based in the Cowboy Way and the Ways of Nature. Thank God for the Colestin Valley community—for without their ties, we would've never ended up with the high-class care we received.

Trying to find concrete information about cancer was frustrating. It was becoming apparent that cancer is still a well-known mystery. Helping us was a small army of intelligent people doing research—some of whom did research for a living. This meant we were receiving current statistics about cutting-edge procedures that some doctors were ignorant of. I'll tell you, doctors hate that!

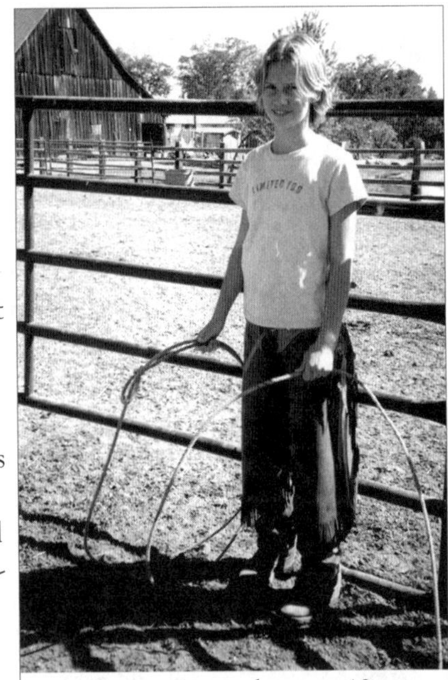

Catie, at a round-up, age 10
Photo: Cindy Warzyn

Cindy had some nursing experience, I am a professional organizer, and Drew is a large cowboy that asks really smart questions, using very few words. Most of our doctors realized they needed to stay on their toes and shoot straight with us. For us, being well-informed was a prerequisite for entering the medical world. Being strong willed and well-connected didn't hurt either.

The Western Way

The more we dealt with Western medical practices, the more it seemed the medical world runs on the principles of politics—it's all about who you know and how much influence they have to pull the right strings. Drew and Cindy's friend and neighbor, Jennifer D., knew the administrative director of a top East coast comprehensive cancer center. This is how, within a few short weeks, we were scheduled for an appointment with "the best of the best."

Dr. Sugarmaker is an amazing surgeon that, at the time of our first appointment, was in the news for his cutting-edge ability to orchestrate multiple organ transplants. Not only did he have experience dealing with children with lung cancer, he worked with a renowned team from three hospitals that worked together like a well-oiled machine. To them, our case was unusual but not unheard of. We may have been up against a challenging obstacle, but at least we knew we had the best tools for success.

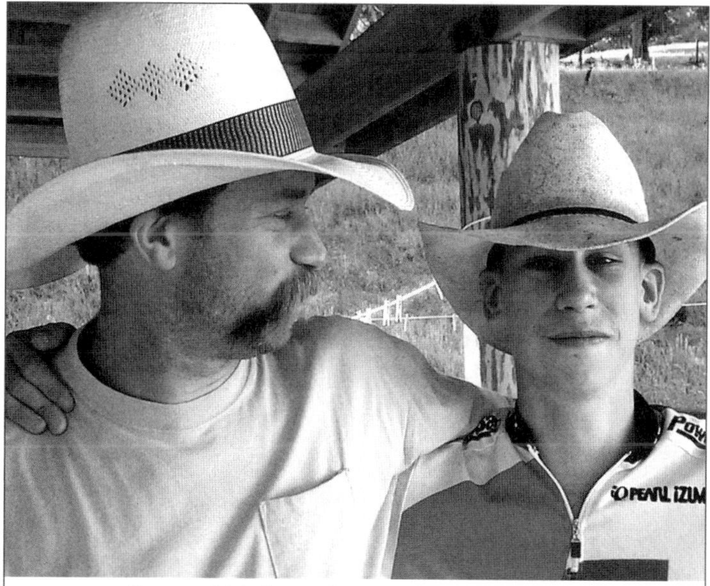

Drew and Marley at their ranch in the Colestin

Photo: Dee Warzyn

Monday, May 22, 2000
Subject: "BOSTON BOUND"

Howdy Gang!

Life's moving at high speed and we're in high gear. Thanks to a well-connected friend of Drew and Cindy's, we now have one of the country's best thoracic surgeons working on Marley's case. Dr. Sugarmaker works with a team of top-notch doctors from several hospitals in Boston. They have agreed to take Marley on. We not only know what river we're swimming in, we're being told exactly what stroke to use.

Some major strings must have been pulled, because I've never seen big wheels turn this fast. It's taken a team of us hustling to keep up with them. Forty-five thousand faxes and phone calls later, we've gathered all of Marley's records and X-rays and sent them via overnight mail to Boston. Our crew has scheduled emergency airfare, "out-of-area" insurance policy authorization, and a housesitting schedule. Believe it or not, we're heading to Boston this Thursday for a Friday appointment. We don't know what procedures to expect. We should know more tomorrow after they receive his records.

Game Plan for Success

• We need to simplify the communication process. Many of you have e-mail. Those of you who don't, but want to stay informed, need to get one or organize a phone tree.

• I need a cell phone and a laptop computer. Can someone help me research this? This will enable me to send out regular updates via e-mail no matter where I am. These messages can then be forwarded to your support networks. We need to limit the amount of calls Drew, Cindy, and I receive daily. It's really hard to repeat the same things over and over again. Thirty phone conversations, each lasting ten minutes, chews through time we could spend doing research or loving the kids.

• While we're traveling, we need people to do fast research on words, phrases, and procedures we don't fully understand.

• Can someone research setting up a trust fund or a stock gift option for emergencies like unexpected medical costs, travel expenses, etc.?

• I'm worried that without physical outlets for Marley's never-ending supply of energy that he may go stark raving mad in the hospital and while recovering at home. He loves building things with Legos, and he is creating a fountain with the pebbles that people have sent as tokens of their love. We need help rounding up Legos and supplies for the pebble fountain project.

• Last, but certainly not least, can someone help find networks and support group contacts for parents, siblings, and young patients with cancer? Sometimes it feels like we're all alone, reinventing the wheel, but I know many other people have gone through similar experiences.

I've never experienced a situation where the phrase "deadline" meant someone could actually die if the job's not done fast enough. There doesn't seem to be much room for error here, folks. Most of you know that Drew and I like to handle our own issues, but I'm quickly learning that there's no way we can do this well on our own. Drew may not agree with my methods of reaching out but...damn...I need your help.

I love you all and thank you for your support.
Jennifer

"Prayer indeed is good,
but while calling on the gods
a man should himself lend a hand."

—Hippocrates

BOSTON GLOBETROTTERS

Ronald McDonald's House

Since the beginning of Marley's drama, my sister Julia had been forwarding my e-mails to her friend Nicky, who lived outside of Boston. Nicky appointed herself our guardian during our time in the city. She didn't ask if she could help, she simply picked us up at the airport, delivered us to the Ronald McDonald House, and said she'd be back for dinner. We instantly fell in love with her no-nonsense approach, and deeply appreciated her help.

The Ronald McDonald corporation has houses located across the country. They're shared community havens for children with life-threatening illnesses and their families. The one we were staying at was a glorious old Victorian mansion that had been converted to accommodate twenty out-of-state families with seriously ill children. It was a ten-minute walk to the hospital, and a five-minute walk to the train stop.

This enormous old house was filled with kids with cancers of every variety. I had not known how many children were in serious trouble. Some were having organs removed and replaced, while others were undergoing gruesome procedures like bone marrow transplants and chemotherapy. Even so, it was a sanctuary—a happy place that offered comfort, camaraderie, and quiet. The entire staff volunteered their time, and every luxury was donated. The whole place was steeped in love and caring. Until Marley got cancer, I turned my nose up in disgust at anything having to do with the fast food corporate reality. But in this case, I've changed my tune—Ronald McDonald's houses are a godsend.

"No matter how much we manipulate, measure, and analyze, life remains wonderfully, terrifyingly mysterious."

—Gloria Karpinski

The kids at this house were amazing. Maybe it was the hardships they faced that set them apart. They were honest, inclusive, and incredibly loving. As soon as we arrived, a skinny five-year-old girl decided that Marley was the best invention since the merry-go-round. Brin was in love with him from the minute we walked in.

She interrogated us about where we were from and why we were there. Then she launched into her cancer story as she led Marley around, showing him where all the cool stuff was. When she pointed to the stack of games and looked up at Marley with her big brown eyes, I knew it wouldn't take her long to weasel her way into his heart. Sure enough, Marley understood her silent question. He playfully picked Brin up, rubbed noses with her, and said, "Okay, you little cutie, I'll play later. Awright?" Satisfied, she scampered off to tell her mother about the new boy.

We had fun exploring the four floors of the mansion. There were gardens filled with flowers, a wraparound front porch with wicker recliners, and a game on every table. Just off the well-stocked kitchen was a private back porch. There was also a parlor with a computer, a living room with a TV, and a cozy basement theater, equipped with hundreds of videos. Marley was especially thrilled with the game room—and the freezer stocked with four different flavors of Boston's finest ice cream.

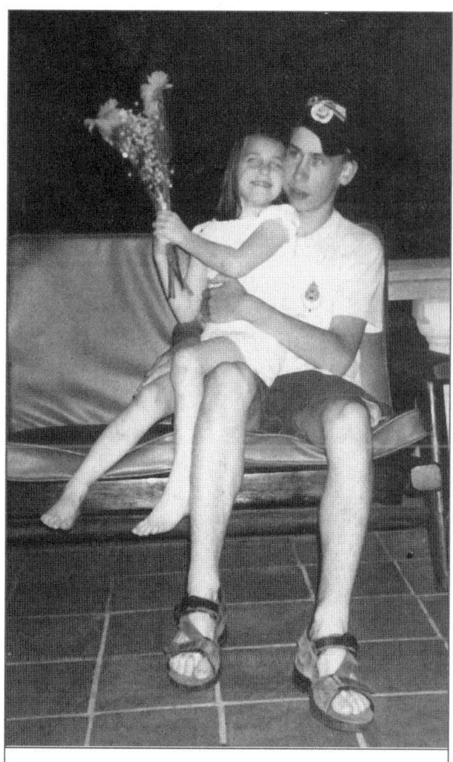

Marley holding Brin at the Ronald McDonald House

Everything's Just Ducky!

Feeling like three country mice, we braved the train and headed to Boston that first afternoon. Drew and I had both grown up in cities, but it had been a long time since either of us had used our city mentality. In Ashland, people look you in the eye and say "hello" as you pass. You don't have to worry about being ripped off, stepping over people sleeping on sidewalks, or becoming a hood ornament while crossing the street.

Once we arrived in Boston, we headed for the tallest building to get our bearings—the Skywalk on the 50th floor of the Prudential Building. What a view! Marley and Drew scared the crap out of me as they smashed their bodies up against the glass walls, trying to look straight down. Marley thought everything was *way* too cool. Then he caught a glimpse of Boston's Duck Boats lined up on the street below. That was the end of our skyscraper adventure. Marley was on a mission.

Nearly frothing at the mouth, he pulled Drew and I back down to street level to see the Duck Boats, up close and personal. There they were, six wartime contraptions lined up in front of him. I thought he was going to have a heart attack from his excitement. The battle-proof vehicles were a cross between a boat and a tank, longer and wider than a bus. These amphibious tour vehicles did a big loop around the city by way of both land and water. These machines were the stuff of Marley's dreams.

We went to buy tickets, but it cost $60 per person for the hour-long tour. Disappointed, we had to say, "Sorry, bud, we can't afford it. If we don't have to stay in Boston longer than planned, we'll definitely go." Marley was no fool; he'd heard that kind of line before. He argued that by the time we knew *that*, he probably wouldn't be physically able to enjoy the experience. He kept muttering about how dumb we were, always putting life off until tomorrow. "Tomorrow! It's always 'tomorrow' with you guys!" He had a good point. He was aware of what was in front of him, so he wanted to cram in the living NOW! He was so good at making us reevaluate our priorities.

The Time Machine

Under the circumstances, the trip to Boston was surprisingly pleasant. Other than in doctor's offices, Drew and I hadn't spent time alone together in over six years. I don't think Drew and I were prepared for what it felt like to be together again. In order to save money on hotel rooms, we had to follow the rules of the Ronald McDonald House, which allowed only one room per "family." That first night, we entered our room and were faced with one double bed and a small cot. After an awkward few seconds, reason prevailed. I was 5'2" while both Drew and Marley were over six feet tall. So, needless to say, I got the cot.

Some things never change. Our habits were cellularly familiar—Drew and I had spent ten years together, after all. And yet this made us even more uncomfortable. Finding myself in the same bedroom with Drew felt downright weird. It was as if no time had passed. I swear he was even reading the same Louis L'Amour western. He still pretended to be awake reading with the book propped against the bedside table as he snored. I had to laugh as I turned his light out. Marley was in heaven. From his perspective, he was alone with Mom and Dad—just like the old days.

After the next day's schedule at the hospital, we had three days with nothing to do but have fun. Drew and I were determined to make this a good trip for Marley. We knew there was a risk that Marley might not be around for long, and we were going to soak up all that life had to offer. Although neither of us liked to admit it, being together wasn't all that bad. He complained that I laughed inappropriately at everything. I had the distinct impression Drew thought I was crazy. Despite our differences, we had a lot of fun together. I'm not sure many other men could have dealt with being with their ex as gracefully—in close quarters and under tremendous stress.

"Sit in the fire long enough and purification does happen."

—Nancy Jane

Thursday, May 25, 2000
Subject: "GOOD NIGHT MOON"

Good Day!

I can't believe we're in Boston!

With only two days notice, we acquired two free plane tickets to Boston and bought the third for $744. (Believe it or not, that was a good deal.) We drove for six hours and flew for another twelve before settling in at our temporary new home: the Ronald McDonald House. Here, we're surrounded by people going through similar scenarios.

As of today, Marley has a new goal in life. From the top of a skyscraper, he spotted Boston's fleet of amphibious tour tanks, called Duck Boats. The ride unfortunately costs $180 for the three of us, and much to Marley's dismay, we couldn't afford it.

Almost forgot…I got to see both Drew and Marley play the giant floor piano at FAO Schwarz—just like in the movie *Big*. What a gas! I almost wet my pants. I thought to myself, "If Marley's going to die, this is how I want to remember him." If I hadn't been laughing so hard I would have definitely cried. Imagine his heavy army boots delicately dancing along the keys of the flat ten-foot keyboard in a crowded super-deluxe toy store—he was a cross between Arnold Schwarzenegger and Fred Astaire!

Marley's courage is an amazing thing to witness. No matter what, I'm incredibly proud to be a part of this family of mine.

It's late, gotta go. Good night moon.

I love you all,
Jennifer

P.S. The hospital's so big, there's valet parking!

Saturday, May 27, 2000
Subject: "INITIATIONS"

Hey Gang,

I'm plumb pooped out from yesterday's adventures—8.5 hours spent in hospital zone. Major stress! We walked to the Brigham & Women's Hospital (BWH) for our 9:30 A.M. appointment. This is one of several *very* large hospitals that are grouped together, covering four square city blocks. This "H-zone" comes complete with its own food court, and never-ending skywalks so you never have to experience nature's elements.

We didn't have to wait long for Marley's vitals to be taken and to have an initial meeting with the Physician's Assistant. But we did have to wait for two very long hours for the head honcho, Dr. Sugarmaker, Chief Thoracic Surgeon. So we took a long nap in the exam room while he was busy doing a kidney transplant. He finally whisked in and spoke to us as we wiped the sleep from our eyes. Then he whisked away, leaving us to talk to his two very skilled Surgical Coordinators. Apparently, when Sugarmaker gave orders, everyone jumped to attention to manifest the impossible. It was amazing to watch.

Dr. Sugarmaker's coordinators sat back-to-back in a very small cubicle. They each had headsets on, and their eyes were glued to their computer screens. Simultaneously, they would ask us questions, input the data, talk to each other, and rearrange 40 appointments to make way for us. We heard undertones of threats and bribes to everyone they negotiated with, but in the end we were miraculously shoved through the system in one day.

Their printer wasn't even finished copying our new, complicated schedule when the coordinators told us a bone scan prep was scheduled—two minutes ago! They pushed us out the door, slapped a map in our hands, and told us to return immediately after the appointment for the rest of our assignments. We had to literally run to the nuclear medicine department. A radioactive tracer was injected into Marley's arm through an IV. The tracer, which would illuminate any abnormalities, would be absorbed by his bones over a three-hour period, in preparation for pictures to be taken of his skeleton later that day.

While the tracer spread throughout Marley's body, we rushed back up to the coordinator's office, where we were told where to go for the next procedures. We were also told how to prepare for the exploratory surgeries scheduled for next week.

Pre-op was next. We had to get blood and urine tests done, meet the anesthesiologist, and get to our next appointment in less than an hour. Our appointment with the anesthesiologist was interrupted because we had to run to the radiology department at Dana-Farber for chest X-rays and an EKG. Afterward, we ran back to BWH to finish up with the anesthesiologist. Between each step, we had to sit in waiting rooms and fill out more forms. Either we were running frantically to an appointment or waiting for one, bored out of our minds and hungry as hell. Remember, all this time, Marley has had this radioactive stuff filtering through his bones!

By now, it was 3 P.M. and poor Marley's energy was fading fast. But, it was time to go back to radiology at Dana-Farber. Fortunately, we had packed PB&J sandwiches and had a chance to stuff our faces as we waited. The bone scan turned out to be pretty cool—we saw Marley's skeleton moving on a monitor (like real life X-ray vision). At least Marley got to lie down for a little bit before the last step. Back to pre-op at BWH to finish the lab tests. We wobbled out of the hospital zone at 5:30 P.M.

Monday is a holiday, so we have a long weekend of waiting ahead of us. On Tuesday, at 1:30, we're scheduled for one more test: a Positron Emission Tomography (PET scan). On

Wednesday, Marley goes in for a surgical mediastinoscopy.

Dr. Sugarmaker will make an incision at the base of Marley's throat, between his collar bones. Sugarmaker will then collect a few lymph nodes to biopsy, look around the *mediastinum* (the space between the lungs, containing the heart) and perform yet another bronchoscopy to remove another sample of the tumor. These new tissue samples will be sent to the pathology specialists, to rule out any previous mistakes.

Thursday will be spent recuperating. Friday, we all fly to New Jersey, where Drew and Marley will fly on to Portland, Oregon, and then drive the six hours home to Ashland, arriving in the middle of the night. I'm scheduled to fly from New Jersey to Chicago for the Book Expo of America, where I have to be an enthusiastic sales person. The timing is enough to make me slip into my designer straightjacket with matching pacifier. I suppose, if I'm smart, I'll cancel my work commitment. If yesterday is a precursor for the rest of our stay in Boston, I think I'll go insane if I don't!

Once we are home, the next step will be chemotherapy to "down-stage," or shrink, the tumor. After that, back to Boston for major surgery—a partial lobectomy (removing the lower half of Marley's left lung). After he recuperates from the lobectomy, they're suggesting radiation and more chemo for an indefinite period.

Now you know pretty much what we know. Will keep you posted on our adventures while trotting around Boston this weekend. I've got to go to sleep now.

I love you all,
Jennifer

PARANOIA

Tools for Success

It felt like Dr. Sugarmaker was making us run around the hospital zone for his own amusement. Most of the tests being done were repeat performances of what had already been done in Oregon. We had worked hard gathering copies of X-rays, MRI films, doctors' files, and radiologists' reports. We had put them all in chronological order, neatly packed them up, and paid to overnight the whole kit and kaboodle to Boston. Only to have them ignored.

It took us a while to understand the rationale behind Dr. Sugarmaker's directives. First, he needed to compare the new film with the older pictures to figure out how fast Marley's cancer was growing. More importantly, we learned that big city teaching hospitals can afford state-of-the-art equipment. A PET scan or an MRI done on a three-year-old machine, analyzed by a small-town radiologist, just wasn't good enough for Sugarmaker to rely on.

Copy Cat

After the tedious ordeal of locating Marley's films and records from two hospitals and four doctors, Cindy, Drew, and I made a pact to start keeping a journal of all dates, weights, procedures, etc. and to get copies of EVERYTHING. It seemed a little over the top, but the first time one of Marley's reports was lost in the mail, we knew we'd made the right choice.

I was always nervous whenever I asked for duplicates of X-rays or MRIs because I would be interrogated defensively. "Why do you want two sets made?" It didn't matter what I said, the nurse would look at me sternly and say in a condescending tone, "Aren't you aware that films are stored at the hospital, and copies can be made *if* you ever need them?" I fantasized about losing control and screaming, "Yes, but don't *you* know a duplicate now is cheaper, easier, and makes for a clearer image than a copy later? Don't you realize that your system sucks?"

Instead, I'd just nod and get the copy anyway.

Tuesday, May 30, 2000
Subject: "PRE-SURGERY PLAYTIME"

Howdy Gang,

This weekend we had no responsibilities other than to have fun. Nicky, our faithful Boston guide, has treated us very well. We went to the Omni theater to see dolphins jumping off the screen in 3-D. It yanked my heart strings. The sleek beauty of the dolphins was breathtaking—and the ignorance of the human race was so embarrassing. The grand scale of technology hit me like a ton of bricks. I cried during the entire movie. (It felt so good to cry.)

We cruised around the Museum of Science for three hours of entertainment. The feature show was about lightning, and was truly illuminating. There was also a computer that took a person's photograph and then digitally aged them over 20 minutes. It was wild seeing little kids turn into 80-somethings before my very eyes. I was thankful Marley didn't want to do this—I'm not sure I could have handled seeing him reach an age digitally that he may never reach in real time. As depressing as that was, I was positively glee-bound when we later discovered the musical stairs. Each step chimed a different note. Drew and Marley rolled their eyes at me when I ran up and down the stairs about thirty times. (Somehow it was different when *they* did it on the floor piano at FAO Schwartz.)

Once again, we have felt the effects of all who are on this journey with us…a band of invisible angels. Because of a recent e-mail describing Marley's desire to experience Boston's Duck Boats, four people responded and said they wanted to cover the cost. Thank you so much for your donations. The Duck ride was everything that Marley dreamed of. I must admit cruising around Boston in a monstrous amphibious vehicle *was* pretty fun. During the second half of the expedition, the vehicle plunged into the Charles River and the guide asked if anyone wanted to drive the "boat." Marley's long arm shot up with lightning speed and he was chosen. Drew and I looked at each other, nodding our heads, silently saying, "Could this possibly be any more perfect?"

Later that afternoon, I bought a book at the Discovery Store that shows each system of the human body in divine detail. It's so graphic that ol' blood and guts Marley even got queasy looking at it. Mom scores!

Yesterday, Nicky picked us up and drove us to her home north of Boston, where her husband Garrick took us sailing. We were all thrilled. Drew and I both love sailing, and Marley had never been on a yacht before. It was a perfect day.

Tomorrow (Wednesday) Marley goes in for the mediastinoscopy. The process begins at 7:30 A.M. when a "cocktail" is given to make him drowsy. At 9:30, they'll begin the surgery. By 1:00 P.M., we should be heading back to the RMcD house, and will spend the rest of the day and probably Thursday being quiet. This exploration, with all the other tests done last Friday, should give us the information we need to make intelligent decisions about what should be done next. If all goes well, we'll be boarding a plane on Friday, returning home on Saturday.

News Flash! My beloved niece, Selene, has chosen not to join a circus in New York, and instead will be living at my place. She is going to help take care of Marley and Catie (personally, I think she's trading one circus for another). Her grandparents, Phil and Liz, have graciously offered to match her circus salary. Yahoo! No worries. Life is looking up!!!!!

I am incredibly thankful you are in my world.
Love you all,
Jennifer

P.S. Catie, I love and miss you!

YOUR WISH IS GRANTED

Ask and Ye Shall Receive

In the e-mail I sent out just before we left, I made a list of the things that I knew we needed help with. The speed with which people moved gave me hope for the survival of our planet, not to mention my son.

By the time I boarded the plane, Jeff, my best friend and co-worker, had provided a briefcase full of research material neatly printed out and filed. At my fingertips was information about cancer camps, new cancer research, Mercy Flights, Make-A-Wish Foundation, and lists of other support networks. It was remarkable.

I was handed a brand new, fully-loaded laptop computer, compliments of the corporation that just bought our publishing company. I know it wasn't a sentimental gift—rather, an evil plot to keep me working; nevertheless, it was shocking how fast an idea made it to reality under the guidance of corporate organization.

JD, our head writer, gave me his cell phone for the journey (although I never did figure out how to use it). JD also volunteered to be the keeper of the master e-mail list while I was in Boston. Maintaining that list was critical—it was the only viable means of communicating with a group as big as Marley's Network was becoming.

While we were in Boston, my brother-in-law, Joseph, took on the responsibility of being the volunteer coordinator. He did an awesome job of trying to keep things straight, as e-mails were firing back and forward at a mind-boggling pace. So many people came forth while we were traveling that he found himself buried in e-mails, relaying to the network who was doing what.

"It takes an awful lot of effort to make everything look effortless."

—Jacqueline Kennedy Onassis

LEARNING CURVES

Keepin' It Simple

Some people that volunteered to help knew what they were getting into, but some realized too late that the task was much larger than it first appeared. We quickly learned the solution to overtaxed volunteers was having better communication skills.

Selene's friend Shannon set up a ListServe—a free discussion list that people can use to receive messages—for Marley's Network. Using the ListServe, an update could be sent using just one e-mail address instead of hundreds. Technology—very useful when used correctly.

Lucky me…I missed the first week of this e-communication technique. What was a simple communication method became a chaotic juggling of techno-education. The task was to teach everyone on the list how to sign up and when to use either e-mail or the ListServe. Frustration and confusion ran high as people were receiving triplicate copies of many e-mails filled with mundane and logistical information. We were at risk of losing a valuable means of communication.

The formation of Marley's Network was a key factor to our continued survival. Having this community greatly reduced the stress on all levels: physical, emotional, financial, and mental. Even on the spiritual level; there were now so many focusing on Marley's well-being that I felt my load became bearable.

Jennifer S. volunteered to coordinate the frequent-flier mile donations, and Dee researched the guidelines for applying to the Make-A-Wish Foundation. Debra, our bookkeeper at the BRI, set up a tax-free donation fund. Selene's sister-in-law, Patty, rallied her Girl Scout troop to make a donation to help pay for the Duck ride.

In a strange way, the money was energetically similar to the pebbles that people had been sending. Marley loved knowing lots of people were behind him. It was also a comfortable way for people to support Marley without getting too personally involved.

Wednesday, May, 31, 2000
Subject: "A COORDINATED EFFORT"

• From: Joseph, my brother-in-law

Hello, all. (Joseph here.)

Here's the latest update from the many people who have committed to being a part of this miracle.

System Suggestions

Our e-mail system needs to be simplified. How 'bout:

1) Jennifer sends Network Updates via the ListServe to all.
2) Network reply e-mails sent to *only* Jennifer and me.
3) Any dialog should be sent directly to specific parties rather than sending notes to everyone on the ListServe. This will reduce the volume of e-mails received by all. It's daunting sifting through the sheer numbers of e-mails we're currently receiving.

Research

Jeff has agreed to be the master of all research files. Oh, great one! Oh, holy researcher. Thank you. Gratitude from all in the village. Yes, continue to make those files. Could those offering information send it directly to Jeff? Aid him by offering your assessments of sites and information available. I think it best to offer Jennifer, Drew, and Cindy (JDC) simple summaries of legitimate options. We're looking for basic information on the strengths and weaknesses of the various choices and treatments, as well as contact information and first steps that need to be taken to learn more.

Stringing it Together

Jay, Marley's uncle, is making Marley a bead necklace. He is requesting that we each send special beads to him so he can make the necklace for Marley using our combined gifts. Nice!

Legos for Learning and Just for Fun
Selene's aunt Shelley moves forward with Constant's idea on a way to teach Marley to read. She has sent out feelers to reading specialists and is checking out Lego sites for educational materials. Yes, ma'am. Keep up the good work.

Marley's Website
Debbie, a long-time friend of Jennifer's, reports that her friend Franco has offered to build and maintain a website for Marley. Thanks, Franco, for your contribution to the Love Fund. This site will become a permanent posting for updates on Marley.

Digital Camera
Patty has offered $60 for a camera so we can have photos of the Marley Man. What a generous soul. Patty, your name pops up again and again, like a heart beat…like a pulse of sweetness.

Continued Research
Jennifer's brother-in-law, Steven, reports that a book, *Grit & Grace*, talks about massive doses of Vitamin C to counteract the ill-effects of chemo. Can researchers find out about Vitamin C and other proven aids cancer patients have used?

Marley $$$$
Many others have offered to make cash commitments once the system for receiving funds is in place. Here are the rules: Each of us can deduct gifts up to $10,000 annually without taxation, while Marley can receive up to $10,000 annually tax free. What do you say? Let's make Marley pay some taxes!

Love, you all.
Joseph

Thursday, June 1, 2000
Subject: "POST-OP"

Hey Folks.

Marley made it through the surgery fine. He took a LONG time to wake up from the anesthesia (four hours post–surgery). We were at the hospital from 7:30 A.M. to 4:30 P.M. He hurts—he says it's like he was punched really hard at the base of his neck. His body seems to be rejecting the pain meds this go 'round. Poor guy, he hurts bad but when he takes the drugs, he throws up and that hurts too. He's exhausted. Me too.

The doc was actually somewhat encouraging when he came to the waiting room to talk to us. He was wearing a blue surgical smock that was stretched taut over a large, round belly. His smock was covered with coffee stains and either dried blood or jelly stains…regardless, we appreciated the fact that he came out to us as soon as he was finished. He said he took samples of six lymph nodes and an additional sample from Marley's lung to re-biopsy.

The plan may change as tests come back, but here's what we think is going to happen. First, we're going home!!!!!!!! Yahoo! Then we're supposed to do two cycles of chemotherapy to make the tumor shrink as much as possible. We'll get more details on what chemo entails after we get home. In about eight weeks, we'll return to Boston for a lobectomy (removal of all or part of the lung that's infected.) He'll also have all the lymphs that are "reacting," or swollen, removed at the same time. Then, after about a month of healing, Marley will start getting radiation which will last four to five weeks. Seems manageable. Maybe we'll be sittin' pretty by mid–September.

That's all I can handle now.
I love you all,
Jennifer

EXPLORING WITHIN

Repeat Performance

This was Marley's fifth bronchoscopy and, other than raw nostrils and a sore throat, we knew the risks of this procedure were low. They were just verifying the results of the previous tests by sampling the lung tissue. The purpose for the mediastinoscopy was to explore the *mediastinum*: the cavity between the lungs, encasing the heart, trachea, and many lymph nodes. This exploration left a two-inch scar in the hollow spot between the collar bones. It's like a tracheotomy—except they don't cut into the trachea, they go into this cavity.

The lymph system is an interconnected network of nodes throughout the body that regulates the immune system and acts as the first line of defense against disease. Of the six lymph nodes they sampled, three of them were enlarged and discolored.

Deja Vu

During the operation, I couldn't keep my mind from wandering to my past. When I was fifteen, my father's lung cancer spread to the lymph system, and within a few months I was being smothered by hugs at his memorial service. Now Marley had exactly the same scar for the same reason. I worried that this disease was going to kill him just like it killed my dad. None of this mattered to anyone but me, and I had to snap out of it and concentrate on my boy, who was waking up from wherever one goes while under a thick blanket of drugs. I was scared.

"Fear is that little darkroom
where negatives are developed."

—Michael Pritchard

My positive opinion of Boston changed dramatically after Marley's surgery. Drew and I were with Marley in "post-op," the room where patients go just after surgery. The post-op in Boston was bigger than the entire Intensive Care Unit in our largest hospital.

We sat beside him, waiting nervously for him to wake up as people hustled and bustled around us.

We waited and waited. And then we waited some more. Eventually even the nurses were concerned. Drew and I took turns falling asleep with our foreheads on Marley's bed. Many hours later, he started to come around. The first thing he did was throw up. Armed with a miniscule pink plastic, half-moon shaped drool catcher, I caught most of what he had consumed 24 hours before. The poor thing spent the next hour heaving, which caused his throat great pain. The nurses were torn between giving him more pain medication; which would make him nauseous, or medicine to make him stop vomiting; which would knock him out again, and take up valuable bed space in post-op. After a few rounds of him sleeping, waking up, and throwing up, Drew and I felt completely helpless. Finally we told the nurse to forget the drugs altogether. We insisted that Marley could handle the pain. We had to stop the vicious cycle and get him out of the hospital—for everyone's sake.

We finally poured our drugged "little" boy into a cab. At just over six feet, and weighing 155 pounds, it was no easy feat getting Marley up to our room on the top floor of the Ronald McDonald House. It was an old house, with narrow stairways, and we had three flights to climb. Drew draped Mars on his back and lugged the boy to bed.

We gave Marley a Percocet and barely had time to kiss him before he was out cold again. He slept through the rest of the afternoon and woke up only briefly, just after dark, for a drink of water and another pain pill. Drew and I sat out on the back porch and had a beer and two shots of tequila. It was the first time we'd had a chance to really talk about Marley's future in a relaxed atmosphere. As exhausted as we both were, it was very healing to debrief each other about the pros and cons of Western medicine, discuss how we felt, and make educated guesses about the future.

After that, we went to the theater in the basement to do the only logical thing left—zone out. We set our emotions and worries aside to watch Bruce Willis in *Die Hard.*

Saturday, June 3, 2000
Subject: "TRAVEL DAY"

Yawn! Jennifer here.

It's four in the morning. Stretch. Groan.

Selene e-mailed to inform me the damned deer are eating my garden. Shoo them away, Selene! Sick the rooster on them! Kill! Save the vegetation, eat a deer!

Leaving Boston now. Don't send e-mails here anymore—transfer to my e-mail at work. Will pick up messages on Monday.

Taking a cab to the airport. Boston to NJ, NJ to Portland. I cancelled my commitment to go to the Book Expo and instead have two flights reserved from Portland to Dreadford, in case Marley's not up to the six-hour drive. Two friends, Mick & Tobin, are meeting us an hour south of Portland to help Drew with the driving. I'm thankful we have options and help—thanks, guys.

If we take the plane from P-town it arrives at 10 P.M. in Dreadford. Jeff, will you pick us up? Will call as we get closer to confirm.

If we drive, we'll be home around 3 A.M. Yuck! I think Marley and I will fly. Drew, Mick, and Tobin can tough it out. Marley's feeling pretty poorly. Spent all of yesterday watching one movie after another.

Thank you so much EVERYONE!
Jennifer

P.S.
Please, give Shannon's new e-communication system a chance. Once we get how to navigate this new process, the ListServe will make life much easier. I promise.

Tuesday, June 6, 2000
Subject: "RETURN HOME"

TRAVELS WITH MARLEY

Lordy be! What an adventure. Nothing went as planned.

On Saturday, we took a cab to the Boston airport, hopped on the airplane, and finally took off after an hour of being grounded due to bad weather in some other city. Once we arrived in New Jersey, the three of us had to run through the Newark airport to catch our connecting flight to Portland. It was already preparing for takeoff. After a heated verbal skirmish with the authorities, they unlocked the door to the plane and let us board. The plane was so full that Drew had to trade seats to sit next to Marley (who felt like crap), while I ended up sitting at the back of the plane.

With our seat belts securely fastened, our seat backs and tray tables in the upright position, we waited for an hour before the plane even moved. (Good thing we rushed!) We finally taxied down the runway and stopped in what looked like a rush hour traffic jam. It looked like New Jersey's largest parking lot. The pilot announced, "Sorry folks, this is your captain with some bad news. We're going to be stuck here until a nearby weather pattern shifts or air traffic control can reroute all flights either north or south. The storm is headed right for us—looks like we may have to wait it out. We're going to be turning off our engines to conserve fuel." We watched airline TV while breathing stale air for another three hours.

Looking out the plane's portholes, we could see hundreds of jets lined up, nose to tail, on every runway. They were filled with thousands of frustrated people looking back at us. It was 5 P.M. when the storm hit us full force. A green-black wave of clouds with high winds and pelting rain shook the planes as if they were toys. I was glad we were on the ground.

Unfortunately, this delay meant that Marley and I were going to miss our connecting flight from Portland to Dreadford. It also meant Drew was going to miss his connection with Mick and Tobin. Sigh. So much for making plans. When we arrived in Portland, just before midnight, all three of us squished into Drew's pickup truck for the six-hour drive home. We finally arrived in Ashland as the sun was coming up on Sunday morning. Hats off to Drew for driving and staying awake the whole way. What was I doing? I was a human pillow for one very tired boy.

Round 'em Up, Yee Haw! Raw Hide!

Drew and Marley went home to attend the Colestin Valley cattle roundup (complete with castration and branding). Even though they hadn't slept, neither of them would dare miss the biannual event and the grand celebration which followed. Selene went to the roundup with Drew, Cindy, and the kids. She later reported that Marley was feeling great and that he gave her an exciting ride on the neighbor's ATV. She was amazed at what a good driver Marley was and thankful that he refrained from jumping any ditches. She kept saying things like, "He sure knows how to have fun!"

I came home to two weeks of weed growth and a very needy cat. I mowed two acres of lawn and weed-whacked a forest of poison oak. During that moving meditation, I identified what's not working in the network's current communication set-up. I plan to make some fixes by rounding up responsible movers and shakers. Selene is currently standing in for Shannon, managing the master lists. Debbie is now managing the design of the website. I'm playing the part of overall communication choreographer. By tomorrow night, some changes will be made and you'll have a new and improved, user friendly path of communication. So don't fret! Simplicity will be the focus.

Good Grades

Just before we left Boston, Drew went to see if he could get any additional information from the doctors. There had to be some report available from Wednesday's surgery. After waiting endlessly for our very popular surgeon, Drew was given some great (but confusing) news.

Before the trip, Marley's condition was rated 3-B (4-C is as bad as it gets). Now, Dr. Sugarmaker is rating the stage at a 2B! There's some conflicting test results, but he seems to feel the tumor in his left lung has not metastasized into the mediastinum. The pathology reports from the tissue samples taken from the lymphs are negative. Except he also reported they are all swollen. Dr. Sugarmaker said he is "quite optimistic." Why the dramatic difference? Spontaneous down–staging? Misdiagnosis? Switched paperwork or wrong X-rays? Who knows…I'm excited but *very* skeptical. Maybe, by some miracle, this boy will be "all better" by Halloween. At least, if a miracle did occur, he still has a few dramatic scars to prove it really happened.

I can't thank you enough for being a part of this emerging healing network. I'm excited about the endless possibilities of what we're creating. Think big!

Joyously,
Jennifer

Follow-up

Several days after our return, the official reports came in from the labs. Those swollen lymph glands *were* cancerous. This changed the hopeful "down–staging." It was confirmed that the lung tumor had metastasized to the lymph system. Marley's cancer was now rated 4-C. According to every book we had, that meant "Do whatever you're going to do, as fast as possible." If you were told that your kid has maybe six months to live, what would you do?

POETRY IN MOTION

Roller Coaster Confusion

Everyone in the family handled the grim news of the official 4-C staging in different ways. Drew and Cindy hustled to finish their house and worked hard at the daily needs of their ranch. They did their best to get the kids to stick around and help, but….

Marley was busy building lifelong friendships with two boys that lived nearby. Luke, Lucas, and Marley had been dubbed "The Coyotes." The boys whizzed around on any motorized vehicle they could get their hands on, stirring up dust and trouble.

Marley's little sister stayed as close to Marley as she could. It took me a while to understand why their connection was so strong. Catie was the only one who was with Marley virtually 100 percent of the time. Every two weeks the kids switched parental units and homes. Their stepsisters and their pets were with them only half of the time, but Marley and Catie were always together.

After our return from Boston, I was kidless. I worked hard and went out dancing and drinking with my crew of close friends, as much as possible. I had a lot of steam to blow off. (Ya think?!)

All of us needed to be close to people who loved us. Connection to our community was the lifeline we knew we had to hang onto in order to survive our doubt and inner pain.

THE LIFE OF A BOY

The life of a boy,
Young with a toy.
The older, the wiser,
And more precious he gets.
Doctors were here,
On with the fear,
That the boy in our family
Might die.

—Catie Pratt (age 10)

Chapter Five:
Networking

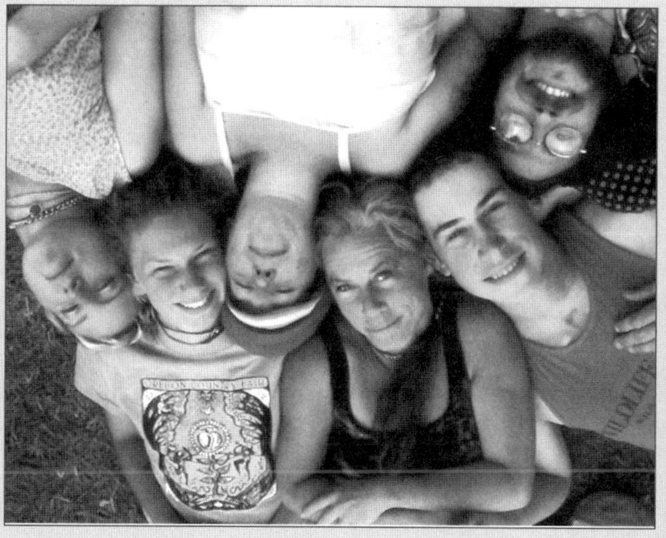

"Six heads are better than one!"
Selene, Catie, Liz, Jennifer, Marley, Jay

Photo: Jay Newman,
Newman Images

COMMUNITY WORKS

It Takes a Village

Community support and networking are the glue binding this story together. While living through Marley's challenge, I've had to look long and hard at the importance I've put on being a strong individual. I know there's strength in numbers, and yet I've spent so much energy trying to solve my problems alone.

> **Definition:**
>
> ***Network***
>
> • A work in which threads, wires, or the like are arranged in the form of a net.
>
> • A complex structure of rivers, canals, railways, or wireless transmitting stations.
>
> • A support system, a lifeline, a tree- or grid-shaped system, a persisting identity of relationships, everyone you know, a structure that knows no bounds, a system of links, and a nongeographic community.
>
> From *Networking* by Jessica Lipnack and Jeffrey Stamps

Until Marley got cancer, I generally didn't want help, didn't much listen to advice, and wanted to figure things out on my own.

But this was too much to deal with alone. Fortunately I realized there were others I could rely on. With relatively little encouragement, a network of loving individuals courageously bonded together to watch over, witness, and participate in our process.

Invisible Glue

I've witnessed other families take care of their terminally ill children with very little help. I have no idea how or why they chose to do this. Although a majority of the families using the aid provided at the Ronald McDonald House were thankful to have their help, I was shocked to learn most of them sought very few other forms of support. They didn't want to impose on family, friends, and extended community networks to help carry the heavy burden of their extraordinary needs. How can this be?

There were two primary reasons I was able to reach out for help. One was that I was well trained by my mother, an anthropologist whose field was the dynamics of social transformation. When my father was dying, she used her professional skills to create a powerful network to form a healing community. And second, I had learned how to create a team while managing the Bathroom Readers' Press. As individuals, we couldn't create and publish several books each year. It took all of us working together as one unit. We didn't work in separate cubicles, doing our individual little piece. We were together in the same space, and everyone knew everyone else's business (professional and personal). Relying on each other was the very thing that made us so strong and successful.

> ***"And it is still true, no matter how old you are, when you go out into the world, it is best to hold hands and stick together."***
>
> **—Robert Fulghum**

Life felt so overwhelmingly difficult that I didn't care if my image of myself as superwoman was shattered. I knew that I could never do alone what needed to be accomplished to help Marley survive. I simply didn't have the skills or the resources. When Marley's Network was first taking shape, it was not well planned, thought out, or organized. I took a risk asking for what I needed, but figured there was at least a possibility I'd get it. It seemed better than not asking and not receiving.

The need for community had been identified by Marley's life-threatening diagnosis. All we needed to do was to find ways to tap its strength. Out of sheer desperation, I made a list of all the needs I could quickly identify. We started by finding out what methods of communication *didn't* work. Together, pooling our knowledge, we came up with better systems that *did* work. I learned all I had to do was invite others to help, and they seemed relieved to participate. We risked only failure. What mattered was we had the courage to think big.

Friday, June 9, 2000
Subject: "PAST, PRESENT, & FUTURE"

Howdeeeee!

Jennifer here. This may be my last e-mail for a while. Hopefully not much will change, but I'll keep you posted if it does!

MARLEY'S CURRENT STATUS

It's hard to imagine how sick this kid is when he's scaling fences, leaping over walls, riding his bike, wrestling with me, or giving his friend Sarah piggyback rides. Last night, we went to see Jackie Chan's new movie, *Shanghai Noon*. It was great fun watching Marley clutch his sides while laughing impossibly hard. He laughed so loud and long, he infected the whole audience. Sometimes his laughter was even delayed because Sarah had to read him the subtitles, whenever Chinese was spoken.

Sometimes he complains that his shoulder hurts or his back hurts along his scar, but there's not a whole lot that can be done unless he wants to stay slightly drugged most of the time. I don't think so! We were cuddling on my bed the other morning and I noticed the left side of his chest was larger than the right. I said, "Don't worry dear, that's the kind of thing the chemo will probably reduce." He looked horrified and replied, "No! I like it! Tell 'em to make the otha side bigger ta match!" (A tumor in the lung: One hell of a way to look buff.)

His response to almost everything these days is, "Who cares?" This worried me, until several other parents indicated this is normal teenage behavior. I can't imagine how he feels or what he thinks about. I don't know what's "normal" or what's related to facing the possibility of an early death. It must be pretty confusing for him, because he simply doesn't feel that bad. On the outside, everything feels pretty normal while on the inside, his body's at war.

RECENT ACTIVITIES

Marley's gone to school a couple of times since we've returned from Boston. He loves socializing and getting lots of love and attention from the students and staff alike. School ends soon, so his schedule is pretty loose. Marley's graduation is next week at Ashland Middle School, just two days after chemo starts. He's really looking forward to it, so we're all praying he will feel up to the event.

On Tuesday, Mike, one of the EPCAM coffee crew, gave an amazing gift to Marley. Mike rented a two-seater plane and a flying lesson for Mars. I thought Marley was going to pop with glee. Marley flew the plane the whole time, except for the take-off and landing. They flew over my house, which was too hidden in the trees to see, and then they flew over the Mount Ashland pass (a very windy and bumpy corridor at 10,000 feet) into the Colestin Valley to buzz Drew and Cindy's house. Afterwards, the instructor thanked *me* for the opportunity to hang with such a cool kid. He also said he wanted to donate another hour in the air whenever Mars felt up to it. Marley was ecstatic!

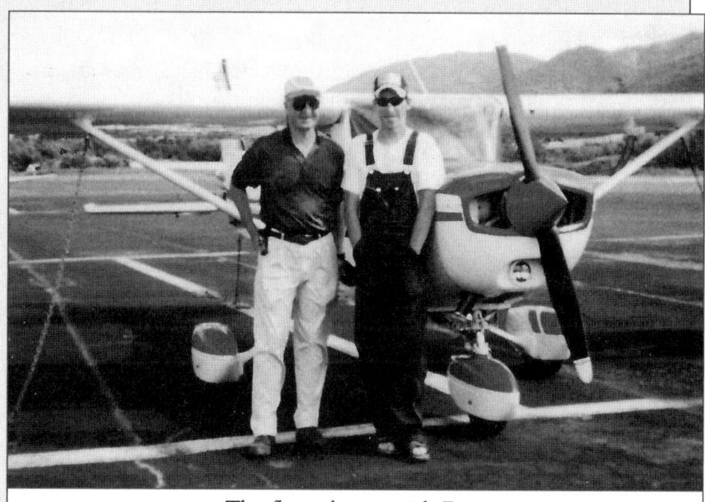

The flying lesson with Don

This Saturday, I'm hosting a party, complete with bonfire. We're a wild and crazy bunch of nut cases who love theme parties. With us, there's always at least one good reason to celebrate something; this time we have five grand excuses to cut loose and dance around the fire. We're celebrating Marley's current vitality (before he starts chemotherapy). We're saying good-bye to Marley's middle school years and to my best buddy Andrea, who is leaving town. We're also honoring Selene's birth twenty-three years ago and the fact she sacrificed her plan to join the circus to come be with her two cousins and me. The theme of this party is "Circus, Circus!" (Marley wants to shave his head and be the strong man!)

ONCOLOGIST'S GAME PLAN

Last Wednesday, we had our first appointment with the Medical Oncologist. He's the specialist responsible for the chemicals Marley's going to be dosed with. During the next few months, he's scheduled for two cycles of chemo (28 days each). This Monday, at 8:30 A.M., the process begins with an hour of education and some pre-meds (two different kinds of antihistamines, a steroid, and Anzimet for nausea). Then he'll spend three hours receiving a slow drip of Taxol. When that's done, he'll spend another hour receiving part two of the chemical "cocktail," called Carboplatin. Afterward, we have to wait for at least 30 minutes to make sure he doesn't react adversely. That same process is repeated 28 days later.

Everyone reacts differently, but we're likely to experience several weeks of not feeling so hot, improving as time goes by. During the second week, he may experience nausea, fatigue, bone and joint pain, and hair loss. For some reason young men seem to react more strongly to chemotherapy than other populations, but there's no telling how he'll react with us behind him, sending our thoughts and invoking healing!

Right now, Marley and Catie are living at Drew's, so the first two days of chemo will be spent with his dad and stepmom Cindy. This Wednesday they start their two-week shift with Selene and me. I'm taking time off from work until I know how these drugs are going to affect him.

Tada! That's the news. Pray that Marley makes it to graduation on Wednesday. That will help his attitude. Let's also focus on not letting him lose too much weight during his time with chemo—he doesn't have much to spare!

I love you all!
Jennifer

P.S. I send a special thanks to Patty, Tom, Dee, Howard, Sue, Tim, and KC for their financial contributions. May the gods and goddesses of Sacred Reciprocity repay your generosity very soon.

"Always laugh when you can. It is cheap medicine."

—Lord Byron

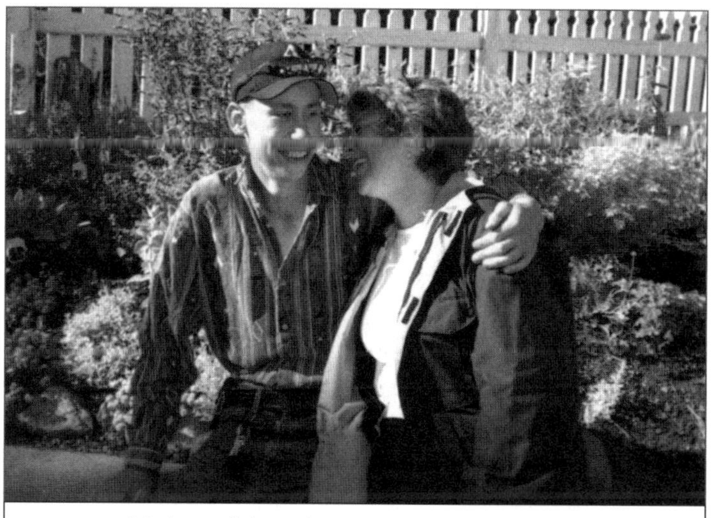

Marley and Aunt Constant at Evo's Java House

HEAD, HEART, HANDS, AND HEALTH

Making the Best Better

Since the kids were little, they had participated in the 4-H club while they were at Drew and Cindy's. The four H's stand for head, heart, hands, and health, and their mission statement is "To Make the Best Better." For the kids, it was a good program. They seemed to learn a lot about being responsible for their critters.

Their specialty was raising rabbits to show. Whenever I went to visit, I'd get a grand tour of the barn. As ten barn cats scattered in every direction, the rabbits would stir in excitement...well...all except Marley's lop-eared bunny. This rabbit was so big that he could barely maneuver in his cage!

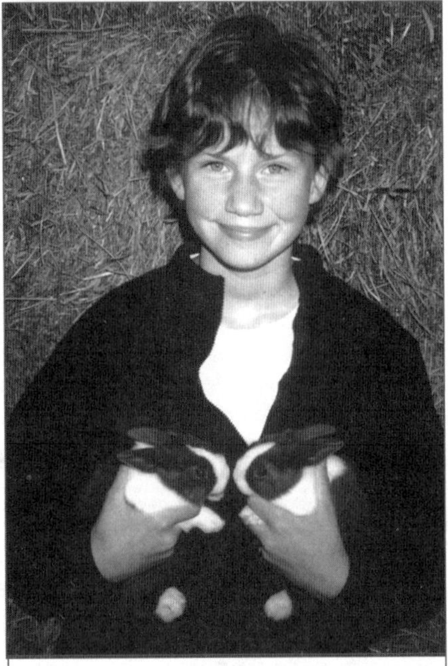

Catie, age 10, with her twin bunnies
Photo: Cindy Warzyn

Hog Heaven

One year, the kids took on raising a hog. I never met Hanky, but I sure heard a lot of stories about this spunky pig. Marley fell in love with Hanky and thought the animal was more intelligent than most of the folks he knew. Hanky entered Marley's life at a time when Marley was focusing on healing rather than going to school, so in a strange way I think Hanky served as Marley's shrink, playmate, and sibling.

The following story was dictated by Marley for a class project.

HANKY THE PIG

by Marley Pratt, age 15

Hanky the pig was a good friend to me. She loved to take walks, which made me feel happy. Walking kept both of us healthy. Hanky was a good listener, and I felt calm when I was with her.

She taught me to give respect when she needed space. Hanky also taught me to be responsible. I fed her food scraps and pig pellets morning and night. She loved apples for snacks. Hanky made me more playful. She loved shoelaces. She quietly walked up, nudged me, untied my shoelaces, and then ran away. Whenever I bent over, she would knock into me and push me over.

I was amazed at how fast she learned new things. She did a great "piggie paddle" in the creek near our house. I trained her with a four-foot-long hog stick, which was a thick stick with a curved top. It worked like a leash. I would tap her to go right or left. She would get down on her knees and crawl across the cattle guard. Sometimes she would run and jump across. This amazed me, and it made me appreciate her intelligence a lot. When she was a baby, I would pick her up and carry her across.

One day my dad called the butcher and Hanky was slaughtered. I didn't really care because I knew that would happen anyway. Hanky made the best ham and bacon anyone ever ate!

"You can complain because roses have thorns, or you can rejoice because thorns have roses."

—-Ziggy

TESTING THE ROPES

Alternative Education

Every spring, as a part of the middle school's graduation preparation, all of the eighth-graders are symbolically prepared for entering high school the following year. This Outward Bound-style adventure, called the Ropes Course, is a dynamic and challenging ritual. Deep in the forest, a full-scale obstacle course set high in the treetops awaited these young people. Their courage and teamwork skills were tested at every turn.

In May, when the Ropes Course date was set, Marley was still healing from the thorocotomy. The incision from his left shoulder blade to his left nipple had mended, but the many layers of muscle were still knitting, making simple movements like raising an arm difficult. Marley had been waiting three years for this event, and nothing was going to stop him from participating. Drew and I were familiar with the ropes course challenge. We knew the physical requirements, the risks, and the psychological benefits. His doctors were saying he was crazy for considering climbing ropes strung between trees 30 feet off the ground. All we could do was nod in acknowledgement and agree to whatever Marley wanted. There's a time to let normal parenting techniques fly out the window.

That was one field trip I decided to attend. If he was going to seriously injure himself, at least I was going to be there. His classmates were so incredibly supportive and tender, my mouth was agape most of the time. As he struggled to climb the vertical rope net, primarily using his right arm, they all whooped and hollered encouragement with every inch he advanced. For all of the high elements, every participant was fully harnessed and safe. Each of them would take turns gripping the lifelines, holding each other's lives in their hands. They completely trusted Marley when he was the one holding their safety ropes. They knew he would keep them alive if they fell. Many of these kids had been with him since the first grade and knew he would gladly risk his left arm and a lung for their safety.

Leap Day

The "Pamper Pole" was the last event, and by far the scariest. I had experienced it before, so I knew what Marley was facing as he strapped the safety harness on. The two ropes connected to the harness went through a pulley, hanging from a wire strung between two trees, 30 feet up. Four of us held each safety rope so if he fell, we could lower him down slowly. The challenge before him was to climb 18 feet up a triangular net attached at one point near the top of the tree. Balance was required to avoid the net dumping him upside down, because at the top of this net ladder the rungs became only inches wide at the very top. The next five-foot climb was straight up the side of the tree using L-shaped brackets drilled into the pole. The tree had been cut off, and attached at the top was a 14-inch wood disk, just a bit bigger than an album. Just to make it even more extreme, this platform, on which Marley had to stand, wobbled and swiveled around!

Once Marley had reached his new perch, he just stood there until he stopped spinning and was completely calm. We were all quiet—frozen in anticipation and readiness—our knuckles white as we gripped his safety lines. The mission, should he choose to accept it, was to leap toward a trapeze that hung six feet in front of him. This was the moment that could make or break Marley's future. One wrong move and further healing could be thwarted completely. He knew he didn't have to prove anything to anyone. I had to trust him completely. He had to trust me completely because I was one of the people holding his lifeline below. I could hear the girl in front of me, who also held his safety rope, whispering to herself, "Don't do it, Marley. Don't do it!" We all held our breath and braced ourselves.

Our necks got stiff watching him just stand on the disk. The platform was no longer turning. He was calm and was aimed in the right direction. Finally, he slowly raised his long arms, like an eagle spreading his wings in preparation for flight. It was as though he woke up from a peaceful meditation. He smiled broadly and just leaned forward in an effortless swan dive. It was breathtaking. We caught his weight and lowered him down. We were all incredibly proud he had not chosen to leap for the trapeze. His judgement was pure, his bravery spellbinding. I cried with complete relief and awe.

The Final Grade

The graduating class of 2004 was now a team, ready to leave the safety of middle school. Their final graduation ceremony took place at the beginning of June, two days after Marley started his first round of chemotherapy. Marley was determined to attended his graduation. It was a really big deal for him.

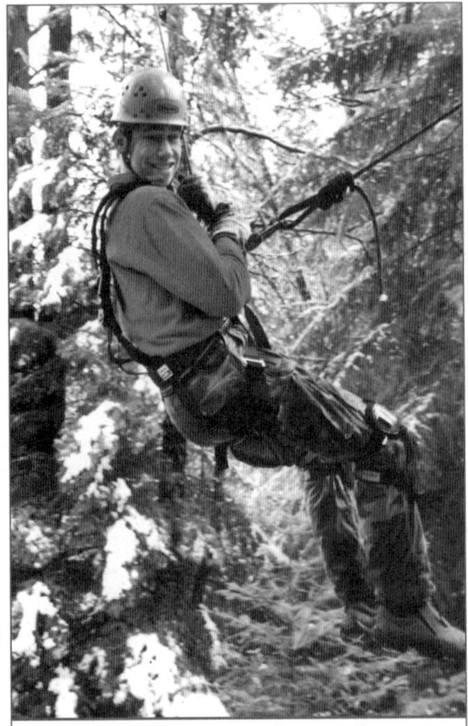

Marley at the Ropes Course
Photo: Shianna Walker

During the time of special commendations, the principal honored Marley's tenacious survival techniques. As he was singled out and praised for living with courage and faith, tears were rolling down the cheeks of hundreds of people. I don't think I had ever seen the boy glow with such pride in front of so many people. As we wiped our running noses, trying to see through blurry eyes, he turned to the audience. He raised his extra long monkey arms, made peace signs, and nodded his head. It was a righteous imitation of Richard Nixon and we all broke out in laughter.

Tuesday, June 13, 2000
Subject: "JOSEPH JUGGLES"

• From: Uncle Joseph

Hi, all. Joseph, here.

Marley went through his first round of chemo yesterday. Keep those prayers flowing. Keep that poison centered on only those areas where the cancer resides. Safeguard all healthy tissue. Pray, people. Reach out and envelop Marley and JDC (Jennifer, Drew, and Cindy), Catie, Laura, and Vanessa. Pray for healing. Pray for each other. Prayer is a powerful tool. Pray to Mother, Father, Beloved, Buddha, Muhammad, Krishna, QuanYen, Jesus, BabaJee, Great Spirit, no matter!

RESEARCH
This area remains extremely important and time sensitive in my mind. What is the best antidote to counteract the poison of chemo? What is the best long-term diet for rebuilding the immune system and maintaining a healthy, balanced physical presence? I don't believe anything needs to be extreme. Given that one man's meat is another's poison, it is my sense that JDC will make choices from among complementary, allopathic, macrobiotic, etc., and will make them quite easily. The key tool arises out of making choices based on initial research. Thus, I ask all researchers: How goes it?

FINANCIALS
Once JDC have shared what expenses have been incurred and how they'd like to address same, donor populations can be offered selections for areas of commitment. Remember, money is an odd energy; the best way to deal with $$$$ is straight on. Know thy expenses and seek for a comparable income.

ASHLAND RESIDENTS
Selene is your checkpoint for hands-on support. Driving. Mowing. Farmhands. Construction. Child care, etc.

For meals: Contact Jennifer's neighbor, Jonnie. Jennifer says having dinners delivered on hard days has been a delicious reprieve.

MARLEY ROCKS!

The Marley Man continues to request pebbles. More and more pebbles to fill his fountain of flowing water—a symbol of what unites us all. As cells of people. In love and commitment.

LEGOS

Send 'em directly to Marley. The word is out, he wants more and more of 'em.

That's it folks!
Love to all,
Joseph

P.S. Jennifer says the necklace that Marley's Uncle Jay made for him hangs proudly around the boy's neck at all times. Thanks to all who sent beads.

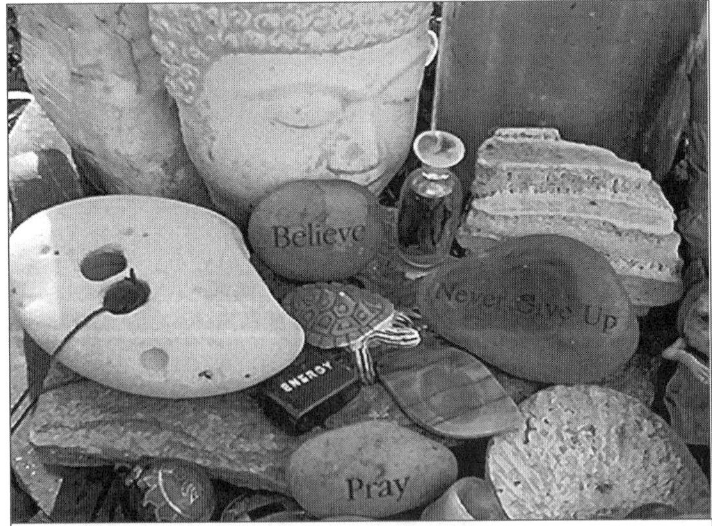

Some of Marley's "prayer stones" for his fountain of love

LEARNING WITH LEGOS

Inventing Solutions

Marley was 15 years old and still couldn't read. Given words from a targeted list, Marley had mastered a whopping 13 words. The symbolic and abstract nature of letters and numbers just didn't go along with Marley's mind. No one knew why. A language arts progress report stated:

> "Marley knows the phonetic value of the consonants and some of the vowels, but sounding out words can still be so frustrating for him that he refuses to continue. On the other hand, Marley enjoys listening to books read aloud, demonstrating that he has an interest in literature. He has an incredible recall of detailed events in stories and can easily relate them to real life events and behaviors."

For years, getting his driver's license was the carrot we dangled before him to entice him to unravel the mystery of the alphabet. I was floored when he figured out how to use the system to get his driver's permit *without* reading. He knew picture symbols, knew the rules of the road, and was loaded with common-sense logistical thinking. Apparently, our system is constructed so drivers don't need to read. Someone can actually read the test to the student and even draw pictures if they need clarification. So much for carrots!

I assumed he was going to be bedridden for extended periods of time and would benefit from learning to read. My sister, Constant, was an educator of educators *and* she personally knew Marley. But he not only had the school system stumped on finding a successful reading tool, he had Constant stumped too, and that's no easy trick. She came up with a great idea but didn't have the time to implement it. That is, until Marley's Network took form. All it took was one e-mail and Selene's aunt Shelley responded. She and Constant fired e-mails back and forth, and soon the inventive teaching tool was a reality.

Marley loved Legos with a passion. Constant figured if she could use small yellow Legos for consonants and red ones for vowels, Marley could grasp the idea of building words. Using all the Legos that had been gathered and sent to us, Constant was sent a supply of red and yellow bricks. She wrote the alphabet on multiple pieces so he could begin a new kind of construction. Marley was deeply impressed with their perseverance, but he never touched the tool.

In the end, he wasn't bedridden for any major length of time and besides, he just didn't see the need to read. Although my bullheaded son never took advantage of this great teaching tool, I'm sure he would like it if someone out there in reader land benefits from it. And I'm sure Constant and Shelley would agree to pass along their idea to help other Marleys in the world learn to read.

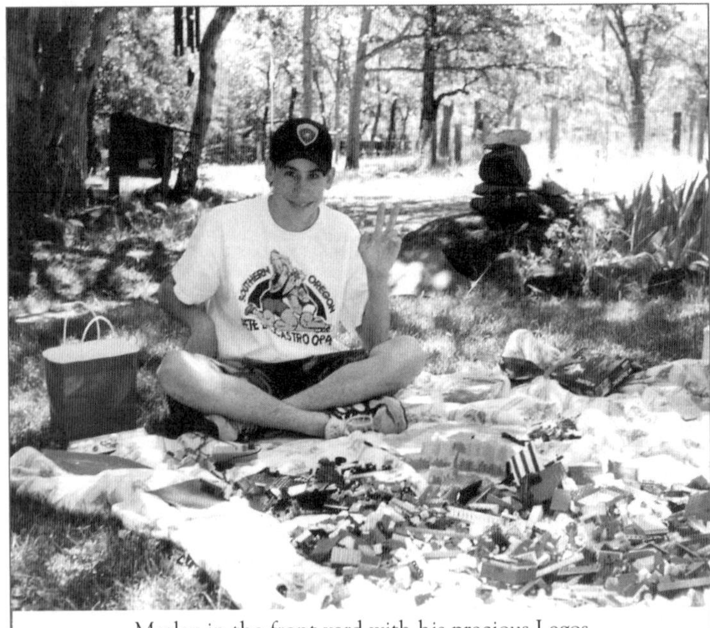

Marley in the front yard with his precious Legos

Photo: Catie Pratt

Wednesday, June 21, 2000
Subject: "LIFE'S A CIRCUS"

Greetings from Jennifluff.

PARTY TIME!
The "Circus! Circus!" party was a success last Saturday. There were fortune-tellers, jugglers, a snake charmer, a belly dancer, and many more. JD clowned around with the perfect outfit, and dear Debbie was a repulsive carny/hobo. (Normally, Debbie's very beautiful, yet her costume made all of us recoil in disgust.) Later in the evening, she stripped off her hobo layer to reveal…a gorgeous lion tamerrr. Wow…what a show!

GOAL SETTING
Marley said there was one thing that could possibly make going in for chemo palatable. "You just don't understand, Mom. The only time I feel frwee—absolutely frwee—is when I'm rwiding my bike." I asked, "What about your dream of having a go-cart?" Through teary eyes, he replied, "That's jus' a dream. It'd be too much wuk, besides I'd have ta buy gas and parts. All I reeeeally need is a BMX (a stunt bike)." He convinced me that I shouldn't get another USED bike because "they get thwashed too easy." It's true, he goes through at least two bikes a year because you get what you pay for, and Mars is hard on bikes! I couldn't help myself; I caved in. $170 from the toy fund went toward buying Marley a very cool, shiny new silver stunt bike. He's one happy camper! Thank you, gang.

COCKTAIL HOUR(S)
He was a bit nervous about getting his first round of chemotherapy. To counterbalance his fears, he popped wheelies and did bunny-hops around the hospital parking lot before going in. He told the nurses he was going to get better really fast so he could ride his new bike.

Marley did not enjoy cocktail hour. His body thoroughly rejected the first dose of therapy. He instantly had a hard time breathing and broke out in hives on his face, neck, and torso. Maybe that's why they give two different injections of antihistamines before the cocktail is given. After more drugs were given to counteract his reaction, he started throwing up. Their final solution was to slow the speed of the IV drip.

The nurses were worried that at the rate Marley was accepting the dose, we would be there long after closing time. Everyone was a trifle testy. In the end, it was decided to split the ordeal into two consecutive days. He was positively miserable and complained bitterly, but he was a champ. This round took eight hours on the first day and five hours on the second day. It was ultimately difficult for him to sit in a lounge chair having to calmly receive his "cocktail" via an IV. I'm very proud of him. He walked away from the experience hating needles and hospitals with a revived passion.

GRADUATION

Marley and Catie came back to Selene and me on Wednesday, the day Marley graduated from middle school. He was lookin' good and feelin' fine! He had a fun afternoon, and later had dinner with a group of friends. Last but certainly not least, he went to the school dance that evening. He was riding high and wanted to party all night. The kid has style but I had had it, so I dragged Marley home. Home, sweet home!

THE SHADOW SIDE

On Thursday, Marley wanted to ride his new bike in town with Catie. We went to Evo's coffee house for our social hour and then the kids rode their bikes to the office. Marley bee-bopped in but within ten minutes he started to feel the effects of the chemo full on. Exit stage left!

He threw up almost every hour until late afternoon on the following day. Our job was to keep him from getting dehydrated.

It was rough, but Selene and I kept him home, poured liquids down his throat, and tried to keep as much food in him as possible to avoid going back to the hospital.

The anti-nausea medications didn't seem to have much effect. We started using Nux Vomica, a homeopathic remedy I used during pregnancy for morning sickness, and it seems to be doing the trick! He finally passed out on Friday afternoon, slept for two hours, and awoke feeling weak but okay. The only other current side effect from the chemo is pain in his joints and muscles, so Selene and I gave him lots of massages. Our best remedy was to make him laugh as a healing distraction.

BRIGHT EYED AND BUSHY TAILED

By mid-day on Saturday, he was ready for action. He's had fun riding his bike in town and swimming in a friend's pool. Later we had another small gathering, because Marley decided it was time to shave his head in a ceremonious fashion. Well, actually, he chose to have a Mohawk. He said his Dad would flip out, but we figured it won't matter much, he's supposed to lose it all anyway. He ended up shaving the Mohawk off too, because he was waking up with his pillow covered with hair. The Marley Man was shedding!

Catie is going to Wisconsin in two weeks. She has the opportunity to go with her stepsisters Laura and Vanessa to Cindy's parents' home, relaxing and playing at the lake. Although I'm going to miss her something fierce, I know she'll be having fun, not having to deal with the rest of what chemo "therapy" may have to offer. Catie is deathly afraid to be apart from her brother, but, after living with him barfing, she's looking forward to a summer vacation. (She ain't gonna get it here!) I'll be doin' my best to keep my nose above the waterline.

I love you all.
Jennifer

JUST SAY NO!

Drugs as Therapy

The kids were out of school and ready for action. Our exciting vacation plans were to fight the cancer by surviving chemotherapy. Everything I know about this "therapeutic" method was bad and it made no sense to me, but every professional in the field agreed that this was the best course of action.

The theory of chemo was to kill all rapidly growing cells. This included not only cancerous cells, but healthy ones too. This was supposed to stop new growth and reduce the size of the existing tumors, making surgery less of an impact. Right after two rounds of chemo were completed, lung surgery was scheduled in Boston at the beginning of August.

We were warned that various smells and tastes might make Marley nauseous, foods might taste different, and that he might lose his appetite. We were told that it was very important to keep him eating, especially high protein foods, in order to maintain his weight and keep him strong. He was most likely going to lose *all* of his body hair sometime in the second week. We were also warned he would be hypersensitive to the sun, and to make sure he wore long sleeves and a sun hat. We could tell this was not going to be fun.

Survival of the Fittest

It didn't take long for Selene and me to understand what we were up against. We had read as much as we could about chemotherapy, but the reality was, nothing could have prepared us for dealing with this. Some things you can prepare for and some things you just can't. The first night he returned to me, he was still Marley, high on completing another year of school, being social, and being a star. The very next day, the kid looked like hell was about to invade his soul. After a few days, Selene, Catie, and I realized hell had the advantage and the battle would be hard won.

Marley was one sick puppy! He could hardly stomach any

food and he was nauseated by most smells, thus he threw up a lot, much to Catie's chagrin. There was very little to up-chuck, except the protein powder that Selene and I had to beg him to drink. The sound of Marley painfully dry heaving sent Catie repeatedly running from the house with two pillows clutched to her head. Generally, I have no problem with caring for barfing babies, but this was different. By the 30th time of the second day, I was at risk of losing it too. There's nothing quite as bad as lovingly holding a bucket for your child to york in, while you do your best not to rudely push his head out of the way so you can throw up too!

"I slept, and I dreamt that life was all joy.
I woke, and I saw that life was but service.
I served, and discovered that service was joy."

—Rbindranath Tagore

A High Price to Pay

Boy was I glad I had insurance when I got the first bill. Each bag of toxic chemical cost $700. (This price tag did not include the visit to the hospital, the doctor's expense, or any of the extra medicines.) In addition to the expense of the drugs, every hour we were there cost $750. Every hour! (No joke.) I guess the high cost was to cover the hospital's insurance. Let's do a little math, shall we? Oh, let's not! I'll just get pissed off all over again and it ain't worth it.

Not only did we spend two months in purgatory, the therapy was in no way effective. Worse yet, four years later, I found out that any patient who was given Taxol during 2000 was allowed a rebate because of the proven health risks. In other words, "Oops, sorry. That was a bad batch. You can have your money back." After living through two rounds of chemo, we all agreed hands-down that even death by cancer had to be better than death by this cure.

"That which does not kill me makes me stronger."

—Friedrich Nietzsch

Tuesday, July 3, 2000
Subject: "DANCING LESSONS"

• From: Selene

Greetings everyone!

There is this image I wanted everyone to have of Marley: Mohawk, camouflage shorts, tight bike shirt and a silver helmet to match his silver bike. Tall and lanky and tan, listening to live music with his arms around two girls. Now his head is completely buzzed, except for a lightning bolt on the side, and he's wearing a black cowboy hat.

Next week, Catie's leaving for Wisconsin. She'll be gone for a whole month and will be greatly missed. Who am I supposed to go to the water slides with? After several trips to the mall, she is actually tired of shopping now. (Here, Jen and I exchange knowing smiles, having planned this shift all along.)

The most recent concern on the home front has been the inopportune decision by one of Marley's wisdom teeth to practically explode into the light of day. It's causing a lot of pain, some swelling, and a low fever. This can be a bad sign during chemo since his body doesn't have the capacity to fight infection. Send some soothing thoughts in the general direction of his lower molars that are erupting a few years too early.

Every day feels like a life, a miniature biosphere, a bell jar of significance, a…o.k., enough Selene. Jennifer is working hard as usual. I started cooking for the Community Food Store. Salsa, the cat, gives us lots of lovin', finding Jennifer's head particularly soft and warm during the night. The rooster roosts on the porch every night, drawn by the shelter of our company, no doubt. And food shows up in the kitchen miraculously.

Bright blessings,
Selene

Thursday, July 6, 2000
Subject: "DING! ROUND TWO"

Hey Gang (Jennifer here),

ROUND AND ROUND HE GOES!
Marley's second round of chemotherapy happened yesterday. It was hardly uneventful, but at least it was done in one day! After several unexpected adverse reactions, the doctor looked at me, shrugged, and said, "Teenagers have such wonderful immune systems." In other words, Marley's natural defense was doing its job, rejecting the onslaught of chemicals being pumped into his body. After much head scratching, the professionals decided to give him enough sedatives that he just didn't care how much his feet, hands, and nose itched.

Selene and I have been working hard in the kitchen. We've learned a lot about nutrition and various alternative cancer cures. We've been using only the freshest of foods, trying to make them look appetizing and be odor free. Until receiving chemo, Marley ate anything (and a lot of it). Not anymore... everything repulses him. Even so, Marley's only lost one pound and his blood count looks good. I just hope we're not keeping him so healthy the chemo doesn't work.

Marley called me last night from Drew's house and said he felt tired but good. Pray for him.

IF YOU GIVE A MOUSE A COOKIE...
HE'S GOING TO NEED A GLASS OF MILK!
In my last letter, I wrote that Marley convinced me he needed a new bike when he said, "You just don't understand, Mom, the only time I feel free, absolutely free, is when I'm riding my bike!" Well, if you give a boy a bike, he's going to need bike jumps! That's just the way it is. What's a mom to do?

THERE'S A BOBCAT IN THE PASTURE

I told Marley he could turn the pasture into a fun zone if he did all the work. Last Saturday, I rented a Bobcat (a small earth-mover) and had six yards of dirt delivered. He's worked with these machines at Drew's, so with very little instruction, he started construction. I was amazed at his skill manipulating that machine. With great precision, he split up small chunks of dirt with the large blade and carefully placed every load exactly where he wanted it. It was fun to see him skillfully doing something that really turned him on. He is designed to work with big tools.

LOSS IS KEY TO GAINING WISDOM

I rented the Bobcat for both Saturday and Sunday, but on Saturday night, all hell broke loose. Leave it to Marley to cut his wisdom teeth at 15 years of age! As soon as the rear right tooth cut through the gums, it became infected. And, of course, it happened on Saturday night. The fever hit and it was a battle to keep it low enough to avoid the ER. The entire next day, the poor guy had to look at the Bobcat just sitting in the pasture. We got some antibiotics in him, and the fever broke on Monday morning, at the same time as the equipment was hauled away.

His tooth was extracted on Thursday with no further infection. Do you really think it was that easy? Ha! First we had to check with the medical oncologists to see if we could pull the tooth. Then we had to find a dentist on short notice. With the help of our neighbor Kim, who pulled a few strings, Marley was in the dentist's chair the next day. The poor nurse came at Marley with a long needle filled with Novocain and Marley freaked! He demanded to be knocked out. Dentists apparently can't do that—only oral surgeons can.

All of my calming mothering techniques could not convince this kid that he could deal with having a tooth extracted while conscious, so I gave up, thanked the dentist profusely, and left. I made an appointment with the only team of oral surgeons available: Dr. Savage and Dr. Slaughter. (I kid you not.) We paid $400 extra to have Marley knocked out, and everyone was happy. A small price to pay. Pray that the other three molars stay put for a few months! No more holes. The risk is too high.

GO GO GO-CART

Last week, our beloved neighbors gave Marley their go-cart! What a gift!!!!! It needs some work, but they told Marley they would help. Marley, his good buddy Ben, and Ben's dad Kevin spent several hours getting the cart to run well enough to drive it to our house. That evening, Marley flopped down on the couch completely satisfied.

The next morning, he and Catie spent another hour getting it to run again. I sneered at it as I walked up to the chicken coop, yelling over my shoulder, "You be careful, that thing's an accident waiting to happen. Don't forget to wear a helmet." A minute later, I heard the engine roar. I looked up and saw Catie going down the driveway (no helmet). All I could do was to shake my head and mutter some not very nice words to myself. Then…I heard her scream. I flew out of the coop and ran across the pasture, hurdling the new bike jumps. Marley was running up our long driveway like a speeding bullet.

When we reached the screaming Catie, we both stopped dead in our tracks. She was so entangled that we had to stand there and discuss how exactly we were to extract her from both the cart and the wire—while she screamed in pain. She had made a perfect—well, an almost perfect—turn. That damned boulder was in the way. She had soared over it, bounced off the big oak tree, and slammed top speed into the fence (three wires with no barbs). Difficulty breathing…possible broken ribs…possible major bruising…but no blood, just wire burns everywhere. I left her crying in Marley's arms to go get the car, prepared to take her to the hospital. Walking away, I turned around and said, "Catie, you realize if this is bad you can't go to Wisconsin. I suggest you focus on instant recovery. You have the power." A look of horror came across her face (she really wanted to go to Wisconsin). Fifteen minutes later, after applying ice packs and arnica lotion, she was as good as new except for a small mark below her eye and three red diagonal stripes on one of her legs—no swelling or even bruises!

The go-cart was taken to Drew's house for repairs and a remodel. I sincerely hope it stays there.

ACTION HEROES

It's time to think about the next phase. We have three weeks to get it together—preparing for lung surgery in Boston. On Monday, our task is to find three free plane tickets. We also have to figure out what questions we need to ask the Boston doctors.

I love you all,
Jennifer

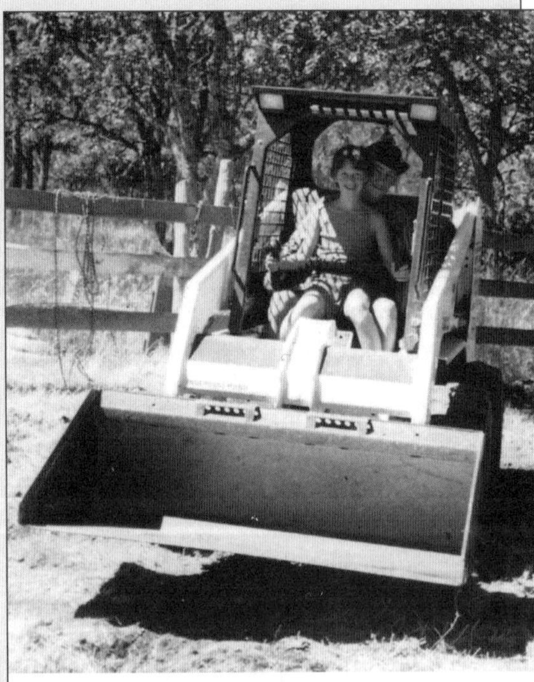

Marley, giving Catie a Bobcat ride

INTRODUCING...THE FENSTEMMERS

Pebbles From Heaven

During the first year of Marley's dance with cancer, we received a large, mysterious box in the mail. It was from Marvin Fenstemmer. We had no idea who this person was. There was no note included and the return address was obviously fake. There were two boxes within, each packed meticulously with glorious pieces of shimmery material. One box was for Marley, the other for Catie. This surprise gift couldn't have come at a better time. We needed help to keep looking at the bright side of life, and a puzzling distraction felt like a reward for persevering.

Marley wrapped his flashy new "scarf" around his neck while he carefully opened his large flat wooden box. Within it were gemstones of all shapes and sizes, each in their own compartment, special little box, or velvet bag. He was in awe and truly touched that a stranger knew exactly what he loved, and cared enough to pack everything so carefully. Catie's wooden box was packed with equal care. It contained scores of tiny, shiny enamel boxes and little carved wooden boxes, each filled with a sparkling piece of jewelry carefully wrapped in tissue paper. We spent the next hour marveling at each and every item.

"Any small, calm thing that one soul can do to help another soul, to assist some portion of this poor suffering world, will help immensely. It is not given to us to know which acts or by whom, will cause the critical mass to tip toward an enduring good. What is needed for dramatic change is an accumulation of acts, adding, adding to, adding more, continuing."

—Clarissa Pinkola Estes

That night, when I went into Marley's room to tuck him into bed, I saw what he'd been doing for the past hour. He had cleaned off his entire desk (a first!) and laid a large piece of leather down on it. This space became his new "altar." He had arranged many of the special new gems on it. A few of the stones were put into his pebble fountain, while the remainder were kept in the original box and stored next to his bed within reach.

Nine months later, we received another large box. This time it was from Mable Fenstemmer with a different return address than on the first package, but from the same state. This one was filled with gemstone eggs and spheres with little carved wooden holders. Each came packaged in their own beautifully unique box. It was just amazing. Who were the Fenstemmers?

After another exciting mini Christmas, we made a thank you gift for Mable. We took a shot of Marley and Catie holding our new baby goats, Gus and Jezabelle. Catie painted a picture frame that said, "Thank you, Love, Marley and Catie." We packed it up, sent it off, and received it back in the mail with "No such address" stamped on it. The mystery would not be solved for another two years.

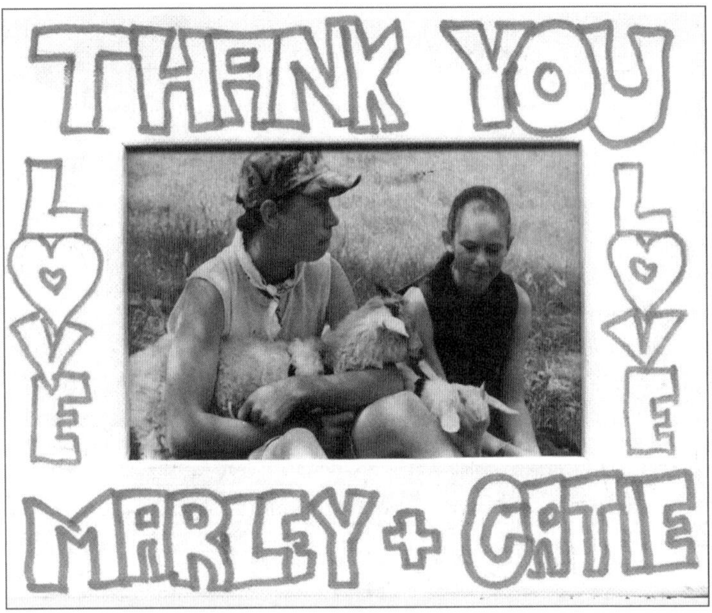

The picture and frame sent and returned.

Saturday, July 22, 2000
Subject: "HAIRLESS IN ASHLAND"

Hi Gang,

What a week! I finally have time to surface.

Marley's doin' pretty well. He's eating, has good color (with occasional dark circles under the eyes), his hair looks like it might even be growing again, although his eyebrows are still thinning. Yesterday, he lifted his arm, pointed, and said, "Look, Ma, no hair!" Indeed, his armpit hair was almost nonexistent—he actually likes it!

Catie is still in Wisconsin, but is scheduled to return next Thursday. YAHOOOOOO! I miss her soooooo much. She's been swimming nonstop, has been to Great America, and goes shopping every time it rains! The poor thing...! She sounds perky and happy whenever we talk.

As for Marley, the boy doesn't stop. He wants to do everything NOW! He's driving me nuts. I took him to see Merle Haggard (old-time country western singer) at the Britt Festival, a classy outdoor concert hall. It felt great to lie on a blanket with my boy and watch the show with the full moon hovering over Haggard. (Thanks John, your extra tickets went to good use!)

Selene and I took Mars for a quick visit to the Jackson County Fair to go on four carnival rides (ones that he simply couldn't live without). Tonight he's gone back to Britt to see an African performance with our friend Eric. I send thanks to Dee's friend who donated the tickets. After another party on Saturday night, I think we're going to head to the coast for a day. Maybe it'll feel more like a summer vacation after that.

Your support makes a big difference. Thank you,

Jennifer
P.S. Remember to look on the bright side of life!

SPACE SYRUP

The Elixir of Life

The ripple effect of the Marley Network always amazed me. Most of the time I had no idea that the waves of our lives were washing up on distant shores in the outside world. But every once in a while, I was reminded that the e-mail updates I sent to a few hundred people were actually being read by hundreds more.

One of the most unusual e-mails I received came from a woman who had been forwarded the Marley Update Letters. This woman changed my life by sending me the following recipe:

Space Syrup Recipe

2 tsp. fresh finely minced Garlic

3 Tbls. Olive Oil

5 Tbls. pure Clover Honey

1 Tbls. organic Apple Cider Vinegar (The more stuff floating around in the bottle the better!)

1/2 tsp. Cayenne

1/4 cup strong brewed organic Green Tea

1/4 tsp. Asafoetida (optional)

> ***Food Fact:***
>
> **Garlic**
>
> While processing garlic, the more air mixed with it (ie: the finer it's chopped) and the less it is cooked, the healthier it is for you.

Mince garlic and saute in oil for 1 minute, add other ingredients. Simmer over low flame for 5 minutes (until bubbly and full of your good, healing energy). Let cool. Pour into glass jar, refrigerate, and serve yourself one teaspoon each day to live forever in grand health with exceptional vitality. If you don't want little chunks of garlic stuck between your teeth, you can always strain it, but I figure if you strain it, you'll only live to be 120!

A Spacey Story

I don't care about the story or where it came from. I know this sounds crazy, but this stuff really works. This elixir energizes me and keeps me healthy. The story behind this recipe was almost as good as the recipe itself. I didn't write this—I'm just passing along as much of the story as I saved. It was an article printed in the *Harmonic Response Messenger.* (The author was cited as "unknown.") It's an interview with a woman who was working alone at her house when "all of a sudden the space around her changed and she spontaneously passed into another state of consciousness."

> "'Seven small green creatures appeared out of the thin air,' she said, 'and they used their huge, glowing eyes to immobilize me. They appeared in the corner of my office and they seemed very loving and concerned,' she recalled. 'They told me they had a great affection and respect for humans and wanted to help us with this gift. I couldn't move or speak. I felt like I was dreaming. When I woke up, the spacemen were gone and the recipe was sitting on the desk in front of me.'"
>
> "Mrs. Ritkiss says she mixed up a batch of the syrup the next day. Because it contained nothing she felt would harm her, she took a teaspoon every day for a month to see what would happen."
>
> "'I couldn't believe what it did for me!' she says. 'My arthritis is gone, my skin glows, even my teeth and hair are different. I feel like a teenager again. Since then, I have shared the recipe with hundreds of people and it had cured everything—acne, heart disease, depression, and even cancer. The syrup is so wonderful, I know I have to tell everybody about it. It's a miracle gift, a token of love from outer space.'"

"Formerly, when religion was strong and science weak,
men mistook magic for medicine;
now, when science is strong and religion weak,
men mistake medicine for magic."

—Thomas Szaszb

Wednesday, August 3, 2000
Subject: "THE MIDDLE MAN"

• From: Selene

Dear loved ones,

They (whoever that is) say it is good to start at the beginning, and yet there no longer seems to be a beginning. So I will start somewhere in between, which is where Marley has been settled now for a while.

The basics first...
Tomorrow he goes to the hospital in Dreadford to get a CAT scan to see if the chemo has reduced the size of his tumor. He is still scheduled to fly to Boston around the 13th of August for surgery.

Jennifer is in the midst of a huge move from one office to another. (A San Diego corporation bought the Bathroom Readers' Institute.) Yesterday she spent a fun-filled day perusing the aisles of Staples, Office Max, and Costco, crunching numbers and dreaming of plush swivel chairs, #2 pencils, and double-sided tape. We envy her not. She will be back with you whenever it is humanly possible. (Despite thoughts to the contrary, I have officially determined her to be a humanoid—stop the presses!)

Rambling second...
It is (surprise, surprise!) hard to know when the chaos will settle into a merely random series of events. Then again, if this whole thing has taught me something (okay, it's taught me a million things, but bear with me) it's that there will always be chaos, there will always be uncertainty, and there will always be tragedy.

These days, I head toward the eye of the tornado. No, I do not sit and spin. I sit still and watch and breathe and hope. And when I'm able to really hold it together, I pray for everyone else out there to find that hollow place of peace. It is there that Marley guns his go-cart, sending dust flying. And it is there that Jennifer, as our friend Eric puts it, "channels the fifth dimension." It is there that you're likely to find Catie painting mountainous landscapes on beautiful pieces of wood, and Drew sitting on the porch of the house he and Cindy built, watching night fall. There, in the center, you'll be in good company.

I wish I could tell you how Marley is. Only he knows that. I think he's tired and wants all this to be over. But I also think he's excited to be going back to Boston, the big city. Maybe he'll see friends at the Ronald McDonald house. Maybe he'll have cute nurses in the hospital.

I keep thinking, if he weren't so young, this wouldn't be so awful. But it's his youth that keeps him so alive, so I'm glad this happened when it did. And I'm convinced it is the invisible support of all of you that keeps this family not only sane, but playful too.

Love and Blessings,
Selene

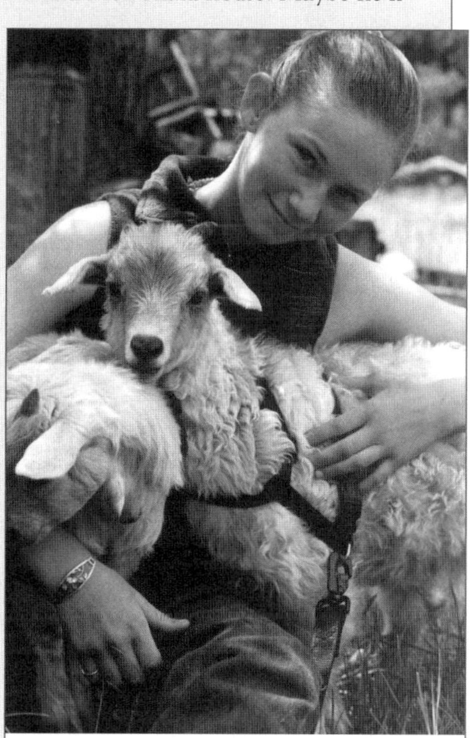

Catie with Gus and Jezabelle

MARLEY'S INSPIRATION

Here's another example of the letters that were sent to us from strangers. It made me have faith that with one heart touching another, sharing our stories, we could become stronger still.

Thursday, August 4, 2000
Subject: "MARLEY'S INSPIRATION"

• From: Rebekah

Dear family,

Although I don't know you, it touched me deeply to read about the journey you are traveling through. The passion and love radiated through your stories, letters and photos. A close friend of my family went through two bouts of leukemia when we were children, and I can only imagine how this has brought you all closer together to realize the important things in life.

In April, due to weather conditions, my little brother Nathanael was in a serious car accident. At the scene of the accident his heart was beating once every 30 seconds, and it took 45 minutes to get him out of the car. He had five blood transfusions in the emergency room, and he was put on life support. Needless to say, things didn't look good, but he was 18 years old and he was strong. Six months later, he seems to be recovering, coming out of his coma. It'll be a long road, but there is so much hope.

Thank you for having a website, and for telling Marley's story. It needs to be told! The love, learning, courage, and support that is apparent through your little "Internet" portal is so encouraging to me.

Hold Marley near and dear. My prayer for comfort is with you.

Sincerely,
Rebekah

Chapter Six:
The Medical Kingdom

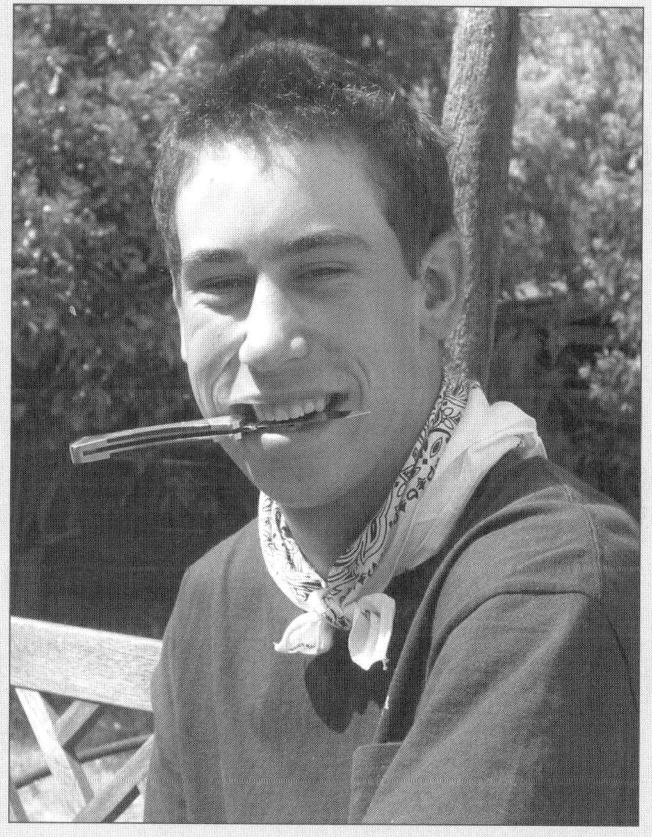

Marley with Buck knife

Photo: Mandy Little

HOW BAD IS BAD?

Going to Hell

Looking back on the days when I had a ruptured disk, during the time Drew and I were splitting up, makes me want to laugh. I thought that was about as bad as my life was ever going to get. But that was a walk in the park compared to the summer of 2000.

For the first time since Marley was born, I had no responsibilities to tend to at home when the kids were at Drew's. My beloved dog Sage was no longer around to take care of me. She had been my constant companion and my best friend for 16 years. She died in my arms the month before Marley got sick, and I was still grieving her absence. The chickens had recently been rudely slaughtered by raccoons. The rabbit escaped, and I let the cockatiels fly away. My only responsibility was my beloved cat Salsa, who was able to fend for herself whenever I didn't show up for a day or two.

So when the kids weren't with me, I worked too much—mainly to avoid listening to the inner workings of my own brain. My life was incredibly stressful. Aside from having a kid with cancer, a large corporation now ruled my work life. They were throwing money at us, which was fun, but their demands were unreasonably high. I was supposed to choreograph moving the entire business to a new location, buying all new equipment, and implementing new systems and programs, all while doing business as usual. It was a logistical nightmare. I can't believe I didn't shoot myself. I think I drank a gallon of Space Syrup a day. Somehow I managed to pull through the transition without missing a beat. Focusing on anything but my personal life was the name of my game.

At night, I would go out with friends and drink too much, trying to pretend there was more to life than pain and suffering. I spent most nights on a couch at the office, crawling under the covers, praying I wouldn't have any dreams. I just wanted it all to go away.

But I somehow kept it together to face another day. I kept remembering the wisdom of my great-aunt, who said, "If you make yourself look beautiful and dress like you feel great, most of the time you will trick yourself into believing it." She was right. Every morning I had a new chance at having a great day. Even when it didn't quite turn out that way, I carried hope and possibility around with me.

Blues, Despair, Agony, All Three...

When the kids were with me, it was like living in the middle of a bad country western song. ...*Deep dark depression, pain, and misery....* (That song from *Hee Haw* was my theme that summer.) Marley was either in a great mood, ready for action, or in a foul mood, demanding attention and spreading a cloud of darkness and gloom. I never knew if the nice Marley or the evil Marley was next to me. I was on guard all the time. It must have been the drugs but, whatever it was, none of us liked it. The worst part was that we had to try to be understanding and nice.

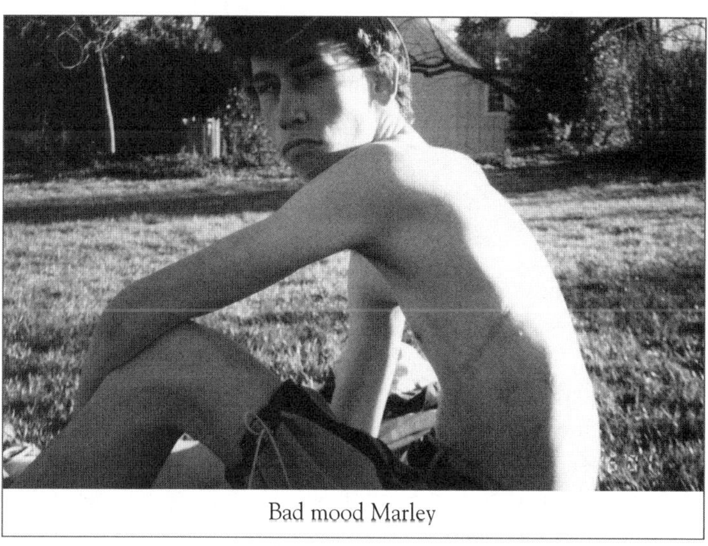

Bad mood Marley

I'm so glad we all survived some of our daily interchanges. It's a terrible thing to admit, but I had visions of sneaking up behind Marley with a knife just to put us all out of our misery. There were times I'd be cooking dinner, pleasantly talking to Catie as she drew pictures at the kitchen counter, and Marley would enter the room. He'd walk past her, kick her chair, poke her in the ribs, and growl at her. I knew what was coming next.

"Mom! Tell him to stop!" she'd squeal.

Trying to stay cool, calm, and collected, I'd say, "Cut the crap, Marley. What's up?"

"I feel like shit. There's nothin' ta do."

"Well, don't take it out on your sister."

Shaking his head at me and sneering at Catie, he'd open the front door and moan, "What the hell's there ta live for?" He'd kick over my tool bucket on the front porch and head for the barn.

Ten minutes later, like nothing had happened, he'd be back to ask Catie if she wanted to play. She'd look at me like he was crazy and turn to him and say, "You've gotta be kidding?" Then it would start all over again.

Catie was lucky enough to miss several of the worst weeks of Marley's chemotherapy. When she returned from Wisconsin, Drew and Cindy moved Marley's bed into the living room so he could be around everyone during the times he couldn't move. There were times when all he could do was throw up. Except for Catie, everyone got used to handing him a bucket and listening to him dry heave.

Drew, Cindy, Laura, Vanessa, Catie, and Marley were living in a trailer while they finished building their new house. The space was tight—there was no privacy—no one could escape the sound of Marley's dramatic yorking technique. My house was larger than the trailer, but the walls were thin and there was still no place to hide. Thank God it was summertime. Marley spent most of his time lying outside on a big blanket surrounded by his Legos, hoping someone would play with him.

When he wasn't moaning, groaning, and growling at us, he was cuddly and quiet. Sometimes he looked like death warmed over, and sometimes he looked like nothing was wrong. It all felt like a bad dream. Fortunately the nightmare ended as summer came to a close and the chemo ran its course.

Wednesday, August 10, 2000
Subject: "MIND MUSH"

To Whom it May Concern,

I'm sorry I haven't had the time to keep you more informed. Unfortunately, you're not going to get much out of me because my brain is about to spill forth all over my glorious new computer. My beautiful niece, Selene, tells me I'm going to turn into a pumpkin if I don't stop working but…but…but….

Bathroom Readers' Press has moved! In four days flat, we're up and running (well, shuffling) in our new location on the other side of this dinky—but beautiful—town. Even I am amazed by me. As of last Friday, we are now officially owned by a San Diego-based corporation called Advanced Marketing Services. I'm pretty sure they'll treat us well…so far so good. Life's going to be intense until this year's *Bathroom Reader* is complete. The pressure to impress is on. We have about seven weeks to get over 500 pages into the hands of holiday shoppers. Please pray for me and my beloved crew. We're going to need help!

Marley, oh dear Marley…. The CAT scan results indicate that the chemo was ineffective. During the last two weeks, Marley discovered a large marble-sized lump on his arm. It was removed by our family doctor, and the biopsy was sent to pathologists in Seattle. Today the results came back inconclusive. They want to compare the "abnormal" cells of this new lump with the most recent biopsies from his lung. Then they will hopefully have a better idea what the new lump is made of. The results will be available right before we're scheduled for surgery in Boston.

Once Dr. Sugarmaker is armed with the CAT scan results, the pathology comparison, Marley himself, and any other lab work ordered, *then* maybe some intelligent decisions can be made. So, for right now, sit tight and know that I'll keep you posted.

There's not much we can do or even think until we have more information.

Meanwhile, Drew and Marley are leaving for Boston on Monday morning. I'm following behind on the red-eye special that night using frequent-flyer miles provided by my lovely sister, Meredith (Selene's mom). Some amazing work was done to try to get us there at a reasonable cost. No easy feat. 500,000 phone calls later.... Thanks to all who helped. Especially you, Selene, you're amazing.

Must leave the office. Must go home. Much to do. Inhale. So much to remember. Where is the box with the yellow folder in it? Exhale. Meet Dee at 10 A.M. (arrrgghh, that's only 9 hours from now). Install the cable modem. Inhale. Inhale. What am I going to do with my cat while I'm in Boston? Exhale. Don't forget to.... Blah, blah, blah.

I love you all!
Jennifer

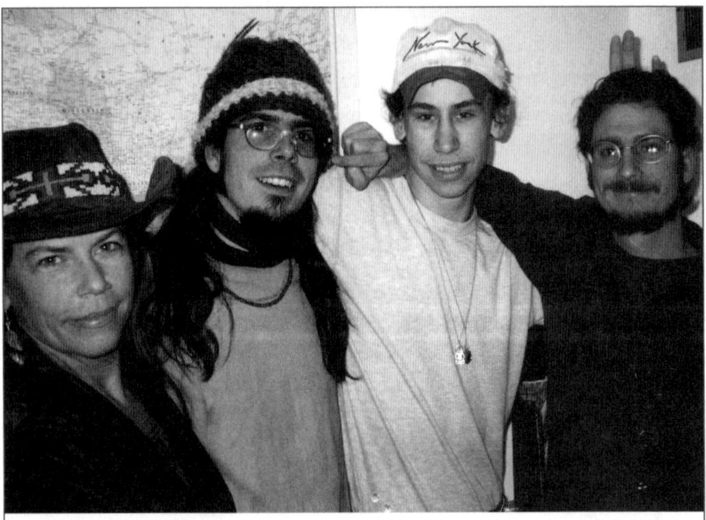

Jennifer, Eric, Marley, and Jay

MACROBIOTICS VS MARLEY

Sisterly Advice

A lot of people were following Marley's story. Whether I knew them or not, my "family" continued to grow in numbers. When I received an e-mail from a woman in Canada and then another from my sister on the same topic, I *had* to pay attention. Their advice about radically changing Marley's diet was right on, but it was Marley, not me, who was sick.

Thursday, August 11, 2000
Subject: "PLEASE DO THIS"

• From: Michele

Jennifer,

I have been quietly reading the progress about Marley and really admiring the strength and support around your challenges with this extremely difficult disease.

The recent news about Marley is very disturbing. I can no longer just quietly read these e-mails. I URGE you to set up an appointment at the Macrobiotic Centre when you are in Boston. These people have had REMARKABLE results in curing and helping control cancer. I know several people who have cured very difficult types of cancer by following a macrobiotic course. You have faithfully been doing what the medical establishment has suggested (and I would do the same in your situation), but PLEASE. PLEASE. SEE THESE PEOPLE. DO IT!

In support of seeing Marley truly healthy and cured,
Michele

"The family—that dear octopus from whose tentacles we never quite escape nor, in our innermost hearts, ever quite wish to."

—Dodie Smith

Stepping Aside

I was reminded of when Drew and I were wilderness quest guides just before Marley was born. Even though we taught people how to stay safe and care for themselves, it didn't mean that's what they always did. Like the time we dealt with the woman who challenged the lightning bolts from the top of a rocky ridge.

This woman had come to us for help marking her independence just after a divorce. She had been warned of the intensity of desert lightning storms and instructed how *not* to die during her quest, and yet she insisted on picking the crest of a ridge to spend her solo time. All we could do was hope she would survive nature's lesson. Sure enough, great bolts of lightning taught her humility as she spent an uncomfortable night trying not to be the tallest thing on that ridge! Sometimes a guide must just step aside and let people learn for themselves.

Marley's identity was wrapped up in the life of a rancher. Drew and Cindy raised beef; they relished eating the critters they loved. Could Hanky the pig be considered macrobiotic? No, but she was organic! If you were to watch Marley's joy as he manhandled a turkey drumstick, devouring it like a barbarian, you too would think twice about asking him to eat only vegetables. I tried to pick my battles carefully. I knew requesting that Marley give up Mountain Dew and beef jerky wasn't a winning proposition. Even if I didn't buy them for him, I couldn't control his intake, especially when he was at school. I had to let go.

"I have found the best way to give advice to your children is to find out what they want and then advise them to do it."

—Harry S. Truman

Friday, August 12, 2000
Subject: "MARLEY & DIET"

• From: Constant

Jen,

Have you heard of the Raw Food Diet? Several folks have mentioned it to me for Marley. I know a couple of people who have cured themselves of cancer with this. If you are interested I could get more information for you.

I'm holding you and dear Marley in my prayers. There are many in my circle doing the same.

Con

Friday, August 12, 2000
Subject: "RE: MARLEY & DIET"

• From: Jennifer

Dear Constant,

I laugh in your general direction! We're talking about Marley. Months ago, I made the suggestion to Marley that he cut back on his meat intake and he almost fainted.

I've done much research on the effects of diet and cancer cells. *I'm* healthier for it! As far as Marley goes, he really needs to decide how much he's willing to risk for life. Does he really want to live? These are tough questions.

I love you,
Jennifer

P.S. Here's one of Marley's favorite quotes:

"Health nuts are going to feel stupid someday, lying in hospitals dying of nothing."

—Redd Foxx

Sunday, August 14, 2000
Subject: "THE BOSTON MASSACRE"

Greetings friends,

Marley, Drew, and I arrived safely in Boston. With very little sleep under my belt, I'm going to try to make this letter coherent and brief.

Marley and Drew arrived last night at 10:30 P.M. and settled in a room at the Ronald McDonald House. I arrived this morning at 6:30 A.M. My sister Julia flew in last night from Asheville, North Carolina. She and her beloved childhood friend Nicky (who was our Boston contact the last go 'round) picked me up at the airport and took me straight to Brigham and Women's Hospital to catch up with Drew and Marley for our 8 A.M. pre-op appointment.

Today he had blood tests, an X-ray, and a physical exam at Brigham and Women's. Then a bone scan was done at Dana Farber Hospital.

At 7:30 tomorrow morning, Marley is scheduled for a CAT scan of his head at Children's Hospital. At 10 A.M., we have an appointment with the big cheese—Dr. Jackson, the chief oncology specialist governing all three hospitals. Our surgeon referred us to Jackson because, as it turns out, Marley's case is unique. Jackson will give us an overview of ways to deal with this new situation.

After lunch, Marley will get a PET scan done. This will be the last and possibly the most critical test before the scheduled surgery on Thursday. This is the test where they inject radioactive liquid into his bloodstream, then wait for it to filter through his body. This scan will, theoretically, pick up any clumps of abnormal cell growth. This will give us a clue as to how extensive the new growth in his arm is.

We'll be done around 5 P.M., at which point Nicky and her lovely daughter Sage will join us for a final feast before Marley begins his pre-surgery fasting. Marley is scheduled for surgery at 9:30 Thursday morning. We'll wait around for a few hours (most likely listening to Marley whine about how hungry he is). At 1:30 P.M., Dr. Sugarmaker will preform a bronchoscopy for one final look inside Marley's left lung. Then he'll determine whether he'll perform a partial lobectomy (removal of the lower lobe) or a full lobectomy (removal of the entire lung). The final procedure is a mediastinoscopy. While inside the mediastinum (the area around the lungs), Dr. Sugarmaker will remove any lymph nodes that appear suspect.

That's all we know now. Some more information will be gained tomorrow and some decisions will be made. Wish us luck. Beam your light.

Marley has been full of fun, loving smiles, and playfulness. He's an amazing soul who seems to be taking this all in stride.

I'll do my best to keep you posted.

Love to you all,
Jennifer

P.S.
Every summer, Steven and Meredith (my sister and brother-in-law) host a family reunion for the Foster clan. These grand celebrations are to honor Steven's birthday and the gifts he has given us. This is the first reunion in many years that Marley and I will not attend, but Catie is going to represent us all. She and Selene will drive to the California desert and will be held by family the whole time we are in Boston. (I love the way this worked out.)

The Butterfly Effect

MY STORY
by Eric Heikell

I met Marley at a Foster family reunion in 1999. He was 14 years old and healthy, but there was no mistaking that he was not an ordinary kid. Tall and gangly, intense in a quiet kind of way, with a strange way of speaking that somehow touched my heart.

I had brought my bright red, inflatable Zodiac with outboard motor to this gathering. As soon as he saw it, he was infatuated. I learned later he was fascinated by most mechanical devices that "went fast." He wanted to be near the boat, operate it, or do with it whatever I would allow. We ended up spending a lot of time together out on the lake, racing around and exploring. While chatting, I learned his parents didn't live together but seemed to have a good working relationship for their kids. He spent a lot of time with both his dad and mom and seemed to feel completely at ease with all of his family dynamics. His soul was an old and a very deep one, with a power to touch the heart that I don't understand.

The next year, at this same reunion, Selene and Catie informed us that Marley had cancer and the outlook did not seem good. He couldn't attend that year, and we were all saddened by this. His absence cast a spell over that year's gathering that still lingers. I followed his progress over the next three years via e-mail updates from Jennifer.

The last time I met with Marley was at his Uncle Steven's memorial (the final and unplanned Foster reunion). We only talked briefly, but he was a fountain of peace to me, floating through the crowd, in love with everyone. He had forgotten who I was until I reminded him of the bright red Zodiac. His face lit up with a grin and he said that had been a fun time for him.

I hardly knew Marley. Yet he's been an influence for so many people. He has brought so many hearts together in sweetness, love, and humanity that it's hard to ignore. I think Marley's gift to me has been his simplicity and his ability to meet me where I am, without guile. He cares only for the moment we're living and the fun we're having while in it. After all he has been through, his life has brought people together, and he has touched each of us. Perhaps we're now connected through our contact with him and his gift of just being Marley. I am blessed by his being, and I would be a poorer man in heart had I never known him, however short and insignificant our time together may have been.

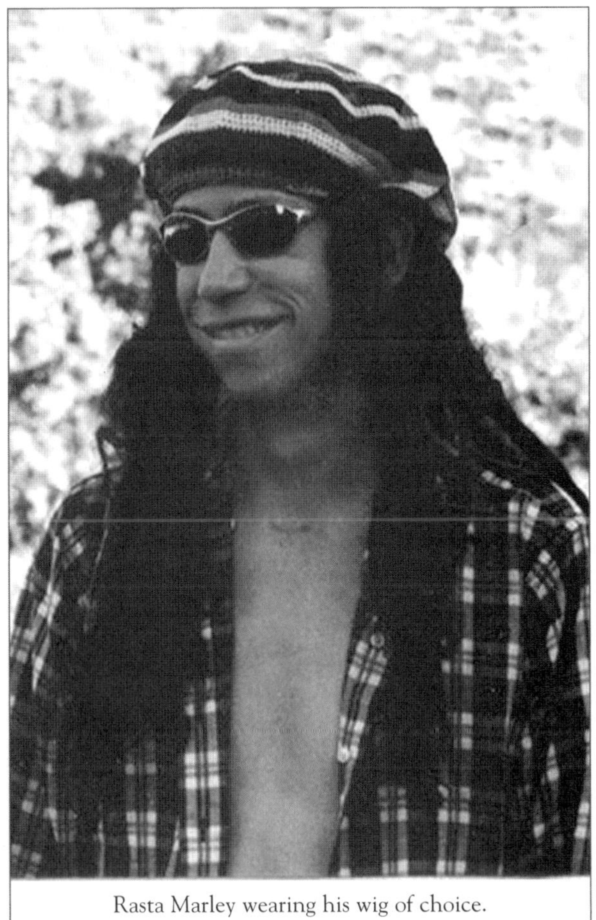

Rasta Marley wearing his wig of choice.

Sunday, August 20, 2000
Subject: "OPERATION REMOVAL"

Hey Gang,

Marley was a trooper on Thursday. We had to be at the hospital at 8 A.M., although surgery wasn't scheduled until 1:30 P.M. At 1 P.M., Marley turned back his watch one hour. Why? He said he wanted to buy a little extra time before surgery. It was an ingenious solution. As it turned out, due to the popularity of our surgeon, Marley didn't go under the knife until 4 P.M. Having to wait was nerve-wracking. We had to stay on hospital grounds so they could find us whenever Dr. Sugarmaker was ready. This delay meant Marley had to go without food even longer than planned. We wrestled, pitched pennies, plucked grass, and wrestled some more. Maybe Marley should have turned his watch forward instead!

After a three-and-a-half hour surgery, Dr. Sugarmaker said everything went beautifully—no complications. Marley is now without his entire left lung. The cancer had been spreading up the left bronchial passage and was fortunately able to be totally eliminated, including a 5mm margin of healthy tissue. They also had to remove half of one rib in order to remove six lymph nodes which glowed on the PET scan. So the boy has been taken apart, cleaned out, and put back together. We still have to deal with the tumor in his arm, but we'll save that for another day—it is not immediately life-threatening.

He has great color, is coherent when he's awake (which has not been often), and has been extremely cooperative with his nurses. Today he actually sat in a chair for 20 minutes with the bribe of a ginger ale. If he can manage to get on his feet and shuffle around a bit, maybe they'll let him "eat" for the first time in three days. (Don't tell him, but I think they're talking about chicken broth.)

He's in a private room, with nurses checking every hour. The care is remarkable. I'm staying in his room during the night. Whenever one of his machines beeps or anything is wrong, those nurses almost beat me to his side. Amazing! The only patients these nurses deal with are thoracic (lung) patients, so they really know their stuff. We're in the right place.

Hopefully, Marley's desire for food will continue to lead him to health. He has much work to do, and this staff will drive him hard. We're expecting to be at Brigham & Women's Hospital 'til midweek. In a few days we'll be moved out of ICU and into a general room in the hospital. At that time, I'll give you the phone number so you can give us a call if you want.

I'm doing really well and am in good spirits, even though my sister Julia left today. It's been so good having her support and her company.

Drew's parents arrived from New York just as Julia was departing. If you want to reach Drew, when he's not at the hospital, he'll be at the Carriage House at the Ronald McDonald House. If you *do* reach him, please be conscious; worrying takes a lot of energy!

If you want to send anything to Marley, send it c/o Ronald McDonald House of Boston, 229 Kent St. Brookline, MA 02446. These folks have treated us very well, and I want to encourage any donations (cash or equipment). I wouldn't be able to communicate with you if someone hadn't donated the computer here. Even the monthly Internet fees have been donated. If you feel generous, toys, movies, blankets, linens, etc. would all be well received by them.

Thanks for your gifts and your prayers,
Jennifer

Wednesday, August 23, 2000
Subject: "LUNGLESS IN BOSTON"

Hello Marley Man Fans!

It's been a busy week. I've stolen a few hours away from the hospital to do some work at the Ronald McDonald House and thought I'd touch base with you, too.

My rosy view of our hospital experience is no longer so bright and colorful. Marley has been caught in another post surgery catch-22 scenario. He's been on a water restriction to keep the lung dry, which makes him constipated. His stomach hurts, so they give him medication to relieve the pain—which makes him nauseous. The anti-nausea medication and laxatives only make matters worse. With no water to flush his system, his stomach was so bloated and tight I thought he might pop! The pain was intense. The poor kid spent most of the time dry heaving. Round and round, caught in this vicious cycle.

Yesterday morning was miserable. It started bright and early at 5 A.M., after just four hours of restless slumber. One by one we were visited by people trying to "help." The night nurse came to check on Marley, the radiologist took X-rays, the IV specialist poked another hole, and then another nurse came in to take his blood pressure. Just as we'd drifted back to sleep, the shift doctors entered, followed by six interns all scribbling in their notebooks. They saw their "quick visit" as a minor interruption. I'm sure they had no clue (or didn't care) that many others had been in just before them.

At 7:30 A.M., Marley and I had a meltdown. A doctor came in to ask if Marley was still nauseous. Marley was sitting in bed, clutching his side, dry heaving. My mouth dropped open as I mopped his forehead, trying to keep him calm. I spat, "You've got to be kidding!" I asked him to leave and to close the door.

Then I barricaded it from the inside and waited for Drew to arrive...he'd know what to do.

Drew and I decided the best thing was to leave the hospital ASAP. (It isn't feeling like a good place to heal.) We fiercely guarded his room and Marley finally got some sleep. After several small battles, the neck IV was removed, the drugs were limited, and the water restriction was lifted. Drew went out and bought Marley a Nerf gun with instructions to shoot anyone that was a bother! I admired Drew's solution. All three of us had fun shooting the gun. By the afternoon, Marley took his first walk, trailing a monitor machine and catheter bag. We also took him for a ride in a wheelchair to a little cafe in the lobby for REAL food!

Today, no one came in until 7:30 A.M. For some reason, they even seemed a little scared. A wonderful night nurse took pity on us and helped to guard the room. Just before her shift was over, she "accidentally" pulled out Marley's remaining IV so he could take a shower and walk without being followed by a beeping machine! Marley also put on civilian clothes which helped his attitude greatly. It's been a very good day.

With any luck we'll be released tomorrow and back at the Ronald McDonald House. With more luck we will be ready to go home on the 30th.

Love you all,
Jennifer

P.S. On the front page of the newspaper today is the story of the first quadruple transplant ever performed. It was done the day after Marley's surgery here at Brigham & Women's, by none other than Marley's surgeon. He's the real deal.

HEALING

In Good Company

When we arrived at the Ronald McDonald House, we were placed on the fourth floor. Julia, Drew, Marley, and I shared a small attic room. It was summertime in Boston, and the humidity was high. Being in the uppermost region of the old mansion meant that it was hot as hell. Drew and Marley shared the double bed, while Julia and I each had a rollaway cot.

During most of our time in Boston, I was with Marley at the hospital. I don't know when, or why, but sometime before Marley was released, we had been moved to the Carriage House (where the carriages were kept in the old days). Julia and Drew's parents had left by then, so Drew, Marley, and I had the place to ourselves. It was a big, newly remodeled, furnished room complete with an air conditioner that worked! It was the perfect place for Marley to heal.

JD had sent an amazing remote control train set, made by Lego, that could be assembled in a variety of ways. While Marley recovered from surgery, we watched TV, played with the train set, and ate home-cooked food. Because we were not in the main house, we weren't a part of the social scene that we had experienced on the first trip. Toward the end of our stay, Marley wanted to visit the main house more and more.

That was when he met a beautiful Brazilian girl his age, who had a different kind of lung cancer. She was there for a similar procedure. She'd had a portion of her left lung removed just days before Marley had. Unfortunately, they met the day she was leaving, and only had a few hours to talk and compare scars. Marley was visibly disappointed he hadn't run into her earlier. She was gorgeous and didn't mind that Marley's speech was unusual because she, too, had a thick accent. After that meeting, Marley didn't feel so alone.

Friday, September 1, 2000
Subject: "LIFE'S A BLURRR"

We're HOME!

(It's Thursday) and yesterday was a loooonnnnnng day. Up at 5:30 A.M. (EST), left the Ronald McDonald House at 6:30 A.M., and were in the arms of family by 3:30 P.M. (PST). 12 hours...3,000 miles...not bad!

(Now it's Friday)—that should tell you what Thursday was like—It's 10 P.M. and I'm done working. I thought I'd finish yesterday's brave attempt at communicating.

Life is a bluuuurrrr. So what else is new? Marley is the most amazing human being that I know. Sometimes I wonder if he's in a total state of denial. Does he understand what he's up against? Does he think about dying? Does he care? Why is he so awesome? How does he heal so fast? What makes this strange kid keep on going? Since he was born it seems he's been struggling against the odds to stay here on Planet Earth. Even as his closest ally, I don't have a clue what makes Marley tick. I *do* know, now more than ever, Marley is one of the greatest teachers I've met (and I've had the honor to meet a few humdingers). I have nothing but R.E.S.P.E.C.T. for this young hero. I am so proud of him.

Back-track...Marley was released from the hospital Thursday last. Drew declared that we all needed exercise and we were to walk everywhere from then on. Seven days after handing over a lung, a rib, and several lymph nodes, the boy walked 15 minutes from the hospital to our little home at the Ronald McDonald House. We spent the next week recovering from our week in the hospital, bored out of our gourds. I've watched more TV in the past few weeks than I care to view in the next ten years.

On Friday, after eight days of recuperating, we had to walk to and from the hospital twice! Drew was a superior drill sergeant. He was always ten paces ahead of Marley and I, saying, "Com'on—why are you walking so slow? You can do it." I held Marley's hand and sheepishly smiled encouragement as he looked to me for help.

The first appointment that day was for a minor outpatient surgery. A plastic surgeon re-opened the place where our local doctor had removed the tumor in Marley's arm. He took out a large scoop of tissue to assure all of the cancerous cells were removed. Marley was given local anesthetics to make the arm numb. I was allowed in to comfort him during surgery, but he was so exhausted from walking, he slept through the whole procedure. I watched the operation in the reflection of the surgeon's eyeglasses.

The second appointment was with Boston's top oncology specialist. This man was like royalty and we were given the red carpet treatment as his patients. We sat in a very plush office on the top floor of the high rise hospital. This doctor shot straight and true—he didn't have to fake wisdom—he was relaxed, calm, and spoke to us as peers. He said there's no other case history to refer to. Our situation is unique and there's no protocol for our boy's case. Marley is the youngest patient with metastasized squamous lung cancer. Because he didn't respond to the chemo in the expected manner, we're left with one option: radiation therapy.

As far as Western medicine is concerned, our goal is to protect the chest area from future cancer growth. It's the most difficult area to operate on, thus the most life threatening. Radiation won't prolong Marley's life, it'll simply protect his chest area. Radiation treatment will start in about a month, and will last for a duration of five to six weeks (five days per week). Side effects: sore throat, difficulty swallowing, weight loss, fatigue, and possible burning of the skin tissue.

At this moment, as far as we know, Marley is free of all cancerous cells. Now it is up to us (ALL OF US) to keep it that way!

Oh, by the way, Marley gained weight in Boston. He's now just over 6' and weighs 159 pounds. And he looks great!

Marley and Catie are at Drew and Cindy's until the 8th, so I'm working my butt off until they return to me. When I'm not working, I have my nose buried in the latest *Harry Potter* book, and I'm happy as a clam under the deep blue sea!

It's late. I love you all,
Jennifer

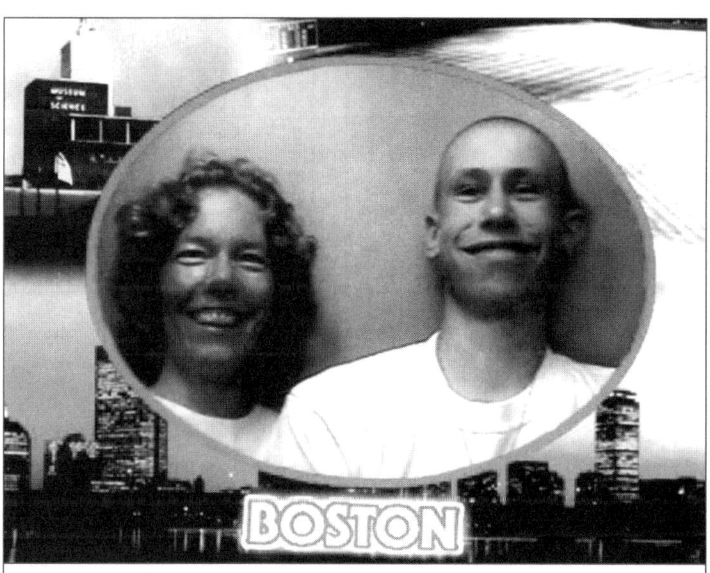

Nicky and Marley

Photo: photo booth

UNDER THE SURFACE

A Small Margin of Error

One of the most significant clues during Marley's journey was the most insignificant tumor. It occurred when least expected—*during* chemotherapy. It was the easiest tumor to deal with. Yet, in retrospect, this little tumor gave us more information about what we were up against than any other tumor—if only we had known enough to pay full attention.

Marley had just received his second dose of chemo "therapy" when he found a small marble-sized lump on the tricep of his left arm. It was just under the skin (*subcutaneous*). We could literally grab the hard little sphere and move it around. Within days after discovering it, we went to Dr Kay, our family physician. He recommended we remove it and send it in to pathology for identification.

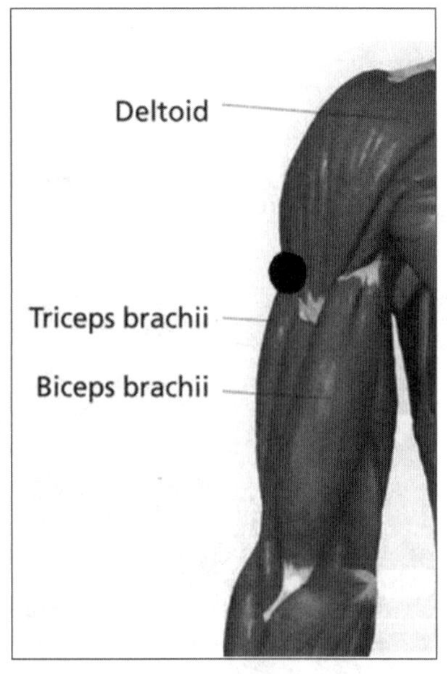

It was a simple 30-minute procedure that was done right in his office. Drew was happier than a pig in shit because Dr. Kay allowed him not only to watch, but to assist with the procedure. Marley walked out of the office with a few stitches holding the one-inch scar together. It all seemed easy enough.

A month later in Boston, we learned a valuable lesson—when removing a tumor, at least a two percent margin around it should also be removed, cancerous or not—to ensure all infected cells are removed, negating the need for a second surgery. Because we had not done this, the Boston doctors reopened that small incision on his arm to remove additional tissue.

The polite little scar left by our family doctor was now three times the length. The amount of tissue removed the second time created a permanent indent that actually accentuated Marley's arm muscles. Had we known more, we would have gone to a surgeon the first time saving money, time, and anxiety. We love our family doctor, but dealing with cancer was not his expertise.

That little subcutaneous tumor was the one that made the bigwig doctor in Boston realize that Marley's lung cancer was traveling fast, and in a curious fashion. The squamous had spread quickly throughout the lung, had attacked the lymph system, and formed an unusual free-floating tumor in his arm while being treated with chemo.

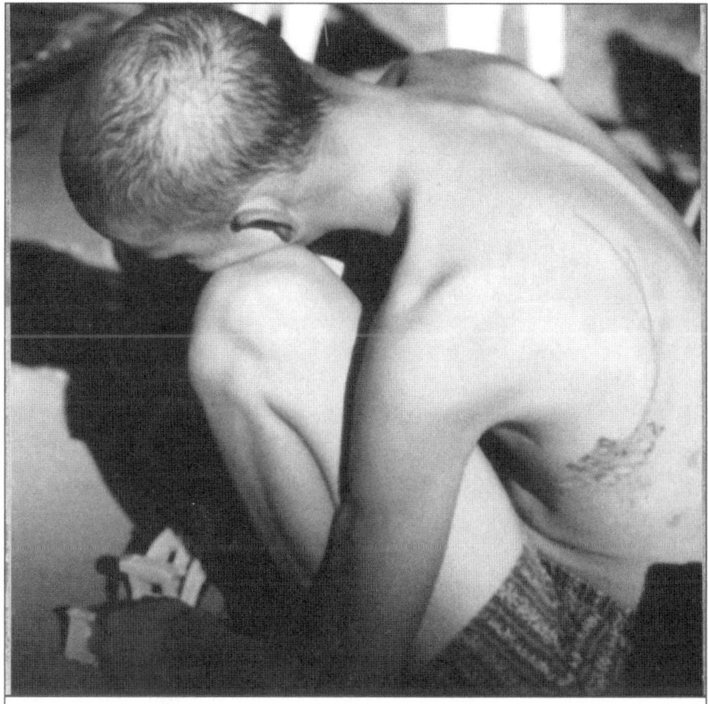

Marley just after his second thorocotomy and arm surgery.

Preparing for the Worst

After we returned from Boston, Drew, Cindy, and I discussed our "worst-case scenario" fears. Cindy said her worst fear was that the cancer would take up residence in Marley's brain. I feared that the cancer, like my father's, would lodge in Marley's spine, paralyzing him. Drew never spoke his fear specifically. I'm not sure if he could allow himself to think about any possibility other than remission and survival.

I guess I knew Marley was not going to survive this disease miraculously. I had to face the facts, and pray hard for mini miracles so we could enjoy the time we had left to love and be loved by him. At this point, I called all the local funeral homes and requested their brochures. I didn't tell anyone but my co-workers what I had done. They thought I was being a bit dramatic, and didn't understand why I was reacting this way. My father had always advised, "If you're prepared for the worst with the right tools, you probably won't need them." It was my ritual for hoping I wouldn't need this info any time soon. If I did, I figured the last thing I would want to be doing is getting quotes from funeral parlors. I just glanced at the brochures and filed them away.

Another thing I kept under my hat was a choice I had to make while visiting the corporate headquarters in San Diego. The CEO was a part of Marley's Network from the beginning, and seemed to be working quietly behind the scenes doing what he could to make my life as easy as possible. When I sat down with the woman in Human Resources, she asked me if I wanted to add a life insurance policy for my children to my contract.

My expression must have been one of horror, because the woman quickly calmed me down, saying, "Look, Jennifer, we highly suggest you do this. The policy doesn't have any pre-existing health requirements, and it will only cost you 25 cents each month. It won't provide a lot of money, but it will surely cover all the funeral expenses." My stomach was in knots—I felt strangely guilty—but all I could say was, "Thank you, I'll take it."

Thursday, September 21, 2000
Subject: "NEWS AND OTHER ILLUSIONS"

• From: Selene

Hello everyone,

Yes, I'm still here. I apologize for waiting so long to articulate current happenings. You could say there hasn't been much to say, but as our lives are continually in flux, there is really always something to say, and yet, why say it when it will all change so quickly?

This thought brings me to one of the greatest gifts Marley has given me: Live the moment. It sounds very New Age, very Buddhist, very…well, I've heard it a lot, anyway. But it takes on new meaning when there is a life hanging in the balance. Some of you may have noticed—you can call Marley in the hospital, perhaps five minutes after he has thrown up everything he has ever attempted to eat—ask him how he's doing and he'll tell you, "Pretty good." It may lead one to believe he isn't telling the truth. However, I have come to understand that his reply corresponds to the exact moment the question is asked, so if he has stopped throwing up and has been able to watch some serious monster truck action on T.V., then he really *is* feeling good.

Sometimes Marley makes fun of me for being a wimp. He'll want to take me on his bike down Mt. Everest or something equally as treacherous, and if I'm reluctant, he'll look at me like I'm crazy. And you know what? I probably am. He's really telling me to follow my bliss (to borrow another New Age-y phrase). Okay, so maybe death-defying feats aren't exactly my bliss, but you get the idea.

The other day he was trying to explain to me why stunts just aren't worth it if they aren't risky. He lives on the edge. You could say he is Prince in the Kingdom of Edge. That's where it's real. That's where you see how precious every moment is. He sees moments flying past…moments he is too tired to go play, moments Jennifer has to work and can't hang out, moments wasted in a sterilized building where everyone keeps asking him how he's feeling…and he gets pissed. I would too.

Radiation started today. Pray for the safety of his body. Pray he continues to build up strength.

Catie started school full time and seems to be enjoying it for the most part. She is astoundingly beautiful and intelligent. She takes my breath away on a regular basis. And after only a few times practicing, she is on her way to a beautiful jump shot.

Jennifer works her butt off trying to get the new *Uncle John's Bathroom Reader* out on time. She is brilliant at pretty much everything she does, I've noticed.

Besides being clearly overwhelmed by my love for this family, I am preparing to go away for a month. I have a job painting murals at a spiritual retreat and alternative education facility just outside Ojai, California. My first paid art job. You can send some prayers my way too if you feel so inclined. I'm a little petrified.

Have a blessed Autumnal Equinox, everyone.
With love,
Selene

"Courage is being scared to death and saddling up anyway."

—John Wayne

Chapter Seven:

Kneeds

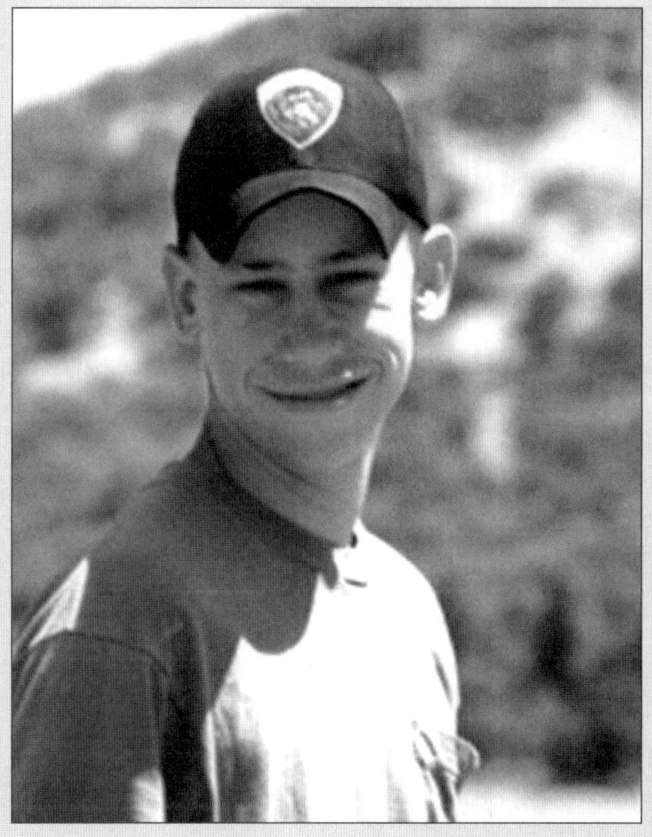

"When in doubt; smile."

Photo: Jennifer

Wednesday, October 26, 2000
Subject: "CATCH UP"

Dearest Marley Network,

I know it's been a long time since you've heard from me. I'm sorry. I'll try to fill you in on the last two months of living.

The Bright Side

We returned from Boston just as school began. Marley's first round of radiation was scheduled during the first weeks of school. We scrapped planning anything resembling a normal class schedule. Can you hear Marley complain? Yeah, right! The poor baby gets to hang out with me at work.

The BRI office has a bedroom upstairs, outfitted with an entertainment center so he overdoses on MTV2, which is okay, 'cause neither Drew nor I have television reception. His room at the office is also set up with the remote controlled train that JD sent while we were in Boston. He's not stuck indoors, though—the BRI is across the street from a cool park. He's a happy camper on an endless summer vacation.

He has healed incredibly fast since the two surgeries in Boston. His arm doesn't bother him much—he says the skin feels like it's been stretched too tight. At the top of his tricep, there's a big indent and a three-inch scar. He loves the way it accentuates his muscles when he flexes. I have to giggle, as he spends a lot of time admiring his new scars.

The Dark Side

If this period in my life is a test from the powers that be, I can say I'm surviving—maybe even thriving—although I can honestly say I've never felt so on the edge of sanity for such an extended period. The waves keep coming and they keep getting bigger. I'm getting used to being pounded and scraped across the sharp edges of the reef. It seems my life is a choice between the painful journey to the beach or continuing to swim among the sharks; so I'm working on growing gills while mastering the fine art of dog paddling.

Meanwhile, I started the annual deadline crunch, getting the newest edition of the *Bathroom Reader* produced. Even though we were working 15 to 20-hour days, we weren't able to finish before the kids came back to me. That first week was easily the most difficult of my entire life. Up at 7 A.M., drive 20 minutes to town, drop Catie at school, and race to meet whoever had volunteered to drive Marley to radiation therapy. I'd grab some coffee and head to work. Sometimes I'd even have time to look up when Marley was delivered back to the office.

One of the last nights before the deadline, Eric came to stay with the kids because I had to go back to town. After trying to explain why I was continuing this insanity, I kissed Marley and turned his light out. Just as I was leaving, he said, "Mom? Just one moor thing." I went back and sat by him in the dark. In a very serious, quiet voice, he pulled me close and asked, "Ma, how would you feel if I died tonight?" Gulp!

Considering there was an invisible knife slicing my heart, I believe I handled it well. I calmly said, "If I thought you were going to die anytime soon, I wouldn't leave." I gave him another kiss and left. I sobbed all the way down the mountain. Hell! With this frantic schedule, *I* was the one at risk of dying!

As payment for putting my kids through this, I've promised them a vacation. It will be the first time just the three of us have gone anywhere special since Drew and I split up in '93. Marley says he wants warm ocean waters.

Marley and Catie are back with Drew now. The finished manuscript was sent to the printer last week. Halloween is just around the corner. Selene's coming home just in time for Ashland's city-wide Halloween party. And radiation ends on

November 7th. After that, maybe life will feel a little less stressed. I can't tell you how much I look forward to spitting firewood, patching my roof, doing laundry, cooking real food, and firing up the generator to watch movies. H-o-m-e!!!!!!!

(Note: "spitting firewood" was the best of many typos in the original Update Letters. Jay loved it, so I promised not to edit the mistake.)

Current Physical Status

Marley has lost weight—he's now at 145 lbs. That's ten pounds less than his pre-surgery weight. He's thin and tall (6'1"). This will change once he's more active and his muscles rebuild. Parts of his torso are numb from where nerves have been temporarily damaged—he says it feels really weird. He's doing great with one lung. He says he doesn't notice any real difference. He gets short of breath occasionally but seems to take it in stride. Marley knows that John Wayne spent most of his career with one lung, and figures if the Duke did it, so can he!

The Radiation Procedure

As radiation approached, Marley battled some major fears. Go figure! Radiation started while Marley and Catie were on Drew's two-week shift. After the first zapping experience, Mars Bar called me and said, "It's just like a giant X-way, Mom...but even coola! It didn't hert one littul bit." Each radiation dose takes only ten minutes to administer, but he has to go in five days a week for six weeks.

He has several temporary tattoos on his body—Xs mark the spots. These targets are on the sides and top of his chest, and where the tumor was removed from his arm. Therapy consists of lying shirtless on a long padded table, holding a foam ring with his arms above his head. A laser beam comes from holes in either wall and from the machine above. Using remote control, the technicians adjust the bed and the machine until the lasers line up exactly with the Xs. Everyone evacuates the room and he's in there with this giant machine that makes funny clunking noises. There's a camera in the room so he can be watched at all times. After they're done nuking his chest, via remote, the machine rotates around to aim at his arm.

This "therapy" is not aimed at killing existing cancer, which hopefully has been surgically removed. It's used to prevent cells in his chest from becoming cancerous. They have done their best to aim the radiation so it won't affect his heart or the remaining lung. Developing a secondary, non-related cancer is the biggest risk. The doctor's theory is that if that does occur, it would take many years for the secondary cancer to show up. "Many years" are odds we're betting on.

Alternatives

I've found Marley's limits when it comes to alternative healing. Meditation is a no-go, as is any major dietary change. "I ain't givin' up bacon, Mom, you should know that!" Noni juice, from Tahiti, which has dramatically helped two other friends of mine, was written off "'cause it smells like shit." Even the wonderful "space syrup" was rudely ignored. He doesn't want to go to an acupuncturist. He calls them "witch-doctors," and "Voo Doo needle pokers." He's 15, what can I say? He calls these things "hocus-pocus" and "hogwash." He says he doesn't need it 'cause he'll be just fine.

Marley will, however, accept massage, energy work, and vitamins (provided they're in pill form). He said he'll even try a *cranial sacral* adjustment (manipulating the plates of the skull). He also believes it's helpful when people pray for him. "The moor, the merrweya!" He loves inspecting the pebbles, carvings, and gems you've already sent. He ceremoniously takes them all out of the overflowing bowl and arranges them around him and retells the stories behind them. That's his meditation.

I love you beyond the beyond,
Jennifer

THE MOMENT OF TRUTH

Life in Balance

There's a constant dance between life and death. I don't know when death will pull me into the unknown, but I hope I know prior to the visit so I can prepare. Maybe death always lets us know beforehand. If only I could ask those that have died instantly if they had any warning—any time, even briefly—to prepare for departure.

If you were to ask me when I first accepted Marley's mortality, I'd have to say it was when he was about six months old. Other than the little polyp on his ear (his supersonic hearing device), there was nothing unusual about this child. Like other toddlers, he wasn't walking or talking yet—everything seemed normal on the outside, but I could just sense he didn't belong here. He was either extremely happy or extremely miserable. My only other clue was how he slept. It was like my baby boy went into a coma every night. Wherever one goes when one is asleep, he went very far away indeed. Every night as I put him to sleep, I wondered if he would still be with us in the morning. I started saying good-bye to him then. That never changed.

I knew Marley was a survivor—for some purpose, every morning for fifteen years he had woken up to live another day. He was also stubborn. He had a battle to fight and everyone was watching him. He wanted to break records, and if it couldn't be done riding his bikes, surviving cancer would do. I knew while he lived he would live well, but I also knew he didn't have long. Although invisible to the eyes of Western medicine, I knew the cancer was spreading throughout his body.

When we returned home from the last trip to Boston, there was a subtle shift in the way I started focusing my energy. I began to live a schizophrenic life, trying to find a healthy balance between many worlds. I worked harder than ever, knowing that soon I would have to take a sabbatical to care for Marley. My goal became to collect as much overtime, sick days, and vacation time as humanly possible. At the same time, I wanted to spend as much quality time with my children as possible. As a parent, I tried to find the balance between tough love and spoiling them. When the kids weren't with me, I played hard. I danced until the music stopped, went to concerts, hosted parties, and dressed with flair. I was learning how to live fully in the present while planning for the future.

"We want to live in the present, and the only history that is worth a tinker's damn is the history we make today."

—Henry Ford

Life Is a Blank Slate

I had the mind-bending task of making sure Marley got the education he would need if he ended up winning his battle. I supported his dreams of the future, helping him plan the steps to make them manifest, never fully trusting that he would have the time to walk his talk.

Marley's Western Rest Home was the perfect example. It was a brilliant idea. He needed to raise funds to buy the property. He knew it would take years, but he started anyway. I deposited money in his piggy bank every time I could. I helped him draw the floor plans, and we talked about buying land in the Colestin Valley. Sitting on our front porch, we would watch the goats play in the yard as we talked about the realities of his rest home idea. I had to plan as though it would happen, while imagining what it would be like to move the sofa after his death and find one of his dirty socks or a missing remote control truck.

In order to do anything in this world, we have to plan ahead —and yet, from one minute to the next, I had no clue whether Marley's health would allow us to do anything. Planning life around Marley's cancer was really no different than before; the odds were simply tipped in the cancer's favor. Buying plane tickets for a vacation is a great example. The reality is, any time any one of us buys a ticket, there's no guarantee that we'll actually get on that plane.

I was living in a world that required plans, yet I was painfully aware that I could no longer assume anything. I was living in a world of limbo. It dawned on me that I could die before Marley. All it would take is a tire blowing out on the steep, winding road I traveled daily. Or, while all focus was on Marley, Catie could be munched by one of the cougars that live in our woods.

I stopped assuming anything, and started living as though the painting I was creating was a blank canvas and the paint was invisible. With every new stroke of brilliant color, I was again starting with a clean slate. For the first time in my life I felt free.

Hello, Good-bye

I started to understand how Marley could be so brave—he had nothing to lose. I watched him greet people like he hadn't seen them in forever. If you were to bump into him on the street, he was genuinely gleeful that he had a chance to hug you again. It wasn't like he just smiled and gave a polite hug. When he saw a friend half a block away, he'd yell their name and quicken his pace, stretching his arms wide for a bone-crunching embrace. Saying good-bye, he was likely to give a hug that lasted longer than average, and then he'd purposely do something annoying so you wouldn't forget him. A poke in the ribs would do, or if his hug hadn't already knocked off your hat and mussed your hair, he'd take care of that. Maybe Marley knew how to live in the now all along and I just hadn't recognized it.

My favorite example: Whenever Selene was due to arrive, Marley would hop on his bike and ride to where our dirt road met the pavement. He would just sit there, sometimes for more than an hour, and wait. Can you imagine how loved that made her feel?

One time, the evening before she planned to depart, I watched him sneak off in the darkness to where he'd stashed his rope collection. He returned with a superior grin plastered to his face. The following morning, I laughed when I looked out the kitchen window to see Selene standing in the driveway, scratching her head, trying to figure out how she was going to get in her car. Marley stood next to me puffed with pride at a plan well executed. He had wrapped her little car with yards of rope, making sure she couldn't open the doors. Marley never made it easy for Selene to leave.

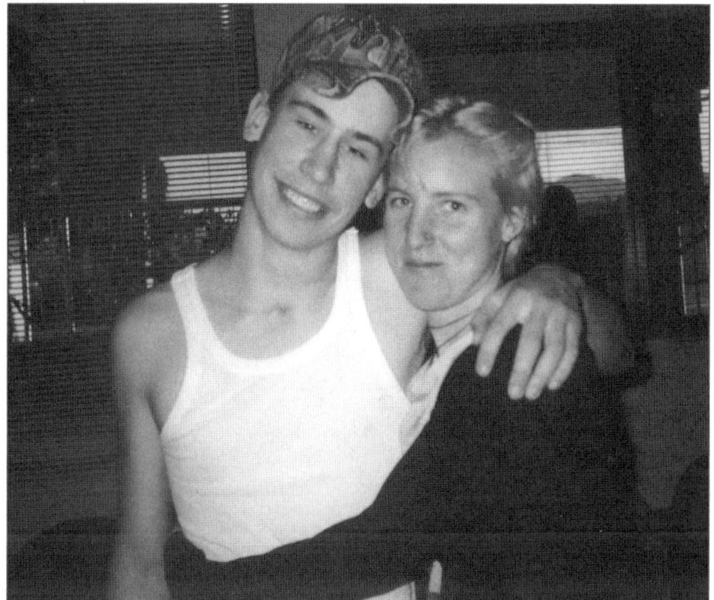

Marley and Selene just before a radiation treatment.

Photo: Nina Davis

As soon as I caught on to the benefits of living in the moment, I took Marley's lead and started driving my friends crazy. They'd say, "See ya later!" and then groan when I'd respond, "Maybe." Instead of simply saying, "Good-bye," I started saying, "If I never see you again, it's been an honor. I love you." It didn't take any additional effort, but it sure did make parting a little more mindful.

"A man should not leave this earth with unfinished business. He should live each day as if it was a pre-flight check. He should ask each morning, am I prepared to lift-off?"

—Diane Frolov
Northern Exposure, All is Vanity

Friday, November 18, 2000
Subject: "A BRAVE NEW MARLEY"

• From: Selene

Hello bright shining lights of compassion, support, and general wonderfulness! It is my pleasure to greet you again, with GOOD news.

I came back from my month away, and it feels as though I have come home. I underestimated how deeply I had dug my heels in during this whole soul journey.

I was in the post office my second day back, and I heard from behind me what could only be the voice of my dear beloved Marley Man. He called my name with an excitement in his voice that made my heart swell. He then proceeded to give me the best hug possible. Yummy.

He looks great! Really great! Who knows what lies ahead of us, but I for one am basking in this glorious respite. Today was his last day of radiation, which has prompted much celebrating on his part. I said, "It's all over!" But he reminded me he has to get PET scans every few months, just in case. He's a realist. A realist who has been through the wringer and come out with a huge smile on his face and the light of a thousand Egyptian suns.

Catie seems to be doing really well too. She's as intelligent and gorgeous as ever, and she's started playing the violin. Jennifer has a nasty cold, but I can feel that she has expanded a bit to let in the comforts of winter nesting and the blessing of having more time.

I love you all.
Thank you for everything,
Selene

THE EFFECTIVENESS OF PRAYER

Semantics

When I was writing to Marley's Network, I went round and round about what terms to use. Some of my most beloved people had an aversion to the word "pray." That little word is loaded with meaning. To be honest, I couldn't find a way around using it without risking the effectiveness of the group's power. The only other phrase that came close was "wish for…" but it somehow fell short of my intended goal.

If I asked you to "think about" me, you might see me with your mind's eye. If I asked you to "focus on" me, you might recall memories of our past experiences together or, if we didn't know each other, you might try to imagine who I am. But if I ask you to "pray for" me, you would probably think about me and focus on creating something specific on my behalf. The difference is subtle, yet immense.

Although the word "pray" is used prolifically in all religions, according to the dictionary, it has nothing to do with the dogmatic practices of any belief; it simply means to ask for something, from someone, with an intent in mind.

When I've asked people, "What's the first thing you think of when I say the word 'pray'?'" most responded with statements like; "God," "Putting your hands together," "Kneeling," "Religion," or "I don't like that word." It also appeared that people with a strong belief system were comfortable with the word, while others seemed to almost recoil when the word was spoken.

> ***Definition***
>
> **Pray:**
>
> • To ask very earnestly;
> • To make supplication;
> • To beseech;
> • To entreat;
> • To implore;
> • In law, to call in aid one who has an interest in the cause.

I'm a Believer...

Dr. Mitchell Krucoff, a cardiologist at Duke University Medical Center, states the reason for his interest in the healing power of prayer and the benefits he has witnessed from touch therapy, music, and guided imagery.

> "The first time you see a nontraditional practitioner take away chest pain, or put a patient in agony to rest, or interrupt a heart attack without adding another drug or device at the bedside, you say, 'Nice coincidence.' The second time, you say, 'This is interesting.' By the third time, you say, 'We need to study this.'"

Dr. Krucoff's experiences prompted him to study the effects of these interventions on his patients. He's not alone. Many professionals are attempting to scientifically prove the effectiveness of prayer (also called *distance healing*, *remote mental influence*, *subtle energy healing*, and *intercessory prayer*). Creating accurate tests has been a challenge, because there are so many variables.

In many cases, the prayors and the prayees are not known to each other, and these tests are sometimes done without the person's knowledge. In one study, eight prayer groups from different faiths, in different countries, prayed according to their customs for the patients assigned to them, knowing only the patients' names and ages and the fact that they were slated for cardiac procedures.

> "Adverse outcomes in the prayer group were 50% to 100% fewer than in the standard therapy group," says Dr. Krucoff. "In the patients who received any of the noetic therapies, including prayer, we found a 30% reduction for every adverse outcome we measured. The therapeutic effect was substantial enough for us to design a definitive trial to confirm the finding."

Thousands of case studies exist, showing consistent results and yet, conclusive results have not been reported.

Tuesday, November 22, 2000
Subject: "GIVING THANKS"

WHAT DO WE HAVE TO BE THANKFUL FOR?

I have you to be thankful for!

My son is alive and kicking and I have a beautiful, healthy daughter.

A very few months ago, I had the impression that Marley was up against a wall that wouldn't budge. Hmmm. Guess what? It budged.

Why? That's the odd thing about prayer and magic. It can't be proven. Too many variables.

Ten years ago, I ruptured a disk. I spent ten months in physical therapy, getting shots of cortisone into my spine, and having acupressure, acupuncture, and vitamin infusions. Blah, blah, blah—nothing helped. I was told my only option was an operation designed to fuse the disks together. I had worked very hard at healing. I felt tired and defeated. I had never been a patient in a hospital. I hated hospitals, but reluctantly agreed to this last resort and scheduled the procedure.

Two days before the surgery, I panicked. I cancelled the operation and called my travel agent. I was booked on the next available flight to Maui. Leaving my six-year-old son and baby girl with their dear old dad, I fled for two weeks. I found a secluded spot and began an eight-day solo while fasting. Armed with a gallon of water per day, I prayed continuously.

My life changed dramatically. I returned with no pain. My back was healed. Pregnant pause....Can I prove that it was the quest? The fasting? The sleeping on the ground? The water? The prayer? One or all of the above? Will the medical profession record it? I don't think so. Do I know it to be true?

Definitely. I could once again pick up my 18-month-old child without crying in pain!

Prayer (or whatever you want to call it) makes a difference. I know it. I hope you know it.

Marley roams this planet like any other 15-year-old (except for some amazing scars). I can honestly say, no human would have come through the traumas he has experienced, with so few side effects, without the amount of support he has had. How can I express my joy and thanks? By sending you gobs of love.

Please, pat yourselves on the back for a job well done. I am thankful you exist. Marley's whole perspective of life is based on surviving the worst-case scenario and knowing he isn't doing it alone. Can you imagine the feeling we'll all have if he lives long enough to graduate from high school or to have children of his own? Regardless of how much time he has left, you can take credit for every breath this boy takes.

We can't afford to slack off yet, but I wanted you to know how I feel. I want to REALLY thank you for praying. IT MAKES A DIFFERENCE. Please continue. Pray for Marley and pray for yourselves. If you have a little extra, pray for me.

I'll be praying for you.
Happy Thanksgiving,
Jennifer

P.S.
If you know someone who's in trouble, let them know what this circle has done for Marley.

"The force will be with you, always."

—Obi-Wan Kenobi
(Alec Guinness), *Star Wars*

THE BRIGHT SIDE OF SAD

Stress Relief

The holiday season of 2000 was a trifle more stressful than normal. Just after Thanksgiving, Marley started complaining that his knee hurt. On the 27th, we took him in for some X-rays. Nothing really impressive showed up. He had wiped out on his bike a few weeks before, but Marley knew that wasn't the cause of the problem. We took him back to our family doctor and asked him to investigate further. Five days before Christmas, we had an MRI and a bone scan done. Sure enough, something didn't look right. We were referred to an oncologist in Portland, and made arrangements to travel north just after New Year's.

At work, we were experiencing record sales. My work load was insane. Fortunately, the corporate gods were pleased with their acquisition of the BRI, so I was allowed to hire on new hands. One of the reasons our little team worked so well was because I hired all of my best friends. In addition to Jeff, Jay, and Jennifer S., I now added Eric and Selene to the team. This made my life much easier and kept Selene as close as possible. I would have died a miserable death without her help, especially through the chemotherapy. I was also allowed to hire an assistant to be my right hand. I asked my favorite waitress, Dylan, and she agreed. She was delightful, and her presence made it possible for me to manage the BRI from a distance. It didn't look like life was going to slow down, but at least there were more hands on deck.

The BRI office was a two-story, renovated schoolhouse, originally built in the late 1800's. It had narrow halls, a very steep staircase, and low doorjambs that Marley had to duck under as he passed through (especially when he was wearing his cowboy hat). Just before Christmas vacation, the pain in Marley's knee had increased to the point that he had to crawl up the stairs to his room. When he slipped once coming down, catching himself with the rail, I moved him downstairs to a room off the kitchen. Now all he had to do was knock on the wall and one of us would go check on him.

For most of that first year, Marley had been at the office, recuperating from pneumonia, two major surgeries, two minor surgeries, chemo, and radiation. I had divided my time between his needs and running the BRI. Whenever I couldn't attend to him, someone else in the office filled my shoes. As bad as my situation was, it couldn't have been a better set-up.

I felt blessed that I had a career that was demanding, yet forgiving of my personal situation. Although I adored my job, I would have quit in a heartbeat if we didn't need the continued insurance. I had never had health insurance before, and now our lives depended on it. Why was I given insurance as a gift a month before Marley got sick? Doesn't that make you wonder how this thing we call reality works? In mid-December, I tallied all the medical costs of the first year. Drew and I had each paid $1,200 to cover the deductible, and the insurance company was paying 100% of the balance. They had covered just over $750,000 in nine months, and it was already looking like 2001 was going to be another expensive year. Even though I couldn't quit, at least I was stuck with a great job and a great insurance policy. Was this luck? Karma? Fate? The will of some expansive creator? Who knows?

"There are no maps; no more creeds or philosophies. From here on in, the directions come straight from the Universe."

—Akshara Noor

Creating Reality

This may sound silly to some of you; but I think we have a lot of control over the events that happen in our lives. I grew up with the phrase, "We create our own reality," and believe this to be true. I really don't want to sound like a New Age kook, but it's a concept I've been exploring since I was a kid. I also believe there's a high-level energy that helps us manifest our desires (a lot of people call this energy "God"). Up until Marley got cancer, I had always felt blessed and figured I had done a pretty decent job of creation. I viewed even the less desirable events of my life as growth opportunities and, if I was patient, everything made sense.

When Marley was a toddler, I pondered my role in creating an "alter-abled" child—one who didn't seem to want to talk or simply to live on planet Earth. Now, at this particular stage in my life, I was again spending a lot of time in confusion. In the privacy of my own thoughts, I wracked my brain for reasons why I had a son with cancer. Not just any old cancer—lung cancer—the kind reserved for old smokers and factory workers. Why him? Why not me? Did I have anything to do with this creation? Or was this Marley's creation? Was I just along for the ride? Why? Did we have some sort of cosmic agreement before he was born? I couldn't help asking some pretty far-out questions.

I realize I can spend the rest of my life questioning the unanswerable. Maybe making up answers—believing there's a reason. Is it a justification or just a way to pacify my aching heart? I'm praying hard that when I die, it will all be clear. Hopefully I'll get my answers and not a whole new set of questions. Maybe I'll never know. Bottom line, it doesn't matter. I thank my lucky stars that I was surrounded by incredible people, that I had health insurance, and that Marley had entered my life.

"I wanted a perfect ending.
Now I've learned, the hard way,
that some poems don't rhyme,
and some stories don't have a clear
beginning, middle, and end.
Life is about not knowing,
having to change,
taking the moment
and making the best of it,
without knowing
what's going to happen next.
Delicious Ambiguity."

—Gilda Radner

CHRISTMAS CHEER

Holy Days

It had been an intense year, and it was coming to a close. The time off from work for the holidays was a blessing. I spent Thanksgiving with my children. Cooking meals to warm the soul during the cold winter season always fed my being. The wood stove was continually tended, so the house was warm and cozy. Pots of melting wax warmed on the wood stove, ready for passers-by to dip candles. Making candles from recycled wax was a winter ritual that doubled as a meditation. It was a constant reminder of the cycles of life, that nothing ever stays whole if it is being used well.

The rewards of working hard were great. Tending to the ever-increasing special needs of Marley was a lesson of expanding. It was obvious; I needed to get bigger, better, and more efficient if I wanted to survive. After tucking the kids into bed, I would stand by the stove, dipping, dipping, dipping strings into wax. I knew it was all worth it. It just felt healthy. Even though my eldest was dying, he was healthy. We were all well loved: by our selves, by each other, and by others.

> ***"The most important work you and I will ever do will be within the walls of our own homes."***
>
> **—Harold B. Lee**

I know how easy it is to lose love, to just watch it slip away. Like tending a wood stove. If I wanted our hearts to stay warm, I had to tend our emotional needs with the same vigilance as I tended our physical needs. The responsibility made me want to crawl in a hole sometimes—to just leave. Going numb and cold-hearted seemed so much easier. The advent of the holidays was helpful—but not enough to fully recharge my life battery. I was secretly worried about me. How much more of this could I take? I had to be mindful about taking care of myself. I knew if, for instance, I threw my back out, we'd all be in serious trouble.

I was a single mom, and during the winter months, my chores at home increased as the temperatures decreased. It often felt like I couldn't chop wood fast enough. Marley was always hungry. I never felt like I could righteously just sit down and take a break. It was impossible to relax in the tub without feeling like I was neglecting something or someone. The only wheel that didn't squeak was Catie. That was the wheel I knew I needed to tend to the most, or I risked losing her to some far-off internal world. Somehow I managed to juggle all the balls and keep most of them in the air.

Stuffed with Excitement

In preparation for Christmas, I usually started making gifts in October, just after the deadline crunch was over at work. This year was no different. I wanted our lives to feel normal and intact. It may have added more to the season's stress, but it also provided energy for my personal power system. It was possible this could be the last Christmas that Marley would be with us, so I was compelled to make sure it was a good one. I made blankets for both kids. With every stitch, I sewed in sweet thoughts and lots of love. This process was healing for me. I could sit down, yet I was still feeding my family's needs. This was how I spent my time whenever the kids were at Drew's.

There was also shopping that had to be done which, normally, I hate due to my opinions about consumerism. But this year, it wasn't so bad. I actually enjoyed it. I used Christmas as my excuse to make sure Marley had cool stuff to occupy himself with while he was healing. I also wanted Catie to feel extra-special by having even more packages than Marley. Doing this for Catie was hard—she had a particular style and was picky about what she wanted. Marley didn't care, and was incredibly easy to please. Giving him gifts was always so much fun because he loved everything. My task each year was to see if I could make him actually cry tears of joy. That always made Christmas something to look forward to.

This year, I had a special trick up my sleeve. I had promised the kids a trip if we all survived the last *Bathroom Reader* deadline.

Because our new CEO was pleased with our performance, we were all awarded well-deserved bonuses. I knew just how to use mine—it was vacation time.

I called Kim, our next-door neighbor and travel agent. She booked us flights to Maui, scheduled so we could spend my January birthday being rejuvenated by sunshine. Yeehaw! I saw a light at the end of my tunnel as I imagined waves endlessly kissing the beach. They were e-tickets, but Kim made them look official and included fancy luggage tags. This was hopefully going to be the gift to make Marley cry. I was excited when I popped the envelopes in their stockings on Christmas Eve. I could barely sleep that night.

Our ritual has always been; when the kids got up on Christmas morning, they could open their stockings without me. This year, my best friend Andrea, who had flown in to be with us, helped me play Santa. Christmas morning, we lay in bed and giggled when we heard Catie climb down from the loft, unhook the stockings, and pad into Marley's room. It's a small house, and we could hear every move and crinkle of paper. Within seconds we had two screaming kids jumping into bed with us, smothering us with kisses and hugs. Marley was too excited to cry. Damn!

Later that day, after the gang arrived, he did end up crying from joy: Wrapped in his new blanket, he opened the box containing his giant new remote-controlled dump truck. Later he almost cried from depression when he opened the gag gift Jay brought him: a game called Operation. The rest of us laughed, but he thought destroying it would be much more fun than playing it. None of us could argue with his logic.

"If you can give your son or daughter only one gift, let it be enthusiasm."

—Bruce Barton

Sunday, December 31, 2000
Subject: "A NEW YEAR BEGINS"

Hi Gang,

Don't have a lot of time; I'm trying to do way too much in way too little time. Some of you are probably saying, "So… what else is new?" But this is serious. I'm topping my own record!

The results of the last MRI indicate Marley's knee is hurting due to a tumor in the bone. 2001 starts with a trip to Portland with Marley, Catie, Drew, and Selene to have a biopsy done to find out exactly what the pictures are showing. Tomorrow morning we drive six hours north, doing our best to avoid people suffering from their first hangovers of the new year.

We have a doctor's appointment on Tuesday morning, and hopefully we'll have time to play that afternoon. Wednesday they do exploratory surgery on his knee to take out a piece of bone to study. He'll probably have to stay in the hospital that night, and hopefully we'll be back on the road by Thursday, January 4th. If I keep it together and do my job, this might end up being an uplifting journey rather than a drag. Catie's thrilled she finally gets to be a part of the action. The plan is to visit friends and go to museums and such.

We're at the BRI office, and spirits are pretty high on the eve of change. Marley's just gone out to "play" basketball with friends. (He just sits on the sidelines, but it makes him happy to be around his friends.) Catie's playing accountant in the freight room while I pack in as much work as possible.

I love you all and thank you so much. For each and every one of us, may this new year be filled with wondrous events and hearts filled to the popping point with love and joy.

Happy New Year!
Jennifer

The Butterfly Effect

WHO CARES?: Thoughts on Marley's Existence and the Impact it has had on my Life.

by Liz Stahlman

I have learned so much from so many, and Marley has been just one of my teachers, no more or less significant than any other, but definitely unique. Marley was not "normal." He talked different, he looked a little different, and he knew different. I'm sure others can more sufficiently explain the fifteen-year-old who couldn't read, but could make almost anyone believe his tall tales—tales taller than Paul Bunyan—which I'm still not sure were untruths or even exaggerations.

Though truly special in many ways, the aspect of Marley that I most admired was that he made being different no big deal. In a world where supermodels have low self-esteem, Marley—a lanky young man who, when he introduced himself to people they often thought he said his name was "Molly"—never seemed out of place, self-conscious, or embarrassed. Whether at the coffee shop with his mom's peers, at school among his own, or among the sterile halls and sterile professionals at the many hospitals he visited, Marley was always Marley. No false fronts, no apparent insecurities. He just was who he was.

The first time I met Marley was New Year's Eve of 2000 at Jay and Jeff's house. He was fourteen then, just two months before the cancer showed up. He must have been six feet tall at least, but there he was, sitting on his mother's lap in a comfy chair in the main party room. I found it odd, and I felt awkward at first, seeing a teenage boy sitting on his mother's lap at a drinking party. Until I took a good long look at the two of them and realized that neither of them seemed the slightest bit uncomfortable, nor were they feigning affection or unhealthily attached. They were just "hanging out," enjoying each other's company.

Oh, for life to be so easy...can you imagine, being a teenager at a party, and sitting on your mother's lap? But what would people think? Would they feel you were being immature? Or would people think your mother was too permissive or overbearing? I can tell you what Marley would say to such questions: "Who cares." I think he said that to me—an insecure, awkward, twenty-something—more than once. And slowly, ever so slowly, it has been sinking in. My insecurities and self doubts melt away one by one, year by year, as I realize the truth that Marley's life taught me: It's not so much that life is short, but that my life is mine, and to waste it away worrying about what others might think makes no sense at all.

"Just because 'they' don't tell you that you can... doesn't mean you can't!"

—Marley Jacob Pratt (age 17)

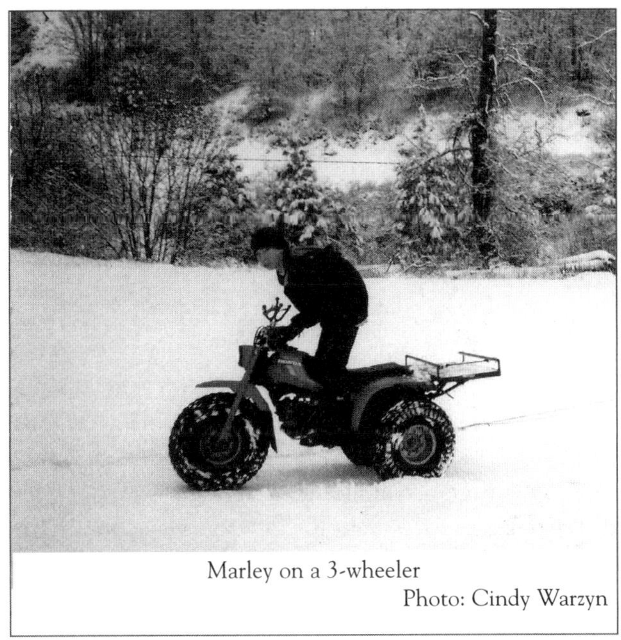

Marley on a 3-wheeler

Photo: Cindy Warzyn

Friday, January 5, 2001
Subject: "DAY BY DAY"

Hi, people who love Marley,

The Portland adventure leaves me with many life questions. I'm confused, yet in awe of how life seems to work. I thought it would get simpler with added years of experience…but no! I seem to know less and question more as time goes by.

RECAP

Monday, January 1st

We traveled to Portland in a mini convoy with two identical little blue Honda "bubble" cars. Marley was in one with Drew at the wheel while Catie and I were in the other with Selene in control. There was an air of excitement upon departure; it almost felt like we were taking a vacation. Our car was filled with the sounds of *Harry Potter* on tape. (Selene and I are obsessed with the series.)

The Ronald McDonald House in Portland pales in comparison to Boston's in terms of charm, technology, and friendliness. But it's literally within spitting distance of the hospital. The medical attention and skill at the Portland hospital is also less than Boston's. All in all, the care was adequate. Drew and I now seem to know the standard operating procedure pretty well. (No pun intended!)

Liz, who had recently moved to Portland, invited us all to her house for a big dinner the first night we arrived. Her brother Eric and Jennifer S. were also in Portland for a music festival, so we all ate heaping mounds of spaghetti and swapped tall tales. Drew and the kids went back to the Ronald McDonald House, to our tiny little room with one queen bed and a roll-away cot. Selene and I opted to sleep at Liz's that night.

Tuesday, January 2nd

We all joined together for an early morning appointment with the Pediatric Orthopedic Surgeon. Our doctor was a grey-haired old fella who shuffled into the room. His age and a few things he said made Drew and me a little nervous, although he came highly recommended. Trust. We were scheduled to have an "open biopsy" done the following morning. We were told a three-inch incision would be made in his knee to see how extensive the damage was.

After an appointment with the anesthesiologist, the rest of the day was ours. We went to the Omni Max theatre (a five-story dome) that was showing "Whales" in surround-vision-and-sound. I got lost in the science bookstore while Marley entertained himself speeding around in the museum's wheelchair. Catie investigated EVERYTHING while Drew and Selene did a good job of simply staying upright.

We ate dinner at a nice Thai restaurant and then went back to the RMcD House to watch dumb movies. There was no way any of us were going to be separated, even if it meant sleeping on the floor sardine style. Marley was antsy that night; his knee hurt and he was scared about the surgery. Finally sleep took control. We woke up bright and early, ready to roll.

Wednesday, January 3rd

Selene and Catie explored the "big city" together while Drew and I talked to the surgeon before the operation. The conversation helped put us both at ease. We agreed this guy was on top of it and would make some good decisions while he was exploring the inside of Marley's knee. Drew and I laughed out loud as Marley was injected with morphine. He did his "Wow, this is Coooooool" routine while trying to track his hand waving goodbye to us as his gurney was wheeled to the operating room.

Two hours later, the doctor sat down with us in the waiting

room while Marley headed for the recovery room. He said there was no question: The tumor was squamous (the same type of cancer cell that was in his lung, lymph, and arm). So the surgeon decided to scrape out the mass while he was in there. He said the places where the cancer had attacked the bone were the consistency of mushy oatmeal. After getting as much mush out as possible, he stitched Marley up and wrapped his leg in a removable blue velcro cast.

The femur is the bone that goes from the hip to the knee. At the knee the femur forms two balls. The interior of one of these balls is now hollow like a bird's skeleton. The risk is that Marley could easily break that extremely fragile bone. Now decisions need to be made, as quickly as possible.

The Portland surgeon outlined two options; amputate from just above the knee or do a full knee replacement. Arrrgh! Under the circumstances, the most logical choice is the prosthesis. This means we'll return to Portland in one or two weeks to replace as much of the knee as we have to.

Thursday, January 4th

Catie, Selene, and Drew slept at the Ronald McDonald House while I stayed with Mars in the hospital. Compared to the surgeries we've already been through, this was a minor one. We wanted to make this a quick trip and avoid any extra time at the hospital. We had learned from the past that we should get Marley off the morphine immediately to avoid the vomiting routine. It was a very long night. He didn't throw up too much, but he did have to deal with the pain. He agreed that getting out of the evil clutches of the nurses was worth it.

As soon as we could, we fled from the hospital like we were escaping from a mental ward. This was no easy trick. We had to wait until the physical therapist came to teach Marley to walk with crutches. He had no problem, even with stairs, and only ended up frustrated with the lady because she talked too slowly. He was ready to go. But…we were told we had to wait for a doctor to sign our release papers and only if *he* thought Marley was ready to leave. After another hour and a half of pacing around our hospital "cell," we were *finally* released.

For the return trip, Catie traveled with Drew, while Marley was neatly folded sideways into the back of Selene's miniscule car. He needed room to stretch an unbendable leg (remember this kid is 6' 1"). Fortunately, he slept almost all the way home, while Selene and I talked about everything under the sun. For us, it was a very pleasant journey home indeed.

I love you all,
Jennifer

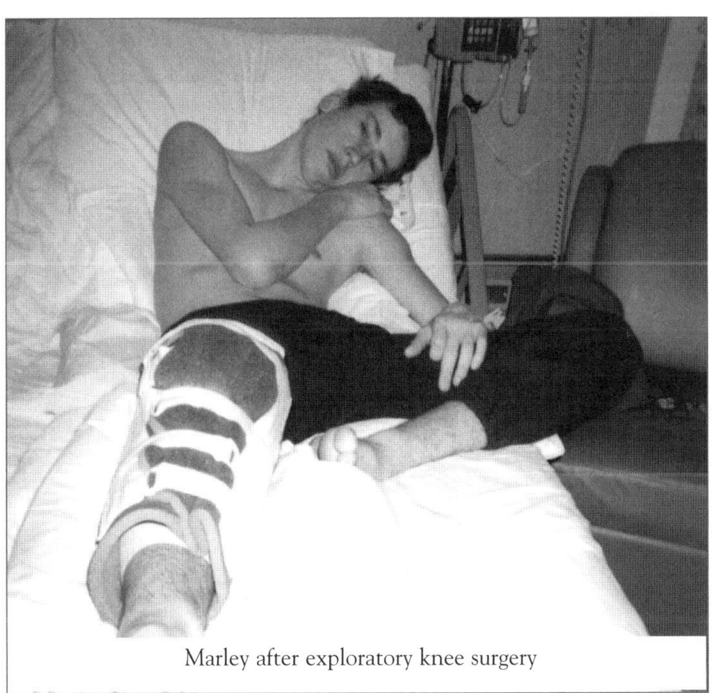

Marley after exploratory knee surgery

CLUELESS IN AMERICA

Exit, Stage Left

Generally, when most of us see a person in a white coat, we assume they know what they are talking about. This, unfortunately, is not always the case. After Marley had the knee surgery, we were ready to go home, but it was a weekend. We couldn't be released without the doctor's blessing, but since our doctor apparently had a life, Saturday was not a good time to reach him. We panicked, thinking we were trapped until Monday.

We "firmly" asked to be released immediately, so the poor nurses paged the on-call doctor to come rescue them. Although he had no familiarity with this case, he had an attitude of superiority that made Drew and I back against the wall. He was spewing facts and directives authoritatively as he flipped through Marley's charts. We listened like good little patients until he said we should do more tests on Marley's foot before his release.

I awoke from my doctor-induced trance to challenge his suggestion. I nearly choked and spat, "His foot? We're waiting for biopsy results to determine whether his leg will be amputated or his knee replaced. Don't you think it would be a waste of everyone's time to study the foot when it might be gone in two weeks?"

After snapping his mouth shut and regaining composure, he scratched his chin and calmly said, "Well, umm, good point. I'll just sign the release forms and we'll be in touch."

Drew and I looked at each other and thought, "Yah, right, you just do that. Thanks for your help, doc." We grabbed the release forms and split as fast as we could. Selene had our getaway car ready to go. We were headin' home, no matter what!

"You take the blue pill and you wake up in your bed and believe whatever you want to believe. You take the red pill, you stay in Wonderland and see just how deep the rabbit hole goes."

—Morpheus (Lawrence Fishburn)
The Matrix

POST PORTLAND

Severance

Drew and I had a hard time with this part of our cancer journey. The reality of how horrible this cancer had become was beginning to really sink in. We were thankful the surgeon talked honestly with us, but hearing the word *amputation* out loud made our heads spin, dizzy with panic. In less than a year, Marley's cancer had attacked his respiratory system, his lymphatic system, his muscular system, and now his skeletal system. We had a sneaking suspicion we were only seeing the tip of an iceberg. The facts were communicated to Marley and his network but, for simplicity's sake, much of the process was left unsaid. Drew had Cindy to brief and emote with, while I relied on family and my tight circle of friends.

I spent some very lonely nights wondering what Marley's life would be like if he were unable to ride his bike. I knew we weren't going to amputate his leg; we'd just have to rely on less dramatic solutions, no matter what the professionals advised. Amputation was simply too radical. Fortunately, the doctors agreed that Marley would suffer too much from having three massive surgeries within a year. Besides, his cancer survival prognosis had just plummeted with the new tumor—taking his leg off wasn't going to help. What we were hearing between the lines of the medical advice was, "Why put him through all that torture when he's not going to live very long anyway?"

Transition

Ah, yes! Choose quality of life as opposed to quantity. We had heard that phrase often enough during the past year, but what did it really mean? For the time being, quantity and quality could still exist together in our lives; but we were getting a taste that at some point in the future, we might have to choose between the two.

Marley was a strong, willful kid. He could take a lot of punishment and bounce right back. He'd proven that during the past eleven months. We couldn't just stand by and watch the cancer eat away at him. Or could we? At least the doctors had a replacement part for the knee. We knew that radical knee replacements were relatively common, and with lots of physical therapy there was no reason why Marley shouldn't be able to get back on a bike...unless something else went wrong.

Reincorporation

The day after we returned from Portland, after a restful night, Catie went to school. Marley came with me to work. After showing off his new incision to the BRI gang, Marley could hardly sit still. After just one day, he had become an expert crutch-cruiser, traveling at very high speeds with his new "toys." He wanted to visit his friends at the middle school, so I dropped him off for a bit of socializing.

I heard many reports of how he went from class to class. All the teachers loved him. Everyone knew he had cancer, and everyone wanted to hear about what it was like. He was honest, up front, and didn't spare any of the gory details when he was repeatedly asked what was wrong with his leg. He sat with the kids, showed them all his scars and proudly told them all about everything.

He later said he wanted to visit sick kids in hospitals too, so he could give some of his courage to them. He said, "I wanna show 'em that it's not always as bad as they think. Like, if I can do it, so can they." Marley was doing a damned good job showing *us* how to be courageous, why not other sick kids? It was a pretty cool idea. I just prayed he got the chance to make this idea real.

I spent the weekend trying to relax and figure my life out. I needed time, precious time, to process the enormity of how serious his situation had become. I needed time to think about what Marley might need after this upcoming surgery. I had to learn more about knees. I also needed to focus on how I felt about all the new information. I needed to sit down and cry a little!

Chapter Eight:
Ceremony

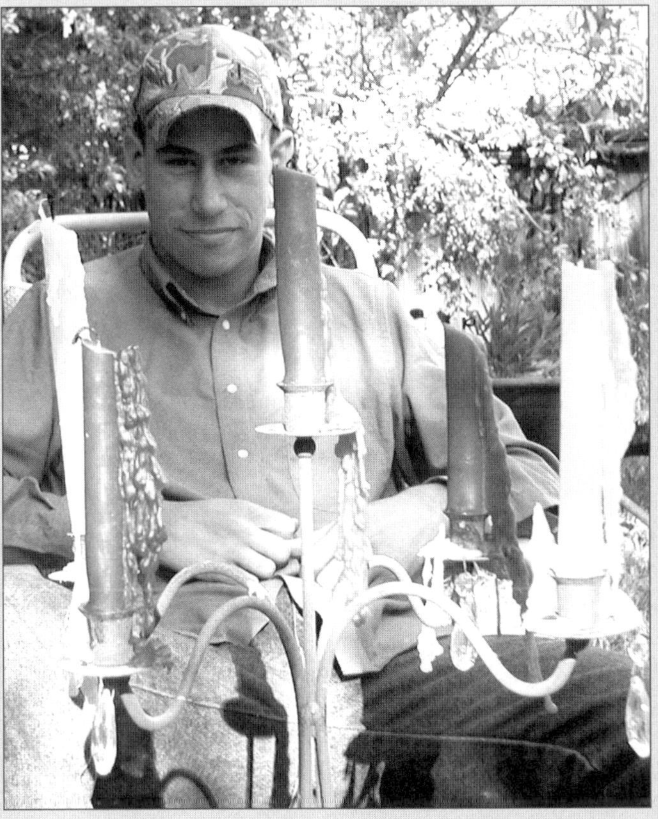

"Burning Bright"
Marley at Jeff's Birthday Party, 2001
Photo: Debbie Thornton

Wednesday, January 10, 2001
Subject: "CREATIVITY –
A BREAKTHROUGH CURE FOR CANCER?"

• From: Selene

Greetings everyone!

There is a lot to say, and a lot to think about, so take your time with this one.

First, you should know that Marley will be heading back up to Portland soon, most likely the week of the 16th, to be blessed by a new and whole TITANIUM knee (it's a bird, it's a plane, it's…). Because there may be a long recovery time when he is unable to get out of bed much, we need to get CREATIVE! Here are some ideas and ways you can help:

Marley loves DOCUMENTARIES—about sports, about nature, about healing. It's amazing how into a program about the Special Olympics—or cancer, for crying out loud—he is. His favorite TV station is the Discovery Channel. He doesn't have cable, so if you could record cool stuff from television, or if you have any EDUCATIONAL VIDEOS to share, please send them directly to Marley. It is important that these videos DO NOT require reading.

Marley has access to a Playstation, so if there are fun games (preferably ones that involve some thinking), let us know or pass them along. He also has a laptop he can use, so CD ROM GAMES would be awesome.

Any creative projects you can think of that he could work on while lying in bed would be great. Any simple meditation techniques that Jennifer could do with Marley would be welcomed too.

Audio tapes, CD's…a portable tape or CD player. These are all things that would be way cool.

If you have any other CREATIVE INSPIRATIONS on how to liven up this kid's life and get him thinking (since he can't do much physical moving) please contact me or Jennifer.

((((((((((((((((((((((()))))))))))))))))))))))))

Marley's birthday is on February 6th. He's turning 16. YEE-HA! There is a big, huge, wonderful CELEBRATION in the planning stages. We want to have a grand and joyous time giving thanks for all we have and all that Marley is. This celebration marks the one-year anniversary of when Marley's cancer trials began with pneumonia on Leap Day. As Jennifer so eloquently puts it, "This will be something for Marley to heal for, and something for us to remember."

LOCALS: We need help getting this party together. Know any great bands that would donate their music? People/restaurants who would donate food? Fun, big locations that would be free?

Other updates:

The Make-A-Wish Foundation is meeting with Drew and Cindy on Thursday. It looks like Marley will be asking for a "MULE," which is a 4-wheel drive ATV made by Kawasaki.

We may have a line on a wheelchair. We'll let you know.

We love you and thank you. I wish I could express how helpful it is to have somewhere to turn when the need arises. I'm sure you all know the feeling.

Blessings,
Selene

"A wise man should consider that health is the greatest of human blessings, and learn how by his own thought to derive benefit from his illnesses."

—Hippocrates

Tuesday, January 16, 2001
Subject: "PORTLAND PREPARATION"

Howdy folks,

Sometimes I feel so on top of things. Sometimes I don't. I'm in awe of my own life. Sometimes I can't believe I'm holding it together. I have a great job at the Bathroom Readers' Institute with a wonderful crew of people that love me. This makes me reconsider smashing my alarm clock to smithereens every morning.

THANKS

How can I possibly thank the people who have been there for me? My beloved BRI crew has endlessly put up with me trying to do the impossible—convince a corporation that small-town business methods are more important than making big bucks. They've also had to endure listening to one-sided phone conversations between me and Drew, who's having a hard time with this whole screwed-up situation. Even as my heart is being ripped from my body, I'm stunned by the beauty of this thing we call life. I have surrounded myself with extraordinary beings of light. For this I am thankful.

BIONIC BOY

Marley, Drew, and I head to Portland this Sunday. He's had another round of brain scans, bone scans, and PET scans. Marley is scheduled to have a titanium knee replacement on the 24th. Recoup time is expected to be six days in the hospital plus a few more before we come home. I realize none of us know anything for sure, so I'm preparing to be in Portland until February 1st.

WORLD PEAS

One thing you can help Marley with is to visualize a skeleton of light and strength, glowing golden with health. Once we've got the skeleton down, each one of us can branch out to other parts of his body, until every cell is glowing with love. It would also be lovely if we can focus on letting the anesthesia leave his body GENTLY and quickly post surgery. He spends way too much energy vomiting after surgery. And because I'm the one left holding the bucket, I'd really appreciate your help!

LUNCH MENU

I plan on buying a new vehicle tomorrow during my lunch break. I don't know what kind, or from where, but it will be BIG and comfortable with great gas mileage. Great Spirit will simply have to guide me. This is going to be a true exercise in creating my reality. Help me visualize the perfect rig.

FUN TIMES

Looks like the trip to Maui that was scheduled for next week will have to be postponed until the end of March. Oh well… something to look forward to. Speaking of which, we're gearing up for a world-class bash scheduled for the end of February. Jay will be writing more about this very special event soon. Scores of people and local businesses have already offered to help us and we haven't even started yet! The energy around this event is astonishing.

I love you all. Keep smiling and loving the people around you. That's the only thing that matters. Feel. Feel my love for you.

Jennifer

P.S. The kids come home to me this weekend before we leave. Feel free to call Marley. He's been going nuts. I'm sure he'd rather talk to you than think about all the things he can't do. Catie could use some extra lovin' too!

P.P.S. Send some love Selene's way; her grandfather (Steven's father) has recently died. They're in L.A. for the send-off ceremony. Selene is as tender as she is beautiful. What a gift she is.

MANIFEST THE BEST

Indispensable Friends

Drew, Marley, and I were planning to drive to Portland in one car. The only problem was we didn't know what car we were taking—Drew's truck was too uncomfortable and my car was too small. Drew was getting a little nervous about this last loose end. I had the money ready. I had been looking, but.... I kept assuring him that by the time we were to leave, I'd have a vehicle.

I knew two things; 1) It had to have four-wheel drive so I could get down my driveway during the winter months, and 2) It had to be roomy enough to contain Marley, who had very long legs, one of which would not be bending for a spell. A tall order. My two choices were limited to a Suburban or a mini-van.

Everyone at EPCAM, my morning coffee clan, knew what I was looking for and they knew time was running out. The day after I sent that last e-mail, I drove to Dreadford and looked at one Suburban. It was all right; the price was right but...I had to think about it. When I returned to the office, I got a call from Sunny. Since coffee, he'd been looking too, and he had a lead for me. I called the number, and immediately went to see it. It was a used Suburban, in perfect condition. It had so many bells and whistles that even Catie would like it. (She wanted a mini-van.) Right after work that day, I bought my new fancy rig.

Drew was shocked that I actually pulled it off. It was the perfect rig; plush captain's chairs, running lights, fog horns, CB and cell phone antennas, and a ladder for climbing up on the roof. Whoever had owned this vehicle must have been ultra paranoid, because it had a security system that took Marley a week to figure out.

I named her Indy because she was an indispensable part of my life. I kept my little Subaru to drive when I didn't have the kids, but, boy oh boy, I loved that rig! I loved the way she came to my rescue, and I loved the way she reminded me that we can have our cake and eat it too.

Thursday, January 25, 2001
Subject: "BIONIC BOY"

Dearest Network,

Wonder Boy Becomes Bionic!
On Monday, Drew, Marley, and I arrived in Portland for a doctor's appointment. We traveled north in my beautiful new Suburban and settled into our room at the Ronald McDonald House. On Tuesday, the day before surgery, Drew and Marley went to the zoo while I worked from my portable office. Later that afternoon, we all went to Powell's Books. Wow! I've never seen a bookstore so big. During two hours of browsing, I managed to cover just one 10-foot section.

Rise and Shine
On Wednesday, bright and early, we rolled into the surgery waiting room at 6:30 A.M. By 8:00 he was fully doped up and was wheeled away into the operating room. At 12:30, we were asked to meet the surgeon in a private room. Gulp. With a concerned look, the surgeon began, "Marley's fine but there was a complication." Imagine how fast our minds filled in the blanks.

Built to Spec
He explained how the procedure was *supposed* to work. First the incision is made and the ligaments and patella (knee cap) are laid aside. Then it is determined how much of the femur (thigh bone) needs to be replaced due to cancer contamination. Four inches of Marley's femur was removed and 1 cm was sawed off the top of the tibia (shin bone) to give the knee prosthesis a flat surface to attach to.

Now comes the tricky part. The parts from a "trial" prosthesis are used to determine exactly which parts are needed for a snug custom fit. They assemble the trial prosthesis and try it out before the surgeon gives the okay to assemble the permanent prosthesis in the same way.

As the final product is being constructed, holes are drilled into the ends of both newly sawed-off bones. Then the holes are filled with cement and the permanent prosthesis is put into place. The ligaments and patella are reattached, they close up the incision and voila! New knee!

The Best Laid Plans

Here's the complicated part. They were missing a part from the permanent prosthesis. Can't you see them all swearing at each other as they started looking under the table, up their sleeves, and in their pockets? Apparently the manufacturing company that sent both kits didn't include all the parts. Ooops!

Plan B: Quick! Put the trial knee back in, close him up, and give the boy more drugs. Run to the phone, order the missing part from the Tennessee-based corporation, and have it sent by courier across the country. Next, go out and explain the bummer booboo to the parents. With his head slightly bowed, he concluded, "Now we have to wait for the missing part to be delivered. It's still early and we'll hopefully get it in time to go back into surgery later today. With any luck, Marley won't wake up." Hmmmm. I'm glad I wasn't the doctor. But at the same time, I sure wish I wasn't me.

A Knee Jerk Reaction

The poor kid. Drew and I were livid, but yelling and screaming at the doctor certainly wasn't going to help matters. We joined Marley in recovery. He was out cold. We had hours to wait before he was wheeled away again so we could wait for hours more. I had to *do* something. This was just wrong.

I left Marley with Drew and found the hospital's patient advocate. The seemingly competent woman jumped into action, calling for an internal evaluation. She scheduled a meeting with the chief clinical blah blah blah, the surgeon, and another blah blah blah, and I was assured the billing would be suspended. It all sounded very official, but I have spent the past six months learning how corporations do business. Needless to say, I'm a little skeptical. The proof is in the pudding. We'll have to wait to see if this meeting actually happens and if any action is taken. At least the complaint is on record, and doing something made me feel better.

Do Not Disturb!

Fortunately for everyone, especially Marley, he basically stayed unconscious and his vital signs remained stable. Everyone tiptoed around us. Everyone was nervous and on their best behavior. I wondered if they already knew this process was going to be investigated.

During the five hours between surgeries, Marley rolled over and threw up a few times, rolling his eyes, trying to focus on Drew and me. He'd attempt a smile before passing out again. At one point, I had my head on my folded arms, resting on the side of his gurney. I felt his giant paw gently take my hand. So sweet. So incredibly loving. Then back into darkness he slipped.

At 6:30 P.M. the same crew came back to wheel him away. Shhhh! Evwyone was vewy vewy qwiet! No one wanted to wake him and have to be the one to explain that he was going back for round two. He stayed asleep. Phew! When he wakes up we'll let him know what he's been through.

Ding! Round Two

The second surgery lasted *only* a little over two hours. But they were very *loooooong* hours. Toward the end, I thought Drew was going to start throwing chairs through the eighth floor windows. I can't believe I even suggested to him that if the news was bad, killing the doctor might not be a very good idea. The waiting room was empty—since 6:30 that morning, we had witnessed scores of patients go into surgery and had shared the waiting room with their family members. They were all gone now. The women buzzing around the nursing station that we had watched all day had gone home for the night. The janitor had finished cleaning. We were alone. Our nerves were frazzled.

We had been told the surgery should take about an hour and a half. Maybe you can imagine what the additional forty-five minutes felt like. We were quiet. I know both of us were going crazy preparing ourselves for bad news from the surgeon. It was truly tortuous. But lo and behold, the surgeon came out saying everything went fine and Marley should be experimenting with his new knee the next day. Exhale!

The Still of the Night

It's very late, and I can't sleep. Today's events seem so far away. My Wonder Boy has transformed into the Wonder-ful Bionic Boy! He sleeps soundly a few feet away. He is completely unaware of what he's been through. Occasionally he moans, grabs the morphine button, and gives himself a booster. They call this practice "PC," for *patient control.* I call it a great invention. Mother's little helper. No pain, great short term gain!! Sleeping is better than throwing up!

I'll keep you posted when some action takes place. In the meantime, thanks for your prayers. We need all the help you can give!

Joyously,
Jennifer

"God is a comedian,
playing to an audience too afraid to laugh."

—Voltaire

A PARENT'S NIGHTMARE

Worst-case Worries

There are simply a few things no parent should have to endure. Unfortunately, many parents have had to survive their child's doctor beckoning them to meet in a private room. Somewhere quiet where they can somberly say, "I'm sorry." Or "We did everything we could." What would I have done? What would Drew have done? I never want to experience anything remotely close to that again. My arms wrap around those of you who have faced worse.

During those long hours in the waiting room, after everyone had left, I played out a thousand awful scenarios in my head. There was nothing else to do while we waited. The words on the pages of my novel were jumping around like they, too, were nervous. I couldn't focus on anything except the hundreds of screaming voices in my head, all competing for attention.

My worst scenario was having the doctor come out in a blood-smeared smock and shake his head "no." Even sitting in my chair, I could imagine how my knees would buckle, the sound of the grief-stricken moan I would emit, and how I would cry. In my mind's eye, I saw Drew lunge for the incompetent doctor's throat, squeezing his neck with all the rage of all the parents who have ever lost their babies. The aging doctor wouldn't stand a chance. Someone would then have to tackle Drew and haul him away to prison for attempted manslaughter. I imagined how I'd feel, left by myself in a darkened waiting room, expected to keep living without Marley and Drew. It was hard not focusing on the worst-case scenarios.

The Real World

The good news is, my nightmare vanished when the doctor said, "Everything went fine." We were lucky. Really lucky. In the middle of surgery, I wanted to burst in and politely say, "Excuse me. We've changed our minds. We've made a terrible choice letting you touch our son. We had a bad feeling about you in the beginning and we didn't listen to our intuition." Maybe I should have.

I'll never know. I'm glad Marley didn't die during that operation. I don't think I would have ever forgiven myself.

The job was botched. In retrospect, I would have advocated for a younger surgeon with more experience in total knee replacements rather than an older doctor with more experience with cancer. I've since seen the scars from similar surgeries and they are half the length and caused half the problems we were to endure. The only good thing I can say about that operation is Marley survived it. But then again…hind-sight is always 20/20.

Follow-up

As it turned out, we were billed for both operations. The second bill was even more than the first! It took about fifty phone calls and some crawling up the ladder of authority, but I managed to make enough noise that they heard me. They bungled not only the operation and the billing, but they bungled on the correction too (in our favor). The insurance company was so confused by the end of the six-month negotiation process that we were charged for only the first operation, but never charged our $2,400 deductible that year!

Weeks later, after the swelling went down, there was a strange bump on the side of Marley's knee. No one ever did identify it. Drew figured it was a bone fragment. It was about the size of the head of a small bolt and it was free-floating, just under the skin. Marley and I would joke, "I think we found the missing part!"

I hope that by now the surgeon has retired. I also hope he forgot to pass his wisdom on to those who took his place. In the future, I shall follow my first impressions of those who hold my life or that of my children in their hands. Little did I know, we would get another chance to test our newfound knowledge.

"Doctors are just the same as lawyers;
the only difference is that lawyers merely rob you,
whereas doctors rob you and kill you too."

—Anton Chekhov

Sunday, January 28, 2001
Subject: "CAUSE FOR CELEBRATION!"

Greetings Marley Fans,

The Marley Man is in the clear. He has had a terrible time since surgery due to vomiting. He wasn't able to eat or drink (other than IV fluids) until Saturday night. But this morning he woke up, after sleeping nearly 12 hours, feeling much better and wanting FOOD! Food glorious food. That means we're outta here tomorrow!

On Saturday evening, we had a wonderful surprise visit. My friends Jeff, Jay, Denise, and Adam drove all the way up from Ashland to see Mars Bar and to party. After joining forces with Liz, they took me out on the town to celebrate my birthday. I didn't feel very social, but today they picked me up again and dragged me back to Powell's Books to restock the library at the Bathroom Readers' Institute. I had fun in spite of myself. Afterward, Drew, Marley, and I settled in for a laid-back afternoon of nonstop eating, watching football, and preparing for departure.

Marley has a beautiful 12-inch curved scar with 25 staples keeping it closed, over a brand new, stainless steel knee (I guess they ran out of titanium). I'm sure it will mend in record time, but there's much physical therapy yet to do. He has to re-train his confused, bruised muscles to perform their old job, wrapped around a brand new hinge.

Next week, Marley will celebrate being on this planet for 16 years. Amazing!

Once again, thank you sooooooo much for your loving support. You make a difference.

Jennifer

Sunday, February 4, 2001
Subject: "MARLEY'S MELTDOWN"

Dear Marley Network,

We're home! Sometimes readjusting back to home life after the hospital scene can be challenging. Last week, Marley finally broke down. It's only the second time during this crazy year that he's actually peeled back a few layers of his onion. His fears were exposed and raw. The tears flowed.

This happened the first night back from Portland. It was a long drive back. We arrived in Ashland at 3 P.M., just as Catie's school let out. Cindy met us at the school to pick up Drew, and then the kids and I were on our own. After filling prescriptions and driving up the mountain, I was faced with a very cold wood stove, and needed to get dinner together. Catie was in shock seeing Marley; he was in a lot of pain and his leg looked like a shark attacked it. I had too much to do and I started to lose it. I just couldn't build the fire, light the candles, cook dinner, and tend to kids all at the same time. I called a few friends. No one was home. Somehow, I pulled it together. As it turned out, if someone *had* come up, Marley and I wouldn't have had the chance to slog through the mire together with such grace. Great Spirit moves in mysterious ways.

Thank God, Cindy had the foresight to hand me a container of home-made—and home-grown—beef stew when we met at Catie's school. Thank God, the pipes didn't freeze while we were away (the temps were low and the winds were high). Thank God, the 40-foot tree that fell and hit the house that night only took the flashing off the roof and didn't break the kitchen windows or smash our precious generator. Miracles all!

After dinner, we tried watching a video. We made it halfway through when Marley said he was hurting and wanted to go to sleep in my bed. Catie had already fallen asleep in my arms. I left Catie asleep on the couch and tended to Marley as he proceeded to completely fall apart.

I was a little raw after a week of sleeping with one eye open, catching a lot of vomit, fluffing pillows, giving massages, and keeping the nurses from doing stupid things. So maybe my counseling skills weren't quite as objective as normal. Here's a slightly simplified version of our dialog.

"Mom, I hate not having contwol. Whatem I supposed to do now?"

"Well, dear, how 'bout figuring out whether you want to live or die. If you choose to live, are you willing to commit to doing whatever it takes?"

Thrash, slam, cover head with pillow…silence…then…, "Like what? What does *that* mean?"

"Like praying your ass off. Like standing on your head for a week if that's what it takes. Like meditating and visualizing stopping the cancer. Like eating pills of Tibetan cow dung and drinking snake venom. Like not just waiting for the next tumor to show up so the doctors can cut it out and put a Band-Aid on the cut."

I'm sure those of you that know me can imagine me massaging Marley's feet, calmly saying things like, "Do understand how powerful you are? Do you get that you're the only one that can heal yourself? Shit or get off the pot, boy, time is a-wasting."

God, I know I can be obnoxious, but I figure in order to be a good guide, I have to know what direction he wants to go. Losing by default is one of his options. I just want to make sure he knows there are other options too. No matter what, I'll be there for him—with no judgement of him (or of me as a reflection of him)—but I have to know I shot straight and offered suggestions.

I'm sharing this with you and, hell, I don't even know who

"you" are. But those of you in Marley's Network, receiving these updates, seem to be interested in this little slice of life. I'm sharing this because it is *not* just about Marley. It's about each and every one of us.

Marley is an inspiration. He's phenomenal. He just stands there, taking life's punches and bouncing back. Although he has murderous thoughts for all doctors, he keeps saying "thank you." He says it to nurses that wake him eight times a night, and to surgeons that cut away his organs and bone. He keeps smiling and loving, annoying his sister, picking on our dear friend Jay, and asking for more hugs. How does he do it? To be perfectly honest, I haven't a clue. I'm 90% certain I couldn't do what he's done. Whatever is keeping him alive and full of love, healing, humor, and Marley-ness must be pretty powerful.

I know he's not ignorant. On the contrary, he's surprisingly savvy about human behavior. Yet, he has always been a mystery. The professionals have never been able to diagnose or accurately label what's different about Marley. He's "developmentally disabled," with an official report to prove it. Yet, this kid is not dumb. He's facing life and death with a strength that blows my mind.

Whoever or whatever he is, he knows something I don't. I'm honored to be able to witness all this firsthand. I am amazed people like you are reading these letters and caring, sharing your support so easily. There has to be a reason for all this, doesn't there?

Well, believe it not, the point of this letter is to say that after two hours of Marley and me "discussing" his future—me watching him rail in emotional pain—he had a revelation. At some point that night, we hit a wall and fell into silence, lying next to each other in my big bed, gritting our teeth. After an hour of staring at the ceiling, the spell was magically broken when he said something. I can't remember what he said, but I considered it to be rude or dumb. I responded, graceful and loving, "Blow it out your ear."

He came back with his classic response, "I don't know how!" We both burst into laughter, turned toward each other, and I listened while he shared his new plan.

"I want the newspapas to pwint my stowy. I want to go to schools and tell kids what I been going thwew and what it feews like. They can ask me questions, and I can ask them what they would do if this happened to them."

Stunned, I asked, "Why?"

He quietly said, "So maybe they can give me some good ideas." Just about then, Catie crawled into bed with us. The three of us held hands and fell asleep wrapped in a blanket of love, inspiration, and forgiveness.

So I've been working on Marley's story for several nights. I've blown through two pens, writing by candlelight next to the wood stove, listening to my many wind chimes. I've stopped to ask for your help. I know the facts, I have a line on the format, but as my beloved "Uncle John" would ask, "What's the story? Find the nugget."

I'm going for gold. I think this is beyond just another wonderful heart-filled human interest story. I just have to find the angle. I think it's the networking aspect, the communication process, and the butterfly effect—that every move we make affects us all. Before I continue, I want your opinion. What's the story here? Write how this is affecting you. Help me tell the newspapers what to print, so Marley can reach out for more clues about his next moves.

I love you more then my mind can express!
Jennifer

P.S. One way to respond is to sign Marley's Guestbook on his website. This way, others can read your wisdom, too.

Monday, February 5, 2001
Subject: "RE: MARLEY'S MELTDOWN"

• From: Gordon (Editor-in-chief of the BRI)

Dear Jennifer,

I just read your recent letter ("Marley's Meltdown")

I have been wondering for some time when you would become aware that you have a story to tell. How fascinating that Marley knew it first. What's also fascinating is that your letter asks us (whoever "us" is) to tell you the nugget of the story. You are the story and you've been telling it. But you want an angle for the newspapers? Okay, I can help.

First, for what it's worth, I think you are a fine writer. Why? Passion and humor. That's what comes across. The depth of your strength, your commitment and love for Marley and Catie, your need to communicate to your friends, and the skill with which you do it are compelling, even breathtaking. I look forward to receiving the letters.

As for the newspaper angle, it's Marley and his (and your) amazing circle of love and support. His strength against all odds is the kind of stuff that makes people kvell (look it up). For example, that the doctors never checked the box of knee parts before the operation, that the parts were couriered from Tennessee MID-OPERATION and he survived is just incredible. I mean it. You just shake your head and say, "how is this possible?" And let's be honest; people—adults and children—are stricken with horrible debilitating diseases every day. Some survive, some do not. What makes you guys different? It's Marley. And your love, faith, and strength. Did I mention your strength? It's incredible.

If you need another angle, it's that you have learned to take it one day at a time, that survival requires a short view, a deep commitment and an ability to, if you'll pardon the expression, go with the flow. Plus there's the very important sub-angle of what you've learned from Marley.

I have to conclude this letter, as people keep calling and interrupting my train of thought. Who are you, again? One more phone call and I'm going to jump out a window (which will be difficult, considering that my office is in the basement and I have to get on a step stool to reach the window).

I'll talk to you later,
Gordon

"Towering genius disdains a beaten path. It seeks regions hitherto unexplored."

—Abraham Lincoln

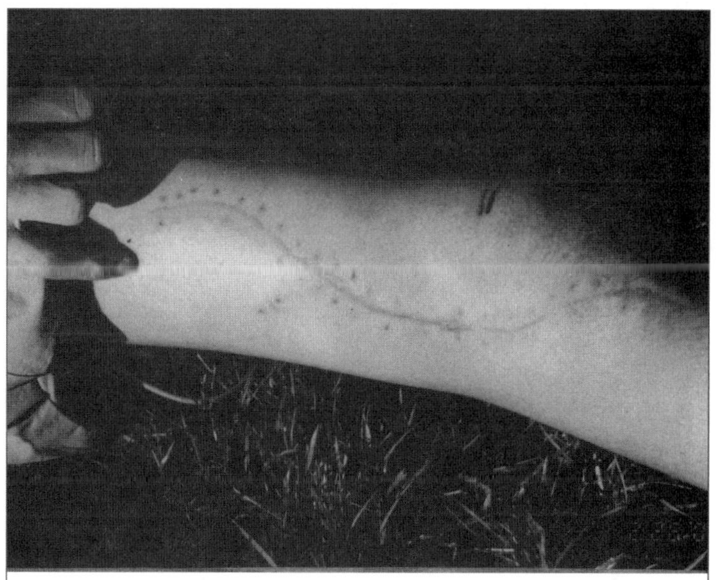

Marley's new leg

Photo: Dee Fretwell

Monday, February 5, 2001
Subject: "MMB: MARLEY'S MONSTER BASH"

• Written by Jay

Greetings and salutations!

About eight of us have met four times in preparation for a great party to honor Marley—this is the combo one-year anniversary of surviving cancer and 16th birthday party. If you have something to add to this party, let us know! A lot of work has been done, and there is plenty still to do. We now have Department Heads that you can contact. (Sounds pretty official, huh?)

CATERING: Jennifer S. has offered to coordinate. She'll need a list of all of those donating foodstuffs. So far we have: the Community Food Store; with a donation of deli stuff, Evo's Java House; contributing coffee and sweets, and the Wild Goose Cafe. But we'll need more.

JD writes: "My parents said they'd donate some pork. (They bought two hogs at a 4-H auction when they thought they were only bidding on one.)"

DRINKS: Caldera Brewery, Ashland Wine Cellar, and Pyramid Juice Co. should be confirmed by week's end. Rhys and Sean are in charge of getting permits to serve alcohol. Jeannie from the Beau Club will happily tend bar.

MUSIC: Eric, our sound dude, will head up this front. Live music includes Little Thom, The Wild Goose Trio, The Riveters, an African drumming group, and many special guests.

GAMES AND OTHER ENTERTAINMENT: I am entertainment coordinator. Debbie and her daughters will be doing face painting. Entertainment ideas brainstormed so far: belly dancing, juggling, the (mostly) Full Monty, and a parade. We still need a clown. (JD, you were a great clown at Jennifer's

"Circus, Circus" party—are you offering to do this?)

DECORATIONS: All of us artsy types should start making signs and banners to honor party contributions. One idea is to tie a rope from one end of the Armory to the other and hang everything from there. Who's got a long rope? Marley?

We also want our invitees to be comfy, so we're asking for throw rugs, cushions, pillows, and anything else nice and soft.

FOUNTAIN: We've decided that making a new fountain for Marley's pebbles will be the least expensive way to go. Rhys, Silver, and Uncle Jay said they'd all pitch in to make it. Debbie will talk to her blacksmith friend about a metal base. We'll also need to transport it. Which brings us to…

TRANSPORTATION: Being the wonderful little consumers that we are, we'll be bringing a lot of stuff to this party, such as: a fountain, furniture, catering supplies, decorations, people, etc. To get all of this stuff there and back, we'll need vehicles. We'll also need someone who can get guests to and from the airport.

MISC: Thanks to Eric, the use of the Armory has been donated. All we have to come up with is the $400 insurance bill to cover the night (so far, this is the only out-of-pocket expense).

EVENT DAY: Very important—those of you with jobs, make sure you can get the 28th off. (Jennifer, can I have the 28th off?)

We have a little over three weeks to make this happen. I know, with all of our gifts and talents coming together into one big ball of love, we can make this the most supercalifragelistic, fantabulous par-TEY ever! Marley deserves nothing less!

Love, love and more love,
-Jay-

Friday, March 16, 2001
Subject: "A MONSTER SUCCESS!"

• From: Selene

Dear dear ones,

Most mornings these days the sun promises itself to us through the translucent curtains and the cracks between the blinds. Most days the clouds come to the rescue, saving me from the itch to be outside, making it possible for me to work and stew and wonder. But there is spring; always it comes, miraculous.

I am writing to tell you, if you don't already know, what a success the Marley Monster Bash was. Each of us who helped to create its beauty and thrill and incredible ease has a different perspective, I'm sure. Mine can only be described as awe. I am still in the process of waking myself up to how great the whole thing was. I mean, did we really pull it off so well? The truth is, we didn't really pull it off at all. It was what you might call an "excitable medium." We catalyzed the evolution, but where it went from there was totally spontaneous and came with the presence of so many good people who all care deeply about life and about celebrating with Marley.

There was a virtual cornucopia of edibles, splayed out on large tables, all orchestrated with great ease and creativity by Jennifer S. There was professional live music the whole night, arranged and inspired by Eric—everything from African drumming to Reggae. There were pictures of Marley at every age. There were hanging banners, and cozy tables with flowers, and rugs and pillows. There were little kids playing, teenagers dancing, people laughing, small quiet miracles of meetings and smiles happening. So many people to thank. Every business I asked to donate something did, from a banner to food to paper plates to beer: an endless stream of generosity. It's amazing how much people want to help when given the opportunity!

One of the highlights was the "ritual," a recognition of why we were all there and the unveiling of the fountain (made by Rob): a huge handmade sculpture of metal formed like petals on a stem, piled with rocks and precious gems. Seeing Drew and Jennifer helping Marley to mark a year of strength and courage, and then watching Marley touch so many people with hugs—while a few hundred of his closest friends stood by—was both sensorily and emotionally a moment to be kept in a velvet box. And of course Marley had to literally kickstart the fountain to get the water flowing…very appropriate.

There are so many gems, and I'll leave it to Jennifer to share a few more of them. So many people have shared with me what a great party it was. You were all there holding it together. Nothing else could explain the fullness we felt. So thank you. Thank you a thousand times around the sun and back.

Marley is presently undergoing another round of radiation, this time on the area around his knee. During which, he and I have had the pleasure of being part of Y.E.S. Training (Youth Empowerment Skills), a weekend of intense bonding and personal growth with 22 other teens, followed by four more sessions. Over the past month, we focused on setting goals and writing a vision statement for our own lives. It's been really good to see Marley around kids his age, talking about his cancer and having the space to express the love and affection he feels toward those around him. Even in the midst of all of the dark, his compassion and desire to "go for it" shines.

Love and blessings,
Selene

"I am committed to being free in my heart and in my mind and being able to connect with people."

— Marley's Y.E.S. commitment statement

EVERYDAY IS EARTH DAY

Celebrate!

I've never met a town that loves to celebrate more than Ashland. Maybe it's because of all the lithium springs that filter through our waterways; just give us one reason and celebration bubbles forth. Downtown Ashland cordons off all car traffic for three occasions: the Fourth of July Parade, the Thanksgiving Festival of Lights Parade, and the Halloween Kids' Parade. Ashlanders love to demonstrate against wars, rally on Earth Day, and celebrate anything from miscellaneous planetary alignments to other nations' holidays. Being a town where every third store is an art gallery or a great restaurant, the first Friday night of every month boasts an art walk. Folks get pleasantly soused sipping complimentary local wines and nibbling hors d'oeuvres as they sample the town's incredibly diverse artistic talent. What can I say, we love to party!

"The only people for me are the mad ones,
the ones who are mad to live, mad to talk,
mad to be saved, desirous of everything at the same time,
the ones who never yawn or say a commonplace thing,
but burn, burn, burn."

—Jack Kerouac

MMB

The group of nut-cases I consider my family would find any excuse to gather in style. Since Marley got sick, we had found innumerable occasions. Marley's Monster Bash was the best event yet. I have never been to a private party like it. It was held at the Old Armory, an enormous building often used as a concert hall. We were lucky as hell to have that place to use. Food was spread out buffet style, under hanging banners honoring all the businesses that made donations. There was a dining area to the right, with round tables covered with linen cloths and flowers. The kids' corner had its own space to the left. The center was lined with chairs, Indian carpets, over-stuffed pillows, and potted palms, leaving plenty of space for wild and crazy dancing. In the very center of the dance floor was Marley's fountain.

Uncle Jay worked all day with Marley to prepare for the unveiling. The fountain was a kidney-shaped goldfish pond. There were two side-by-side three-foot towers with metal tubes in the centers that water could be pumped through. Each tube had three circular platforms welded to the core. On the day of the bash, Marley and Uncle Jay spent hours placing all of Marley's stones and gems in it and trying to get the two water pumps to actually work.

Four hundred people came and went. The music was great—each band had their own style—there was country, funk, jazz, drumming, and reggae. We all danced. It felt so good to let go and have fun. For the first time in a year, I saw Drew and Cindy looking truly happy as they danced in each other's arms. One of the last songs was Bob Marley's "Three Little Birds," and when the chorus of "This is my message to you ooo ooo...Don't worry 'bout

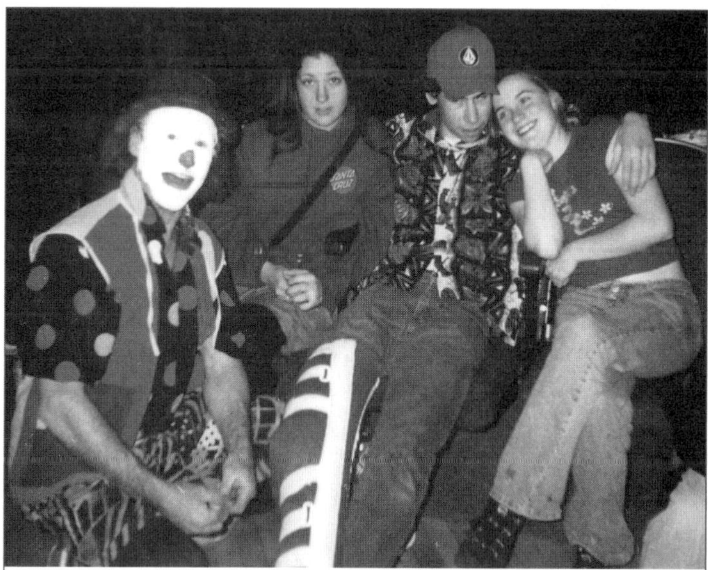

Marley at the Monster Bash, soakin' up some love.
Photo: Debbie Thornton

a ting, every little ting is gonna be all right…" played, we all whooped and hollered and danced even harder.

The diversity of people at the party was amazing. On this night, Marley was the glue that stuck us all together, and he loved *everybody*. Marley was that kind of guy. As far as he was concerned, it didn't matter who you were, what you did, or what you believed. None of it mattered, especially during party time. What was important to him was that people got together and shared themselves.

He was always trying to play matchmaker for me. I loved being single and didn't want that to change, but Marley had other plans. All night he kept nudging me towards the one man that intrigued me. Rhys was something special, but my plate was full, and I wasn't really looking to add a new boyfriend to the menu. I think, in truth, it wasn't for my benefit that Marley was so intent on hooking me up with a fun guy. It was because *he* wanted another live-in playmate.

Nine Nine Ninety-nine

Five months before Marley got cancer, on September 9th, 1999, I had thrown a three-day party. Why not? The numbers would never line up like that again! I lived off highway 99. So we started the party at 9:00, and everyone was asked to bring nine things. It was a free-for-all, and ended up being a great party where I met a lot of new people. Rhys was one of them. Before that, I had never put much stock in fate or love at first sight, but this man seemed too good to be true. During those three days, we danced around each other and with each other. Both Marley and Catie fell in love with him. All of my friends loved him. I loved him, but I guess the timing wasn't right.

Then Marley got sick and my life was swept away. It wasn't until the planning of Marley's Monster Bash that Rhys came back into my life, up close but not yet personal. A month after the Monster Bash, the buds started popping and the layers of winter clothes started peeling off, as the sun brought everything to life once again. Spring fever! Party time!

Earth Day

I think Earth Day was invented for Ashlanders. Everyone came to Lithia Park to celebrate the warm weather, a possible future. That was the day Rhys swept all three of us off our feet…again. During the festivities, he and Catie lay next to each other on the grass and called each other on cell phones. They giggled and laughed while Marley and I wrestled. When it was time to go to the band shell for the day's entertainment, Rhys gave Marley a piggy-back all the way through Lithia Park. This was an act of love, because Rhys and Marley were the same height. It was a pretty funny sight. I nearly wet my pants when I looked over and watched Marley with his arms slung over Rhys' shoulders. As Rhys marched with his heavy load, Marley was lovingly gazing at his own arms. He flexed his muscles, admiring his strength, all the while being carried by another man.

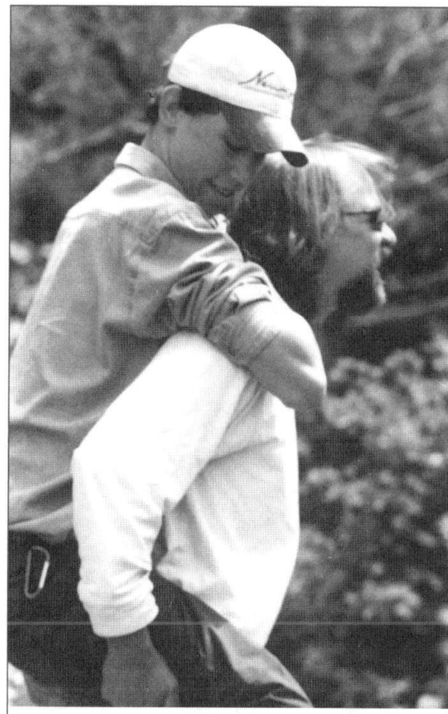

Rhys giving Marley a lift on Earth Day

The whole town was in a good mood. Gallons of glitter and face paint must have been used that day. Marley was still having a hard time walking, but that didn't stop him from climbing to the top of the 40-foot high band shell. When we heard his whistle, we looked up to see him peeking over the edge with an ear-to-ear grin on his face. If he had fallen either way, it would most likely have been fatal, but all I could do was wave and smile. It made me think about the time when he was a towheaded little kid and he climbed up the ladder to the barn roof. Nothing much had changed. He was a lot bigger but he was still the same ol' Marley.

> ***"I want to stay as close to the edge as I can without going over. Out on the edge you see all kinds of things you can't see from the center."***
>
> **—Kurt Vonnegut**

It was one of those days that everything felt right and so easy; I almost forgot my son had cancer. I think I'll remember that day when I'm on my deathbed. Except for the cancer, both kids were healthy and happy. My relationship with Rhys was deep and true, like we'd been together for a hundred years even though we hadn't yet connected as a couple. It didn't make any sense to anyone, including us, but that was how it was and it was good. We just had to trust that somehow the All-That-Is knew what they were doing. Nothing was pressing. Everything just felt simple. It felt good to breathe deep and enjoy the day.

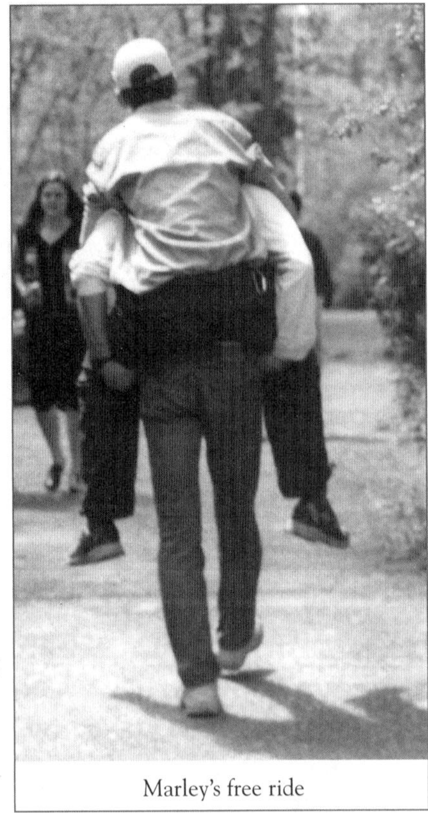

Marley's free ride

Chapter Nine: Life's A Beach!

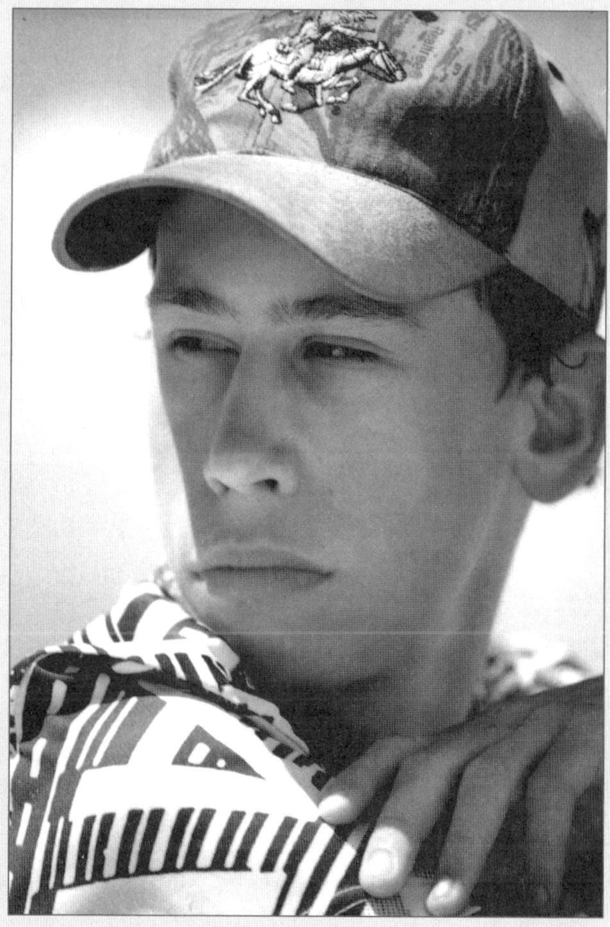

Mars in Maui

Photo: Jennifer

Saturday, March 31, 2001
Subject: "BACK IN THE RING: ROUND 5"

Hi Gang,

Round 5.

Ding!

On your mark, get set…PRAY!

I'll give details later. In short: Marley has a new tumor in the shoulder bone (acromion). Catie, Marley, and I are vacating to Maui for a week to heal from the knee surgery before we do anything else. Exit, stage left! Be back on the 11th.

Jennifer

"Run away! Run away!"

—Monty Python and the Holy Grail

THERE'S A TIME AND A PLACE TO…

Run Away!

There are only so many times that this one small, deserving family could postpone paradise. We weren't going to put our trip to Maui on hold again. It seemed like as good a time as any to exit gracefully. Even the doctors gave us their blessing. So we consciously entered a blissful state of denial. We were going to simply ignore the implications of the new test results.

"Never knock on Death's door: ring the bell and run away! Death really hates that!"

—Dr. Mike Stratford (Matt Frewer), ***Doctor, Doctor***

Tuesday, April 3, 2001
Subject: "PARADISE"

• From: Selene

Dear Ones,

In the dark of the early morning, I dropped Jennifer and the kids off at the little Dreadford airport. There had been a snowstorm the night before, but the morning was clear for their takeoff. They must be in Maui now, basking in the glory of this earth. It makes me feel good to know that.

It seems all I can do these days is just breathe through it all, one inhale at a time, and try and be sure I am exhaling enough of what I take in. There is a Buddhist meditation I have heard about, where you practice breathing in all the pain and suffering of the world and breathing out all the joy and love you have inside you. The more we put out there, the lighter the air, the brighter the skies, the cleaner the rain; or so I tell myself.

I just wanted you to know that through all of this, Marley has remained the rebel, the trickster, the hero, and the sweet love. Catie is blossoming like the flowers of spring, so alive and expressive and intelligent. As I told Jennifer the other day, the more I get to see the human in her, the more I accept it in myself, and the more I love. These are hard times, but I am putting my trust in where it will take us.

I think now is a good time to pray especially hard for those guys, while they are in a place where they can be a little more open to receiving it. Let's bombard them with vibrant, colorful, expansive, pervasive waterfalls of well-being, ease, healing, and bliss!

May you all be well.
So much love,
Selene

Sunday, April 15, 2001
Subject: "RETURN FROM MAUI"

Dear Marley Network,

I'm in the office catching up on some work, and I thought I'd take time out to communicate with some of the finest people on Earth.

Maui

Marley, Catie, and I left for Maui on the 3rd and returned very late on the 11th. (This vacation had been postponed since New Year's, due to the tumor found in Marley's knee.) He had just finished the month of radiation after his knee surgery, and we figured we had a window when it was safe to vacate. But, alas, the week before we were scheduled to leave, we found out why Marley's shoulder had been bothering him. These tumors grow fast, so it was a tough call whether or not we should be traveling. Everyone agreed: We should go for it. So I packed the kids up and left all the "doctor talk" to Drew and Cindy.

Believe it or not, our travel plans went without a hitch—not even a ten-minute delay! We even saw an entertaining movie on each leg of the journey. The weather in Maui was superb. Truly a paradise. This is where I have gone to heal in the past, so I knew the lay of the island. I plotted the trip to include many of the different aspects and ecosystems of this amazing little island, hoping to make the most of our eight days.

The first day, we stayed in a hotel on the beach in Kaanapali (a tourist mecca). There the sand is white, the turquoise water is warm, and the waves are gentle. We climbed into our wonderful convertible rental car and got a tan while driving along the north coast, past fields of pineapple and breathtaking views. We found a great beach, with perfect, curling four-foot waves. We had fun "surfing" with our new boogie boards, then went back to shower before our scheduled Luau experience.

Unfortunately, as Marley was getting out of the shower, he slipped on the wet tile floor. His naked, wet body hit the tile hard and he yelled from his depth. It was a sound I hope will soon leave my soul. I can't fathom the pain he must have felt. He said it felt like the prosthesis in his knee had pulled out of the hole drilled in his femur as it bent sideways. This mechanism is designed to bend up and down, not side to side.

Catie and I made a temporary bed for him right there on the bathroom floor. A thousand thoughts flew through my head. Was the knee surgery done properly in the first place? Do I call 911? Do I drive him to the hospital to get an X-ray? Should we just pack up and catch the next plane home? Or should we forget panicking and just relax and go to the Luau as planned? The worst part was, I couldn't dose him with painkillers 'cause I needed to know how bad it was. I could have screamed as I watched all the physical therapy of the last month slip down the drain. Welcome to our "vacation."

We decided to just calm down, move Mars to the bed, and assess the damage done. In the meantime, I notified the hotel manager and filled out their accident form, just in case. We ended up going to the Luau—at Marley's request—and we actually had a good time. We had the use of the hotel's wheelchair while we enjoyed the incredible food and dramatic entertainment.

The second day wasn't so much fun. Marley's mood was foul—he was mad at everything and everyone in his path. We went to Lahaina—Maui's oldest tourist town, filled with restaurants and art galleries. (This excursion was a dumb idea on my part—oh well, live and learn.) We did, however, go to an amazing magic show that evening, which helped his outlook. On day three, we went to Goodwill to get some crutches and checked into the historic Pioneer Hotel in the heart of Lahaina. Day four: We set up camp at a great campground right on the beach. We had fun, until…Marley caught a wave wrong while body surfing, and jarred his shoulder. Now, his right knee *and* his right shoulder hurt. He couldn't use his crutches to take the pressure off his knee, because the crutch put too much pressure on his shoulder. Damn!

I was about ready to scrap the trip at this point, but the kids wanted to continue. So on day five, we broke camp early and drove to Hana, on the east side of the island. Driving the Hana highway felt like a two-hour carnival ride as we monotonously wound in and out on a thin road we had to share with oncoming traffic. Fortunately, the scenery was so majestic, it took our minds off our stomachs and brains sloshing from one side to the other. High lush cliffs and waterfalls were on one side, while on the other, sheer rocky cliffs disappeared into the crashing, smashing waves far below.

Marley was a trooper, but on the sixth morning, he admitted he couldn't camp anymore—it just hurt too much. So, after relaxing on a beautiful black sand beach, we once again survived the Hana highway to make our way back to the civilized south side of the island. Our hotel had a superior ocean view. We had our own little beach, 20 feet from the room, a cool pool, and swaying palms—the whole bit. Marley laid low for the remainder of the trip, watching "Bay Watch–Hawaii" and "Walker Texas Ranger," while eating endless pizza. Catie and I went exploring, shopping, and swimming.

The grand finale, on our eighth day, was a boat trip on an enormous catamaran. We sailed to Molokini, a small island that is the exposed rim of a volcanic crater. We watched migrating whales and saw sea turtles swimming right next to the boat. We snorkeled for a few hours and saw millions of colorful fish and coral.

It filled me with pride to share the ocean world that I had grown up with. It was like going back home. Catie was glued to my side like a remora to a shark. My heart swelled and memories filled my soul. It was just like the way I used to stick by my dad's side while snorkeling. Being next to him in that watery underworld is what I think of when I need to feel safe during this perilous journey I call my life. I hope she feels as safe by my side as I did by my dad's.

Make a Wish

While we were in Maui, Drew told us that the Make-A-Wish Foundation had finally come through with their promise. A shiny new Kawasaki Mule (a powerful flatbed, four-wheeled, ATV-like vehicle) was waiting for Marley at Drew's. While in Maui, Marley lost the full use of his right arm, but after this bit of good news, instead of whining, he spent his time designing a ball to attach to the steering wheel of the Mule. He figured if he has one of these balls, he can drive with only one arm. That's what I love about Marley.

One foot in front of the other, we'll figure out what the next steps are: more radiation, more surgery? Tomorrow.... Sometimes not panicking is a very healthy thing. Today we concentrate on the beauty of spring, new beginnings, and growing things. Trust. I simply trust. Everything is as it should be.

I pray I am given the wisdom of the Great Mystery to guide my children on their journey so they can feel the massive amounts of love available to them. Then I know they will have the tools to bravely cross the threshold from life to death. I hope they will die knowing they've lived whole.

I hope you will help me. Hold your palm open. While you do that, wish that I am able let go, able to wrench my heart open and feel and express my emotions. Wish that I can learn to be like Marley; taking that next breath, that next step, and doing whatever it takes to keep living my best... until it's time not to anymore. Now blow your wish off your palm and know that it will come true.

I'm pleased to be a part of your circle, a part of this miracle. I thank Marley for bringing us all together.

Blessings,
Jennifer

P.S. Marley's tutor Kathy thinks a video camera would be a grand tool to help Marley do his upcoming report on the Colestin Valley. She also gracefully hinted we should record these precious days with the Marley Man. She's absolutely right, but I know nothing about these cameras. Anyone willing to help with research?

"Live to the point of tears."

— Camus

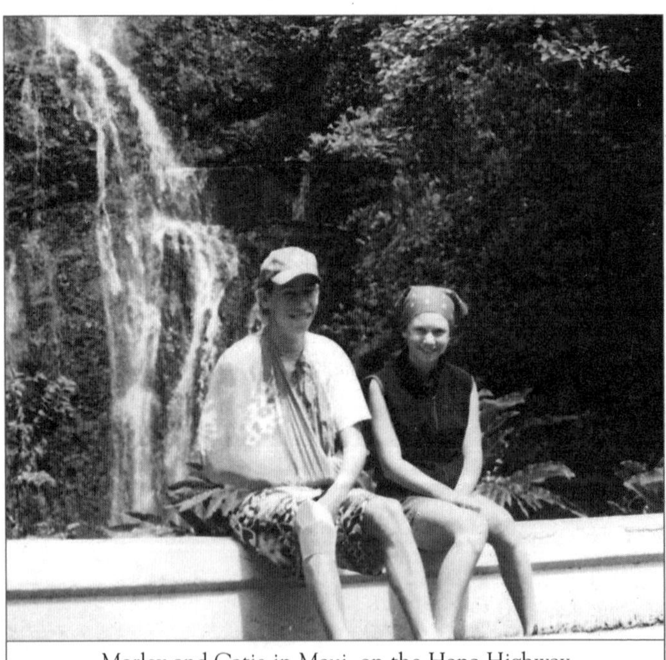

Marley and Catie in Maui, on the Hana Highway

MAKE A WISH

Patience

There are several wish-granting organizations that cater to kids with serious illnesses. Examples of common wishes: a new computer system, meeting a favorite celebrity, a trip to Disney World, or to have their bedroom remodeled. Eligibility, rules, and the wishes granted vary, depending on the organization. Many of them, like Make-A-Wish Foundation, require verification listing the kid's condition as "life-threatening" or "terminal." There are a few organizations that don't require imminent death to grant a dream. Our lives were radically changed by having Marley's wish granted, and I'm extremely thankful these foundations exist.

The guidelines for Make-A-Wish Foundation seemed pretty simple at first. Proving that Marley had a "terminal" illness was not an issue. Marley knew he wanted an All Terrain Vehicle (ATV)—one that was fast and BIG! Once the paperwork was complete, it was our job to wait. Waiting had never been Marley's strong suit. Drew and Cindy were the ones who filled out all the forms, did all the follow-up, and suffered the brunt of Marley's whining. As payment, I agreed the ATV should stay at their house. (After my experience with the go-cart, I had no problem with this.) It took many months, phone calls, and endless hours of being put on hold and talking to clueless representatives before Drew was finally told that the delay was because they do not grant wishes that could be dangerous to the recipient.

Plan B

Drew found an alternative vehicle, a Kawasaki Mule. A Mule is safe, rides lower than a regular ATV, has four wheels, and has a steering wheel instead of handlebars (like a golf cart). The new request was resubmitted and the waiting game started once again...much to Marley's chagrin. In his mind, the hoops we adults jumped through on a continual basis were a perfect definition of insanity.

Eight months after the process had begun, Drew was informed

that they needed a written request for this most unusual "last wish" directly from Marley…in his own handwriting. We all moaned. Marley didn't know how to write. This seemed an insurmountable mountain to climb. Marley worked hard on this project. He wanted this Mule—and he wanted it bad enough to jump through a fiery hoop.

One month after that, just as Marley was preparing to have his knee replaced, Make-A-Wish said they had paperwork that needed to be notarized. Another month after that, Drew was notified that the request had been granted, if, and only if, a form was signed releasing the Foundation from any liability. Yeah, yeah…another big hoop, complete with flames. After much cursing and head banging, this form was drafted, signed, and witnessed by a lawyer (at our expense).

"Once you hear the details of a victory, it is hard to distinguish it from a defeat."

—Jean-Paul Sartre

Another month after that, Drew was told Marley's new Mule was going to be ceremonially presented at the Kawasaki dealership in Dreadford. Drew, Cindy, and I nearly slithered out of our skin with excitement, but Marley had been disappointed so many times that we kept it to ourselves. On the big day, Marley and Catie were with me. I made up a story about needing to go to a store near the Kawasaki dealership. I said Jay, Selene, Jeff, and Liz were coming with us. Marley and Catie thought a group shopping trip was a little weird but, then again, I'm weird and they knew it.

When I drove past the turnoff to the store, Catie yelled, "Mom, you missed it! How could you miss it?"

I faked embarrassment and said, "No worries, we'll just turn around up here." Marley's eagle eye spotted Drew's truck and horse trailer parked at Kawasaki. I asked innocently, "Hmmmm. What do you suppose he's doing there? Let's go find out."

Marley started quivering in the seat next to me. Catie wanted to go shopping and groaned about the delay, while Marley flew out of our rig, grabbed Jay, and took him inside to browse. Drew pulled me aside and blew off some steam about how this supposedly seamless transaction was hopelessly unraveling. The Make-A-Wish rep hadn't arrived and, apparently, she hadn't notified the dealership. We could taste another disappointment heading our way. I switched gears and told Marley that Drew and Cindy were in Dreadford with the horse trailer because they were on their way to buy lumber. Yeah right! (It was the best story I could come up with on short notice.) Anyway, Marley kept his mouth shut and had a grand time drooling over all the Kawasaki toys.

The representative finally showed up, and Drew pounced on her to find out why the Mule wasn't on-site. Drew informed me, through clenched teeth, "Apparently there was a communications error and no one told Kawasaki to have the Mule ready so this…this…*woman* could ceremonially give the damned thing to Marley." There was nothing left to do but go shopping.

Another month after that (we're talkin' April—one year from the initial contact), Marley got a call from Drew while we were in Maui. Poor Drew wasn't taking any chances on a repeat performance, so he waited until the Mule was actually parked in his driveway to tell Marley his wish had been granted.

Gratitude

Drew worked really hard to give Marley the ultimate gift, and he was rewarded for his perseverance. The experience was a hassle. It tested the limits of our patience; we feared that Marley would die before he got his wish. But in the end, Marley was ecstatic, probably more thrilled than if the process had been simple and quick. Maybe there really is a higher power that knew exactly what Marley needed to hang on to life just a little longer.

"There is no medicine like hope,
no incentive so great, and no tonic so powerful
as expectation of something tomorrow."

—Orison Swett Marden

The Mule was exactly what Marley needed. It had a flatbed that could haul bales of hay, dogs, and an assortment of people. It had the size, power, and stability to go where other vehicles wouldn't dare explore. And…it was safe! It had a bench seat that fit three skinny people, two of which could be seat-belted. The reality was, safety wasn't the point; Marley's last wish was. If Marley had died driving the Mule, I knew he would have died happy—really happy.

The Make-A-Wish Foundation will forever receive our undying gratitude for buying Marley an incredibly expensive, big boy toy that gave him much joy and independence. We had no idea that Marley's future mobility and status as one of the Colestin Coyotes would depend on this rig.

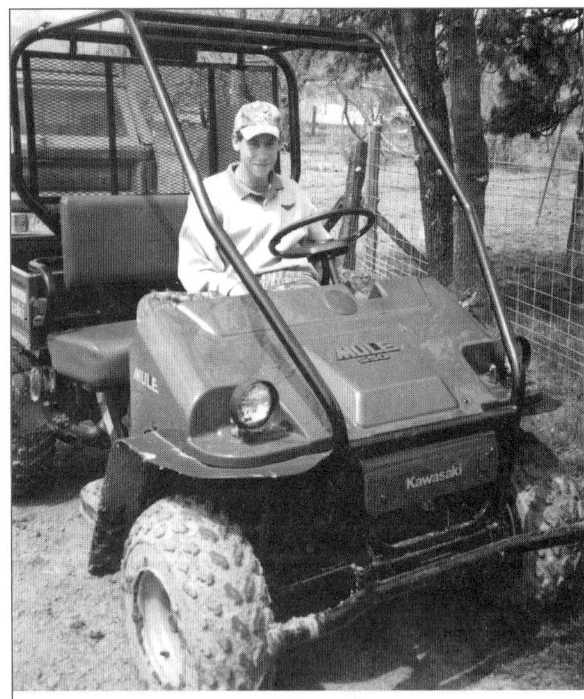

Marley on his brand new Kawasaki Mule
Photo: Cindy Warzyn

Tuesday, May 8, 2001
Subject: "HEALING"

Hi Gang!

Just checking in to let you know what's shakin'.

Marley is in his last week of radiation for the tumor in his shoulder. We didn't have the option to do surgery on that part of the body, because they haven't yet invented a replacement part for that particular bone. Even if we could, too many surgeries too fast could do more damage than good. So we'll sit tight with nuking the cancerous bone tissue with radiation.

Meanwhile, the knee is healing slowly. It can loosen up only as much as this beloved, stubborn 16-year-old will force movement in the joint. As it turned out, the fall in the bathroom in Maui broke the adhesions that had prevented him from bending his knee. Okay, so it hurt a little, but he gained many degrees of flexibility.

All we need to work on now is the straightening of his leg. I joke about waiting until he's relaxed with his leg outstretched on the coffee table, and then jumping on his knee to break more adhesions. Hmmmm. An evil fantasy!

His new best friend is of course his Kawasaki Mule. I'm told they're inseparable. The kids come back to me on Friday, and poor Marley will have to do without it for two whole weeks. Maybe it's time for him to try school again!!!!!!

Catie is jazzed to be going to middle school next year, and we're busy trying to plan summer activities so she doesn't go nuts. In the meantime, wish us luck!

Love you all,
Jennifer

The Butterfly Effect

THE BIRTH OF THE COYOTES
by Lucas Morgan, age 15

One morning, I was awakened by my alarm clock. It was six o'clock. While making breakfast, I felt I needed to get something done. So I got on my quad and rode. Sunglasses on, the wind flowing through my hair. The sun was two and a half hours over Pilot Rock—its radiation beaming through the atmosphere in such a way that the valley's hills shone like seashells on the shore. After riding all day, I decided to pay a visit to my old friend, John.

As I was riding up his driveway, I saw a Kawasaki Mule enter the road ahead. I passed it and the two men standing in the back waved, and the young man in the driver's seat tipped his hat. I thought to myself, "Isn't that, that Marley guy? I hear he's got lung cancer or somthin' like that." I wave, not knowing that this older teen would have the biggest impact on my life since the death of my father.

After my visit with John, I was riding down the driveway and I saw three figures walking up the road. Two stood straight while one kind of limped and hobbled to the side of the road. I asked them, "Any trouble?" The teen said, "Weew thtuck in a mud ho and we weuw gonna get sum halp from Johnny." I said, "I can tow you out." And he replied, "I dunno. Ya think that fuckew can pool out my Mule?" I looked at my quad and said, "Aw, hell ya."

When we got back to his rig, I could see it wasn't stuck too bad and I pulled him out after only a little struggle. After working, I hung out with them for a while. He told me his name was Marley and introduced the men that were with him as Jay and JD. I was amazed at how much this guy had to say, and I was already starting to like him.

He had me follow him up the road to his house. On the front porch, there was a man with a weather-beaten face and a red mountain-man style mustache wearing a big worn-out cowboy hat, standing in the doorway. He said to Marley, "Well, who's the guy on the four-wheeler?" Marley yelled, "That's Lucas!" After greeting this man named Drew, I met Marley's three sisters.

I noticed that these girls were very, very beautiful! Vanessa: With a playfulness in her voice that would bring the strongest man into a weep of pleasure. Laura: With a soft shy appearance. But when talking to her, I noticed a mysterious beauty that lives in her heart. Catie: With a royal and elegant charm. Her golden-green eyes burned through my body like the warmth of the sun in the canyons on an August day. A few weeks later, Marley brought me to his other house where I met his mother and discovered that Catie had her same eyes.

It didn't take long before my uncle, who was the fire chief, got all of us teenagers to do the fire training for the Colestin Volunteer Fire Department. The first night, before we had the meeting at the church down the hill, we met for dinner at the little restaurant in Hilt. In the Mule, Marley and I followed the line of cars heading for the meeting. It was dusk, so the high plain's scenery was bathed in a dark orange color. My Uncle Steve looked up the hill toward the Mule. All he could see was the silhouette of the buggy, me, and Marley with his cowboy hat on. My uncle said to my sister Andrea, who was standing next him, "Those coyotes!" Those are the famous words that made Marley, our best buddy, Luke, and me "THE COYOTES."

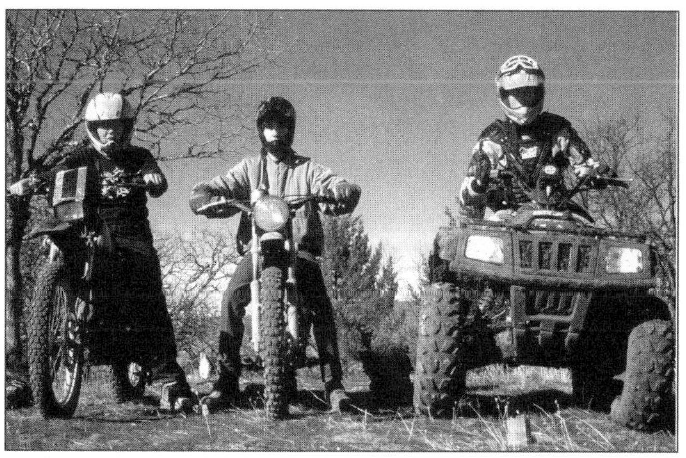

Luke, Lucas, and Marley ready for action!

Photo: Jay Newman

Saturday, May 26, 2001
Subject: "SUMMER PLANS"

Greetings all,

As you've probably figured out by now, no news from me is usually good news.

Marley keeps cruising through life. A few weeks ago, he completed the round of radiation aimed at the tumor in his shoulder. The effects (low energy) are just now wearing off. He looks good, his attitude is much better, and no new tumors have shown up. Thank God.

Now all he needs to do is continue to work his knee so he can run, jump, and ride his bikes. It's going to take hard work and lots more physical therapy which, I might add, he's not too thrilled about. Surprise, surprise!

Summer is just around the corner. Planning for this time is rather daunting for me, and I could use some help. Creative mothering, under these circumstances, and while trying to work, scares me. I seriously don't think I can do this alone. The first half of the summer is covered. My brother Tim and his family are visiting from New Zealand just after school lets out. We have fun things planned in July, including a circus camp for Catie, a trip to the Oregon Country Fair, and visiting with my sister Julia, who is coming from North Carolina.

August and September is when it will be critical for me to have support, because it will be crunch time again at the BRI. We'll be finishing this year's 522-page book. My kids are always sorely neglected during deadline. I want this summer to be far better than last year's disaster. Help!

Anyway…I love you all and hope that your summer is all that you dream of.

Jennifer

THERAPY SUCKS

Under Pressure

Sometimes it's a good thing to heal remarkably fast, and sometimes it's not. Throughout Marley's life, whenever he cut himself or wiped out on his bike, I was always amazed at how fast his wounds healed. It was like he had aloe running through his veins. The downside to this was he also scarred more than the rest of us. His hands were crisscrossed with scars that never faded. When he was little, whenever doctors were investigating his unusual disorders, I always tried to highlight his speed-healing as an example of Marley's oddities. No one thought this weird little clue was important enough to pay any attention to.

After all of his other surgeries, his unusual ability to rapidly heal was of great benefit. It meant in no time he was up and around, bouncing off walls and jumping his bike. It was a good thing, making all of his caretakers proud (as if we had something to do with it). But the knee was a different matter. His body saw the prosthesis as a foreign object and did its best to create scar tissue around the metal hinge. Physical therapy was critically important because it kept the joint flexible as his body tried to heal itself—keeping the army of cells from creating thick tissues (*adhesions*) between the moving parts.

I think even if Marley did do everything he was told, the mobility in his knee still would have been limited. But *this* we'll never know, because if you add a lackluster desire to exercise with a system that heals double-time, you get a battle with nature. The fall he took in Maui might have been a saving grace. If he hadn't broken the adhesions in the early stages of healing, he might have a knee that couldn't bend at all. The trick was to keep his knee flexible without killing him in the process!

He hated doing physical therapy. It was almost worse than school. Fortunately, he loved George, his therapist...well...um, he loved George, the human, but passionately hated George, the therapist. If Marley saw George in the grocery store, he'd hop-run over to him and give him a giant hug, but when George greeted him at his office three times a week, Marley would growl and nip at him like a mad dog. It was so embarrassing. I always felt sorry for George.

The weather was glorious, and Marley wanted to be riding his bike, not visiting George. Marley would stick his fingers in his ears when I'd say, "The fastest way to get back on your bike is to do whatever George tells you to do." I might as well have been convincing a circus lion that his cage is protecting him from all the nasty people. I felt like the mother in the *Peanuts* cartoon that never said anything other than "Wa, wah, wa, wa, wah." Every time I dropped Marley off at George's, he'd pick from any of the following responses, "Blah, blah, blah!" "Yeah right!" or "Whatever!" We were lucky if that's where the "conversation" ended. Usually, it was just the beginning of a verbal skirmish.

"Come on, Marley, you know you have to work the knee or it'll never be able to bend." I'd blunder ahead, "If your leg stays stiff and you have to keep rotating your hip like you do, your back is going to get totally screwed up. I've been there. When your back hurts, everything hurts."

He'd bite back, "Evewything alweddy hurts, Mom. So what else is new? This isn't helping. It just pisses me off. You just want to see me suffer mowa, is that it?" He knew just what buttons to push.

I'd launch into some silly argument like, "Give me a break! Sometimes we all have to do things we don't want to." (Translation: "Wah, wa, wa, wah, wah!")

Little did I know that while falling prey to these parking lot battles, I was helping to make his therapy session with George a little shorter. After I realized Marley's intelligent tactic, I felt really stupid. I had to hand it to him.

No Rest for the Weary

Marley was full of surprises that spring. Maybe I was just noticing more of them because this was the slow time at work and I was focusing my attention more on the kids. One day I went back in their little den at work to check on them. Catie was making cards with the laminating machine and Marley was sawing a slit in the top of an oversized clear plastic bottle that popcorn had come in. When I asked what he was doing, he said he was making a donation holder for his rest home idea.

When Marley had first gone into the hospital a year and a half earlier, the folks that ran the Hilt store in the Colestin Valley put a plastic jar next to the register for people to put donations in. (Hilt is the name of a "town" on the California–Oregon border. The Hilt store and the owners' home behind it make up this town.) It's the only store in the Colestin Valley, and this is where everybody swaps gossip about everyone else in the valley. It's a gas station, liquor store, and old-timey soda fountain and grill. The owners loved Marley and knew they had the perfect spot to gather donations for Marley's benefit. More than a thousand dollars were collected in loose change, from thousands of travelers who took the time to help a kid they'd never meet. From this experience, Marley knew the concept and hoped the bottle-bank project he was working on might actually help.

He hadn't mentioned the rest home idea for a long time. He didn't see the need to talk about something just to talk about it. He figured he needed to take matters in his own hands and start collecting the funds for the down payment on the property. "What property?" I asked him. He responded, "Dunno yet. When it comes up for sale, we'll be weddy."

Therapy comes in all shapes and sizes—sometimes I forgot that emotional therapy was far more important than physical therapy. He didn't care much about his knee being as stiff and gnarly as an old fence post. Why bother? He didn't have to depend on his bike anymore, he had the Mule. If he wanted to run, he could. It looked a little funny—but do you think he cared?

"I am not dying, not anymore than any of us are at any moment. We run, hopefully as fast as we can, and then everyone must stop. We can only choose how we handle the race."

—Hugh Elliott

Monday, June 11, 2001
Subject: "PLAYTIME"

• From: Selene

Dear ones,

I am about to embark on a grand adventure to Mt. Olympus and back, including many points between. I wanted to touch base before I disappear for two months. Not that I've been all that present lately.

Last weekend I went out to visit Marley and Catie at their dad's house in the Colestin and was met by Marley and his Mule on the road. He was just chillin' on the edge of a field, gazing out across the valley at the mountains beyond. He had been putting some finishing touches on a video project for school, and I was struck by how grown up and settled he is. If this journey has done anything for both Marley and Catie, it is to spirit both of them into a raging and beautiful groundedness.

I was blown away that day by their compassion and vision and presence. But more than that, by their sweetness. Marley and I went on a kick-ass ride through the woods to a gorgeous stream. We just sat and talked about how beautiful it was there.

So to me, they feel good. Despite fears surrounding the healing of Marley's knee, there is a humor and lightness to him. And I literally can't say enough about how wondrous Catie is to me, as a cousin and a friend. And Jennifer…I won't even try, because I know you know.

There are a billion families in the world, and I admit this is only one, but I am convinced that if the world were to go dark, and all lights were extinguished, together their circle would glow and light up the edges of the leaves on the trees and the bugs on the ground. And scattered across the country, all of us would give off a faint illumination too, having fed their light and ingested it ourselves.

Go swiftly into the space and brilliance of summer and send prayers out while you play. Play! *That*, I think, is the best way to create healing now, for everyone.

Blessings and love,
Selene

"America is an enormous frosted cupcake in the middle of millions of starving people."

—Gloria Steinem

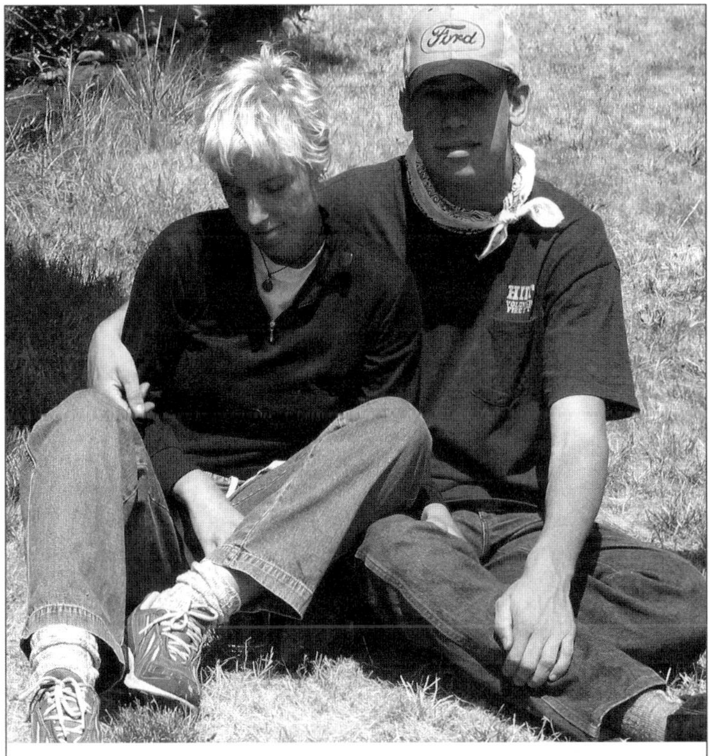

Selene and Marley

Photo: Mandy Little

SEEING IS BELIEVING

Pointed in the Right Direction

Following the advice of Marley's tutor, I did end up getting a video camera that spring. I figured I would use it to get as much of Marley on film as possible. But I never got a chance to use the thing. Marley scooped it up and started working with it like a pro from the start. I always hated it when he did that. I sat next to him reading the instruction book and I looked up at him to see if he was paying attention. By the time I had gotten to the part about how to install the battery, he was all set and ready to go.

As his final project for his freshman year at high school, he used the camera to film his report on the Colestin Valley. I didn't pay much attention to the process because he did this whole thing with his tutor Kathy, and it was all done while he was at Drew's house. Kathy had told me how talented and focused he was. Then his teacher called and invited us to the last of three school presentations. He was shocked by what Marley had created and how well he was presenting it.

Marley had posters with a timeline of the Colestin Valley, dating back to the 1860's. He couldn't read, so he must have memorized everything he pointed to as he told us of the Colestin's remarkable history—a story of a thriving town, owned by the Dole corporation, that disappeared overnight, leaving barely a trace.

I was amazed. He had a really good eye for both photography and filming. I left his school thinking of possibilities; all we had to do was to give him the right tools and a subject that he loved. Other than making stuff with duct tape and putzing around with bike parts, photography became the closest thing Marley had to a hobby. He was inspired, which thrilled me to no end, because it gave me hope there was actually something that he might be able to make a living at—if he stayed alive long enough to have to worry about money.

"What does education often do?
It makes a straight-cut ditch of a free, meandering brook."

—Henry David Thoreau

THE OREGON COUNTRY FAIR

The Rites of Freedom

My non-kin family join the kids and me in celebration of as many rites as possible. We celebrate Halloween, a few Christian holidays; Thanksgiving and Christmas, as well as Pagan holidays; Beltane (May Day), spring and autumnal equinoxes, and summer and winter solstices. None of us are drawn to any particular religion, but there is one annual event that I consider the closest thing in my life to a religious event.

On the second weekend of every July, 10,000 people, young and old, join me in celebrating the freedom to dance and be different. The Oregon Country Fair is special—there's nothing else like it, anywhere. Drew and I discovered it the first year we moved to Oregon. We packed up our six-month-old baby Marley and stepped into another world, filled with tie-dye, mud-covered bodies, and elaborate costumes. This community, which exists solely for this three-day event, caters to musicians, artists, inventors, and earth lovers. It is not a Rainbow Gathering, Renaissance Faire, or County Fair. It is all of the above and beyond.

The Country Fair is located in the woods and is completely kid friendly. The layout is a giant figure 8 with semi-permanent structures and tree houses that line a wide dirt path on both sides. Stages, booths, food vendors, and performers of all varieties take up every square inch on either side of the path. There's only one way in or out and it doesn't matter where you are, there's always something mind boggling to watch and fun things to play with. There's no way to remain an observer—everyone, in their own right, becomes a performer.

When Marley was little, he would prepare for the Country Fair by packing up a red wagon full of rocks, trucks, stuffed animals, and toys. While I and baby Catie would be dancing to the endless line-up of great music, Marley would be displaying his goods on a blanket, inviting everyone to barter with him. At the end of the day, he would pull his red wagon all the way to our campground and show me all the new stuff he received during the day of trading. It was pretty cool. No one else did this, and he could spend all day interacting with "strangers" doing something that his language skills didn't interfere with.

Alter-abled

One of the reasons Marley loved the Country Fair was he was never seen as handicapped. No one looked at him like he was strange—everyone was strange. At this event, the emphasis was on the freedom to express. Marley could wear the most outlandish combination of clothing; bark, growl, or lovingly nuzzle strangers; and no one would question him. He was accepted for who he was and he loved it. In the past, there was nothing that really set Marley apart from the other participants. But this year, he was obviously handicapped (or as the folks there call it, "alter-abled").

It had been a rough summer and the boy was not going to sit by and watch fun slip away. He was determined to go to the Oregon Country Fair even if he had to maneuver around the rough terrain in a wheelchair. "Don't worry, Mom, just bwring some pain-killas for me." Whenever I doubted the intelligence of doing this two-day extravaganza, Marley would poke me in the ribs and say, "I'm only gonna live once, Mommy, be bwave. Live dan-gaously!"

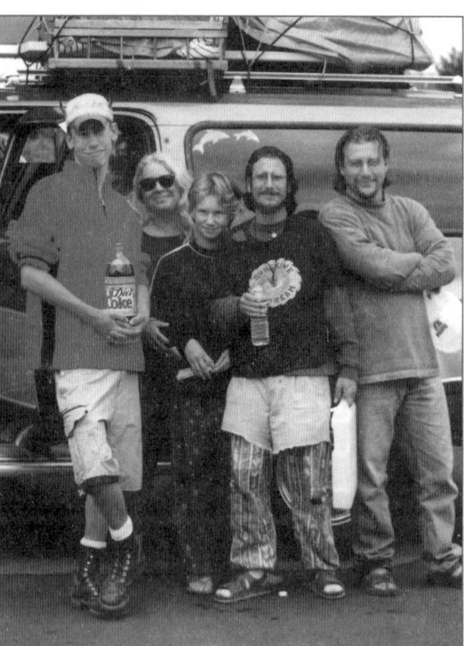

Marley, Andrea, Catie, Jay, and Jeff—ready for action!

Andrea, Jeff, Jay, Catie, Marley, and I piled into "Indy," the Suburban, with all of our camping gear on the roof and the manual wheelchair strapped on the back. We were ready for an adventure and Marley was leading the way.

Because this event takes place in the middle of our very hot and dry summers, all of the pathways are sprayed with water to reduce the dust. Which, of course, makes mud. On the wooded paths that were inaccessible to water trucks, they laid thick layers of straw instead. Marley discovered that his wheelchair tires had absolutely no traction on the straw and that it covered protruding roots. With great enthusiasm, Jay pushed Marley at a run along the path until they hit the first hidden root with the chair's footrests. The wheelchair stopped dead in its path and Marley was nearly catapulted out of his seat as Jay slammed into the back of the chair. As disastrous as that could have been, the rest of us couldn't stop laughing at their antics. We all had our turn doing similar stunts, and the laughter soon turned to cursing.

Marley managed most of the day on his own steam, which took incredible amounts of upper body strength. Toward the end of the day, after the paths had been repeatedly sprayed, Marley's main issue occurred when he was cruising along and would hit a mud hole. The lurching motion was painful, and the crowd behind him would all bump into each other trying to stop fast. It also took great effort to avoid colliding with baby strollers or gouging holes in people's ankles with the metal footrests.

We were all exhausted that first night. Marley took advantage of his painkillers as soon as we got to the campsite. It was then I discovered something about drugs and Marley. When Marley was in fourth grade, we had tried giving him Ritalin to calm him down and help him focus. The theory being, if you give speed to a speedy person, they slow down. It worked great, but Mars rejected the drug after two weeks because the new-found clarity confused him. The opposite rule seemed to apply for downers. After taking a Vicodin, Marley babbled nonstop about miscellaneous engine parts, the speed of an 100,000 horsepowered snowmobile, and the damage a .7,000 calibre bullet would inflict.

In preparation for the second day, Marley decided the dangers and hassles that came with the wheelchair's attached foot- and armrests weren't worth it, so he stripped the chair down to the basics. There were pros and cons to this choice, but Marley made a smart decision. He moved swifter and safer through the crowds, often maneuvering only on his back wheels. People would point at him spinning and rolling along doing wheelies and think he was a part of some act. He was a ham and loved showing off his strength. The down side to the decision: He had to support his bad leg with his good leg crossed under it, acting as the footrest. He was one tired puppy on the final night. When he asked for a painkiller, I decided to split it in half, spreading out the effects. We had a great time. The pleasures were well worth the pains. On the way home, we all talked about how much we we looking forward to next year's adventure at the Oregon Country Fair.

***"As a well-spent day brings happy sleep,
so life well used brings happy death."***

—Leonardo da Vinci

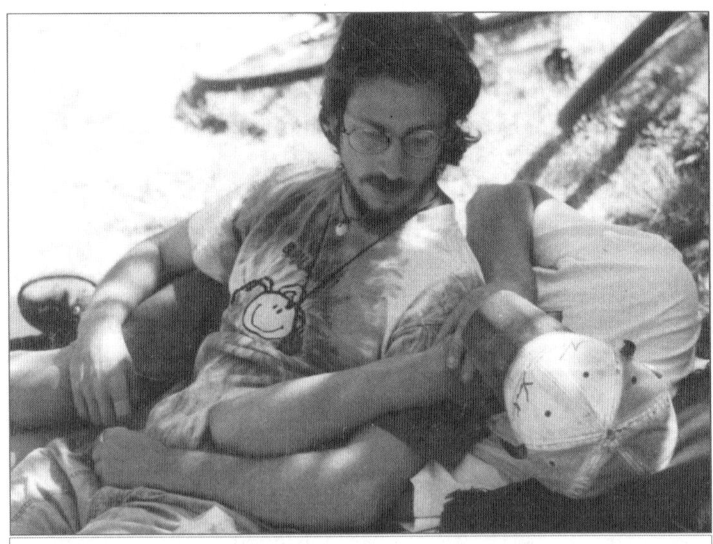

Jay and Marley (with horns) hanging out at the Country Fair 2001

Chapter Ten: Between a Rock and a Hard Place

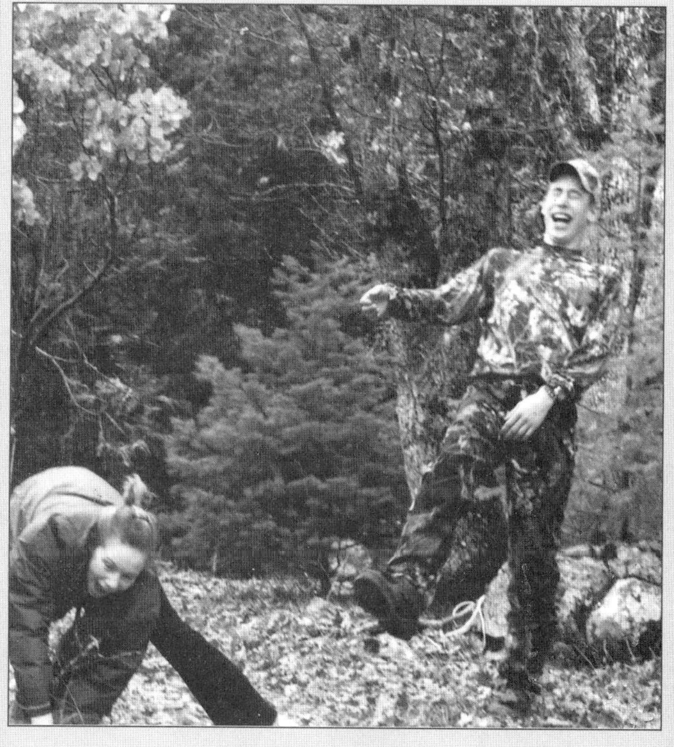

Fall 2001
Catie's landing after trying to jump into Marley's arms.... He dropped her!

Photo: Jennifer

Monday, August 20, 2001
Subject: "SUMMER'S END"

Hi Y'all,

After dealing with one tumor after another for so long, it's turned out to be a wonderful summer vacation. The last major update was in May, right after the tumor in his shoulder was nuked. Marley is now 16.5 years old, 6'2" tall, and weighs in at almost 150 lbs! It's been a long haul to get back to the weight he started with last year. He is some kind of skinny, but damn, he looks good.

SUMMER FUN

He's been busy dawn to dusk putzing around on his Kawasaki Mule, visiting and helping neighbors while at Drew's. He loves the freedom of mobility while he's there. It's not so easy when he's with me, especially after his mountain bike was ripped off. (His shorter stunt bike is difficult to use because he can't bend his knee well.)

In July, he did an amazing job of maneuvering around in his wheelchair on dirt and gravel amongst 10,000 crazed people at the Oregon Country Fair in Eugene. We just returned from a two-day journey to Redding, California, where we picked Catie up after she went to Las Vegas to see Cirque de Soleil with my sister Constant. We also had a great week-long visit with my brother Tim and his family, who were visiting from New Zealand. And in July, my sister Julia flew out from North Carolina to hang with the kids. Julia always shows up at just the right time and does all the right things.

And last, but certainly not least, we had the opportunity to do The Edge—a challenging, day-long wilderness rite of passage located at the same place where Marley did the Ropes Course. Shianna, one of the guides, also works at the high school and has taken a sincere liking to Marley because of the way he is dealing with his life. She and her husband Dean offered their services to our family and the crew at the BRI. It was perfect! I had done this event several times before, but never just with my closest folk. It was such an amazing day I'm compelled to describe it.

Indy proved her four-wheeling ability as we drove straight up a mountain on mud-washed, rocky trails. We parked in a beautiful meadow just below the wall of rock where this event took place. Before we made the slow climb up the cliff (The Edge), we shared our fears about the challenge before us—leaning out over a cliff, a mirror of the fears we have in our lives about scary things we face. It was most touching when Catie—the one who usually keeps it so together—simply lost it and wept, sharing her fears about experiencing Marley in so much pain and being unable to do anything to help him. There wasn't a dry eye in the circle.

The climb up to the cliff was a stretch for Marley—it was dangerous and it was painful—but he *had* to reach The Edge (his edge). Ahhhh! Imagine standing at the top of a 60-foot cliff with your toes just at the edge of it with a beautiful valley below, mountains looming on all sides, and hawks flying *below* you. Close your eyes and listen. All you hear is the wind in the trees behind you. You're wearing a harness attached with two safety lines in the rear which are secured at two trees. There's no obstruction and nothing to grab on to in order to feel safe. The other participants sit in silence behind you on the hill, witnessing your process from a respectful distance.

Are you ready? Inhale. If you are, say, "Go." Your guide feeds out the line so you begin to lean forward over the edge. Say "STOP" when it gets so scary you can't breathe and your legs become jelly. You worry about looking dumb, even though you know everyone behind you loves you. Breathe, figure out how to relax. Screw looking bad, all of a sudden, when you fear most that you're going to die, find a hidden well of courage and

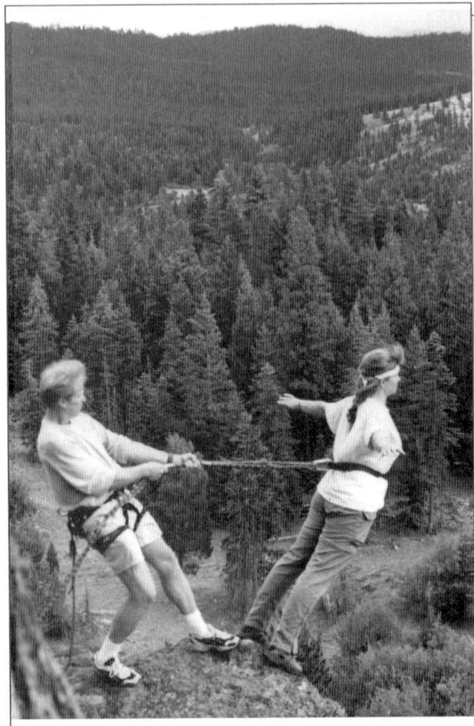
Dean and Shianna at The Edge

then say, "MORE!" You let go and lean into your fear. Take your time, lean as far out as you can handle. No. Further than that! Spread your arms wide and feel the incredible sense of freedom. Pray, yell, cry, or simply breathe. Feel the uncompromising strength of experiencing total lack of control. When you're ready to stop, just say, "Edge!" Then be received by those that love you and have witnessed your courage.

PHYSICAL UPDATE

It's been seven months since Marley had his knee replaced. He was in physical therapy until the last tumor in his shoulder showed up. I think he feels defeated, as well as tired, and he lost all desire to work his knee (not that he had much to begin with). He still cannot straighten his leg, which makes for a major limp. The limping is stressing the hip to the point that he's now feeling pain shooting down his leg (pinched nerve?). But it also hurts to the touch on the flat of the right pelvis (new tumor?). He can't use crutches because his shoulder has started hurting again (another tumor?). Aaaarrrrghhhhh!

Last week, he finally agreed to get X-rays. He said he didn't want to because if anything new showed up, he feared he wouldn't be able to go to school in a few weeks. He REALLY wants to be around other kids again. The X-rays were inconclusive (terrible shots) so he's going in on Wednesday for an MRI which should show us what's causing the pain.

CURRENT STATE OF AFFAIRS

Marley keeps going like the Energizer bunny. Most times we don't notice him wincing in pain. He keeps challenging the edge. His desire to move and be active outweighs the pain, but he pays a price for pushing himself so hard. After a long day, especially during the last few weeks, it's hard to avoid his growling, cursing, and moaning. The boy has definitely been hurting and it's hard to watch. The pain is wearing him down. He complains that he's falling apart slowly as he hops to the nearest place to lie down, exhausted.

He wants to hug and be close. He wants people near him. He wants to talk about his bike-riding days as if they're still happening and how much fun it is to hang with friends even though his friends haven't been around much (except for our neighbor Ben). The most consistent complaint is, "I'm bored!" Yet, he doesn't want to develop new skills. Life is simply too hard. It's frustrating for us all.

MAGIC HAPPENS

My experience leads me to believe that what I have been taught about magic is true. The three stages of creating magic are: 1) Identify the desired outcome, 2) Concisely speak the desire, and 3) Do something physical to symbolically make the desire tangible. (Think it. Speak it. Do it). Making a toast is a good example of this process.

Problems usually occur in the first stage—identifying the desire. Assuming that what is desired will become manifest, then we need to pay close attention to what we ask for. Let's say we pray incredibly hard for speedy healing. In response, could his body actually try too hard to heal a stainless steel knee, seeing it as a "foreign object," creating adhesions too great to break? Or what happens if praying for a long life isn't in his best interest, causing prolonged misery? Gulp. Because I know this to be a powerful group of magic makers, I now ask that all of us take note of the importance of our words and be conscious of what we are trying to create.

For Marley, I have personally started to pray for grace and acceptance of Right Action on the highest level. I ask that he feel little or no pain. For Catie and her stepsisters, Laura and Vanessa, help me ask for courage, honesty, and openness. Pour your love and energy into Drew and Cindy so they have the ability to discern between when it's time to fight and when it's time to release and simply love. May their love for each other keep them strong so they can love each other no matter what.

On a purely selfish note, I need help juggling my life, my work, facing another winter, and whatever Marley has planned…all while staying open to my emotions, being gentle, and continuing to be in awe of Life. For me, I pray for perfect health and to live in a state of fearlessness. My prayer for you is that you are kind to yourselves and that you remember how sweet life is. Soak it in so you can pour it out.

If I had the energy to experience regret, I'd feel terrible about not sending "thank you" cards to the scores of people who have sent amazing boxes of gems, homemade CDs, videos, and donations. I would personally thank my kind neighbors who have snuck in during stress times, filling my fridge with dinner and placing flowers on the table. I hope you all feel my love and thanks.

I love you all,
Jennifer

P.S. When I look outside the window at Marley's rock-filled fountain, I can feel you all right close. Thank you.

KEEPING IT TOGETHER

Friends

This was a summer I hated to say good-bye to. Everything felt so normal, like we were a real family with a future in a sane world. We spent a lot of time glued tight to friends and family; there was always some fun event going on. The kids joined my morning rite at EPCAM for a bit of socializing. Kids rarely hang out at Evo's Java House, so it was a refreshing change for everyone. It was the perfect place for Marley to share his tall tales. Hell...why not? Everyone else did. Some mornings Marley would babble with the best. Whenever the conversation got deep or cosmic, he'd just listen and flip through his *Four-Wheeling* magazine or the newest *Cabelas* sporting goods catalog.

Sticking Together

There are four things Marley preferred never to be without; *Four-Wheeling*, *Cabelas*, a knife, and duct tape. Constructing something with duct tape was one of his favorite ways to pass the time. I bet if I had all the duct tape Marley had used in his life, it would wrap around the globe at least once. Marley would duct tape used batteries together for paperweights and door stops. He made holders for water bottles, patched his jeans, made wallets, and covered his bike helmets, shoes, and cane with the silvery stuff. One day he entertained himself by making cardboard wings and a nose for his bike, wrapping it all up in duct tape so it looked like an airplane. Some days he spent hours just making round balls. The resonating sound of duct tape being pulled from the roll was a part of our daily lives at the office. I figured buying endless rolls of duct tape was a good investment; besides, his wallets *were* pretty cool.

Whenever he was bored, he'd clump over to my desk like a pirate with a peg leg, bending down to give me a kiss as he took control of my purse for money. "What are you up to?" I'd ask.

He'd grunt, "Need mowa tape, Mama," and with a cock of his head and a giant pouty lower lip he'd slip some bills into his pocket, smile, and give me another kiss.

Marley stored most of his bikes at the office. He never let me get rid of any of his old bikes, even if they were totally thrashed. He explained his rationale, "You neva know when ya need extwa parts." He would pick out one of his bikes depending on how his body felt. Recently, he had been relying on his smaller stunt bike because he discovered that he could use his long legs to push the bike along without having to use the pedals, kind of like a scooter with a seat.

If he was lucky, he would convince Catie to join him on his adventure. They would head to the hardware store down the street to buy more tape. Well…that was the excuse, anyway. The hardware store didn't just have tools; they sold hot dogs and ice cream too. But what Marley really loved was the people, who, like him, seemed to make excuses to go buy something just so they could catch up on the latest gossip.

Contractors, plumbers, ranchers, and electricians would gather there. At any given time, Marley would run into several of his favorite folk, including Cindy, who would take her coffee breaks there. But, then again, Marley never went anywhere in town without bumping into at least four people he knew and loved. I never knew until much later how many people really loved him. He was a social critter and it kept him alive and happy.

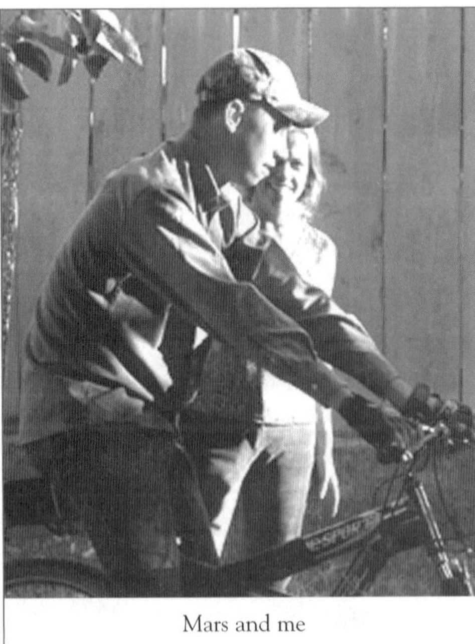

Mars and me

Friday, August 24, 2001
Subject: "HIP HOP"

Howdy Gang,

I'm drained, my eyes are tired from staring into a computer screen all day. I want to run, screaming, out of the office because it's Friday and the weeks are seeming VERY long (especially this one). But first, I need to communicate the recent findings. Bad news—sit down.

THE HIP

According to the pathology report, a large tumor is "eroding and destroying portions of the sacrum and the iliac wing and involving the gluteal muscles and portions of the iliopsoas muscle. This involves the right side and probably incorporates portions of the nerve roots exiting from the distal lumbar region [lower spine]." The good news: the femur (leg), spine, and remainder of the pelvis appear to be free of disease.

Like the shoulder, they have not yet invented a replacement part for this particular bone. So other than chemo (which we refuse to do) we have but one option: 20 days of radiation (5 days/week) which will begin this Thursday.

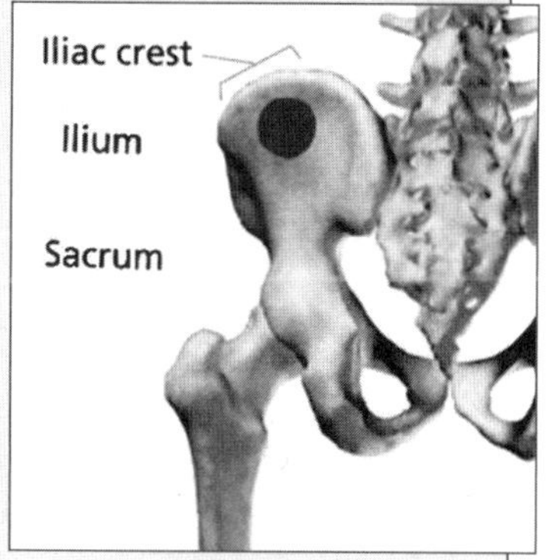

Symptoms usually appear two weeks after the treatment begins. He may end up with a permanent sunburn on the side of his butt, as well as fatigue, possible diarrhea, and nausea. The colon and the intestines will also be nuked in the process, but they try to spread the effects from the radiation over a larger area.

The objective is to reduce the size of the mass which is affecting the nerves that run from the spine across the flat of the bone under those muscles. We want to stop the shooting pains that run the length of his leg. Hopefully, he'll regain some of the muscle strength in that leg too.

THE SHOULDER

The results are not as clear-cut as they are with the hip because he's already had a tumor in the same spot and it's already been nuked. So, looking at the pictures, it's hard to tell what's new growth and what's scar tissue. The pathologist's "easy to read" report states: "Patient has an intramedullary, almost cystic appearing process presumed to be necrotic neoplasm." The doctor's helpful translation is: "A marrow-like substance in the inner core of the bone which looks like an abnormal membranous sac containing a semisolid substance." (Aren't you glad we all speak the same language? It seems, the less they know, the more covert the lingo.) My translation: we're looking at continued tumor growth which is continuing to kill other cells.

The remedy is fourteen days of radiation beginning this Thursday. They have prescribed less radiation than for the hip, because it'll be the second time the shoulder has been nuked. They're trying to find the balance: reducing the pain and killing the cancer without doing too much damage to healthy tissue and remaining bone.

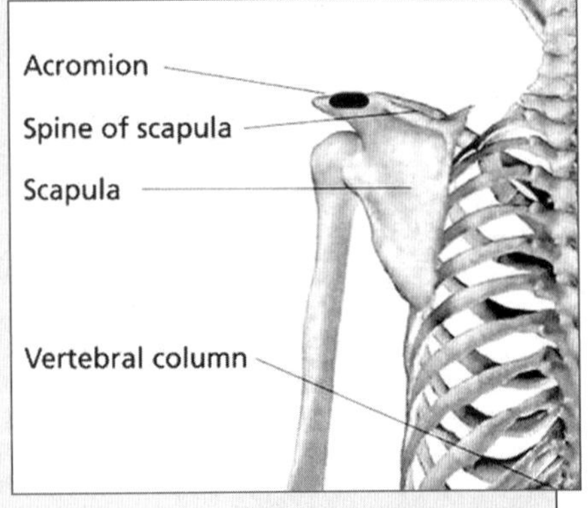

The possible side effects are a permanent "sunburned" look, arthritis, and fatigue. Fortunately, there are no major organs between the skin and the tumor which is going to get blasted. They have to be careful to keep a margin of his arm radiation-free so the circulation of blood still has a pathway that his body doesn't read as "under attack." The thing we need to watch for is any unusual swelling of the arm. The concept is to reduce the number of cancer cells to reduce the pain.

ACTION PLAN

On Wednesday morning, Marley goes in for *blocking*. This is when they do a CAT scan to give them precise dimensions to create a virtual 3-D image that they use to simulate the angle of the laser. Blocking also includes creating molds of his body, so every day he lies down in EXACTLY the same position. This will be a three-hour blocking process, because we're dealing with two different areas. It could take longer if they screw up, the machines are testy, or Marley moves. That would mean they'd have to start all over again. These events have all happened in the past, but I'm not sure he could handle a mishap this time, because lying down has become as painful as standing up.

Next weekend, Marley, Catie, Laura, Vanessa, Drew, and Cindy are going to go camping at the coast. Living the ranch life doesn't allow them to take vacations often, so I'm hoping they have a WONDERFUL time frolicking in the sun.

I'm looking forward to a productive yet relaxing weekend. My goal is to get my generator running again (my only source of electricity). Then we can watch movies while charging the 12-volt system so we can read at night. I'm also going to research ways Marley can be mobile (other than the manual wheelchair) and find a REALLY COOL cane. Currently he's using the hog cane—strong, but not exactly a fashion statement!

I love you all,
Jennifer

"When sorrows come, they come not single spies, but in battalions!"

—Shakespeare

RADIATING PERSONALITIES

Visiting Jackie Sue

Going to radiation had become a routine part of our lives. It had been more than a year since the first time we were introduced to the folks at the cancer center. Because the machine was large and "hazardous," it was located in the basement of the hospital. After six rounds of treatment, each lasting anywhere from one to three weeks, we knew the routine.

With each new round, the first step was a visit with Jackie Sue, the admissions director. She would look up as we entered her office and moan, "Not again!" Marley would flash her a cheesy grin and throw his cane up, catch the bottom of it, and slap it on her desk as he announced, "I'm B-a-a-c-k!" She'd laugh at his dramatic showmanship as he hop-skipped around her desk to give her a big squeeze. By this time, she knew what he was going to ask for next and wouldn't delay—she'd open her drawer for the bag of the rootbeer candies Marley loved. He'd take the bag to fill the candy jar in the lobby then pop a few extras in his jean pockets before handing it back. Those two had a special relationship that required very few words.

While waiting for his treatment, Marley would grab one of the wheelchairs in the corner and start practicing his stunts until someone would yell at him. Then he'd grab a magazine and limp over to the back of the couch and leap over it like a pole-vaulter, landing in a relaxed, lying down position. Others waiting in the lobby would stare at this kid who acted like he owned the joint. Catie would settle in a chair to do her homework or join me at the card table where there was always a jigsaw puzzle in progress. By this time, I had done most of the puzzles at least once, but it didn't matter. I loved having the time to focus on something completely neutral.

Most people who came for treatment didn't become a fixture like Marley. Most people who went there were also over forty. Although there were twenty-five chairs and the long, overstuffed couch in the lobby, there were never more than five people there at a time. Usually there were old couples and middle-aged women waiting for their turn to be zapped. When Marley, Catie, and I would enter, I knew they all assumed I was the one being treated for cancer. I was used to watching their eyebrows go up when Marley was the one to go through the door with the "Danger: Radiation" sign on it.

King of the Hill

Because everyone who worked there knew and obviously loved Marley, he secretly didn't mind the process of getting radiated so much. When his name was called, Marley growled at the technicians, slapped the magazine on a coffee table, and pretended to nip at them as he passed. One of the technicians in charge of blocking was a big man in his early thirties who always kept a professional air and a straight face, but I caught them behaving like brothers a few times, elbowing each other while walking down the hall when no one was looking.

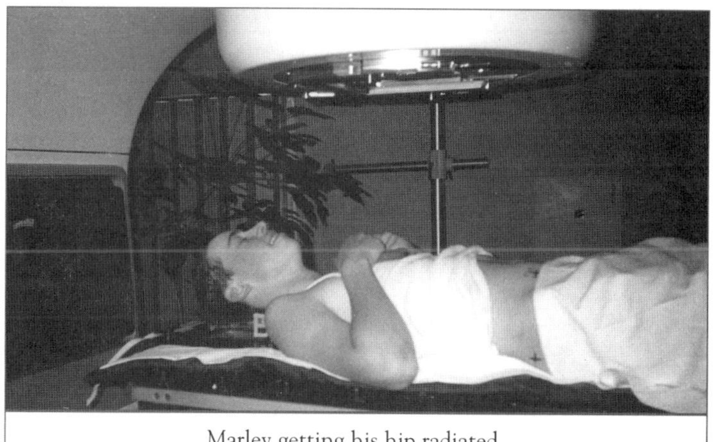

Marley getting his hip radiated.
Photo: Selene Foster

The other technician was Edie, a tiny, red-haired woman. She was the one in charge of the radiation machines, making sure the line of fire was exactly what the doctor ordered. She must have been in her fifties and looked like if you blew on her hard, she'd fall over, but she knew what she was doing. I loved watching Marley with her. He towered over her, but when she would look at him sideways with a silent order, he would shut right up and submissively follow her directions.

The people at the cancer center didn't work with teenagers often, and they didn't usually have extended relationships with their patients. I think there's some sort of code about not getting close to patients, because I'm sure a staggering percentage of them die. Unfortunately for them, they didn't stand a chance of remaining professional with Marley around—he just wouldn't hear of it. Every party we had, Marley always invited the cancer center crew, but no one ever came. Jackie Sue crossed the line of professionalism one day when she pulled me aside and asked to be a part of Marley's Network. She kept saying, "I don't know what it is about that boy, but I do love him so."

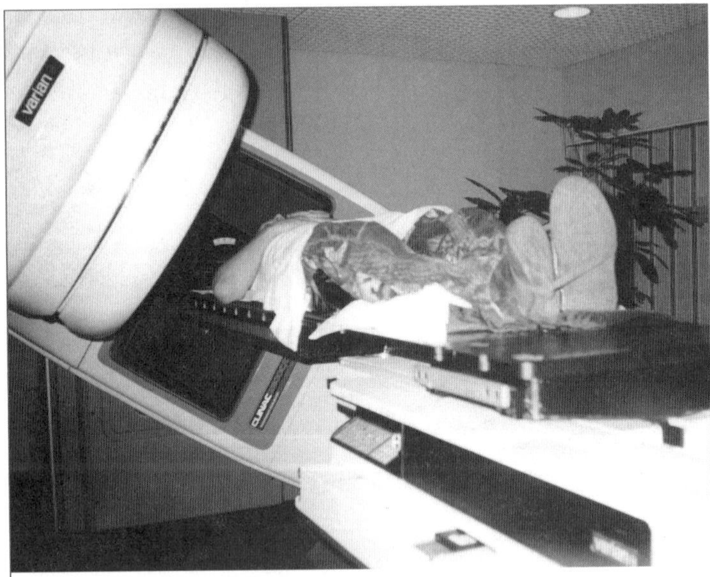

The radiation machine turning to aim at his hip.
(Note the different angles of his legs and the rubber band on his feet.)
Photo: Selene Foster

Thursday, September 6, 2001
Subject: "BACK TO NORMAL"

Hey Gang,

Marley and Catie have both started school. Everything seems rather "normal" in a weird sort of way. Catie is incredibly excited to be in her first year of middle school, and Marley, who hasn't really been in school for a year and a half, seems to be looking forward to the perfect tenth grade school schedule: two morning classes and lunch!

Cousin Selene is back from her two-month journey to Greece—just in time for our annual deadline month at the BRI. She is acting as surrogate mother, taking care of the kids while I try to slam in as many hours as I can at work. After lunch, she picks up Marley and drives him to Dreadford for his radiation therapy and back to Ashland just in time to pick up Catie after school.

Marley is doin' well. He's on a new arthritis medicine called Celebrex, which is stronger than ibuprofen but gentler on the stomach. I know I sound like a pharmaceutical advertisement, but this drug seems to be working very well. He's hardly moaning at all these days when he wakes up. Until recently, he complained about the pain when trying to move his fingers for the first fifteen minutes of each day. I also bought him a memory foam mattress pad that he coos and talks to every night. I think he's in love! Anyway, he's sleeping through the night and wakes up in a good mood.

I'm proud to announce that Drew replaced the hog cane with a "real" one. (It was painted with a flashy metallic gold paint until Marley wrapped it in duct tape.) We're working on getting Marley a very cool motorized wheelchair with the help of the insurance company. And my sister Julia, her husband Joseph, and their three boys, Winston, Peter, and Rawley, are all coming from North Carolina to visit the first week in October. They are going to help me get the house ready for winter.

As if I can somehow add more to my life without tipping over the edge of sanity, I'm trying to get an additional home loan. I want to add on to my little cabin so, in case it is needed, Marley has a room he can get a wheelchair into. The new addition will also include a room for Catie so she can move out of the loft and into a room she can actually stand up in! I can't believe I'm even thinking about adding more to my plate, but something tells me the intensity of my life isn't going to ever get lighter than this. (That thought makes me want to jump off a cliff!)

So breathe easy, keep praying and know we're doin' all right!
Jennifer

"If everything is under control, you are going too slow."

—Mario Andretti

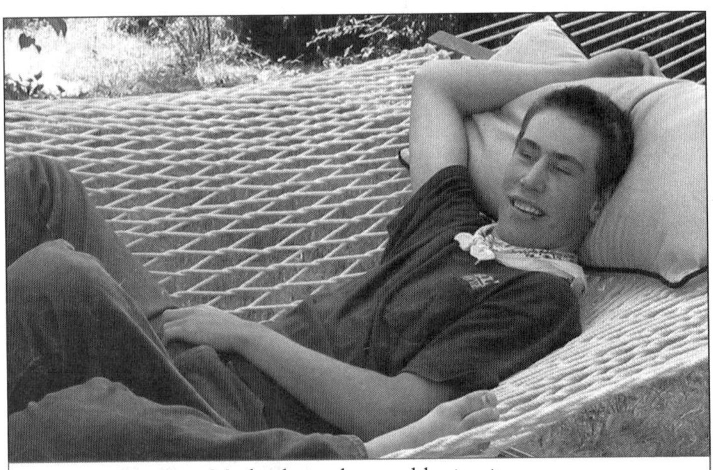

Marley being lazy and loving it.
Photo: Mandy Little

MARLEY'S VIEW ON CANCER

Interview with a Survivor

Reagan was one of Marley's special ed teachers when he was in elementary school. She had been hooked by Marley's special brand of love. If anyone had borne the brunt of Marley's frustration with conventional learning, it was Reagan, yet she and Marley remained best friends long after her job was done. Reagan was twenty years older than Marley, but they had made a bond beyond the beyond.

Reagan was taking a film class at the college, and decided Marley's uniqueness would be the plot for her documentary. She would visit him at school, and take him to lunch to interview him on various topics, using her video camera. One day, she got some great footage of him working in the lunchroom before taking him to a Mexican restaurant to talk about cancer.

Reagan: "Do you ever get angry about the cancer coming back over and over?"

Marley: "I just kinda took it as life. But when anyone says I'm not gonna make it, I just tell 'em, then and there, that they're full of dog shit."

Reagan: "How do you think you've survived it?"

Marley: "I dunno. I'm still trying to figea that out."

Reagan: "There must be something that's helped you. Does it help to have parents like yours?"

Marley: (Nods and then bangs his head back against the wall.) "Friends too. You've hung out wif Sunny—you know how hard-headed he is. I think he's gave me some of the best knowledge. He always says, 'Give the nuses the most gwief possible.' My dad got me a Nerf gun in the hospital one time. As soon as a nuse stuck ha head in the room I'd blow ha head off!"

(Smiling ear-to-ear, he bangs his head again as if it'll help him think of other answers). "Goin' out fo-wheelin', blazin' twails.

That's my life. I fogget about evurwything. People ask me if I take drwugs. I say, 'Yeah, I take one dwug; adrenaline.' They say, 'That's not a dwug.' And I say, 'Damned stwaight it is. There's more wedemption in that than anything.' When they ask if I wead the Bible I say, 'Yeah, *Cabelas*!' Now, *that's* good weading!"

(Pauses to stack the dirty plates and remembers one more thing that's helped him survive.) "Catie. Catie's the little hounddog in the family. If anyone's gonna start a fight in the family, it'd be Catie and she'd be the one to win. She's a sweet, little innocent girl but she's feisty. She wins!"

Reagan: "How do you feel about getting radiation?"

Marley: (Using two knives as drumsticks, he talks while trying to keep a beat). "I hate it. I hate going to Drweadford evaweeday, baaaack and fowth."

Reagan: "Do you have to stay in the hospital?"

Marley: "No. It's just boom boom and you're done."

(Stops drumming to chew on a callus on his palm, notices some dirt on his middle finger and scratches at it). "Since I've had canca, the one thing I can't stand…that's tofu. Can't stand it! Used ta eat it all the time." (Remembering how he felt about chemo, he looked at the dirty plates and pushed them away even farther before he continued.)

"Ya know, I like adventure and I've fwipped three-wheelers. Like once, when I thought I was gonna kiss the gas tank…. But I walked out of it! I'm mowa careful now cause I wanna walk. I think havin' canca has halped to keep me alive."

"Believe that life is worth living,
and your belief will help create the fact."

—William James

Friday, September 14, 2001
Subject: "WON'T YOU BE MY NEIGHBOR?"

• From: Selene

Dear Web,

The sky is just beginning to get light and the crescent moon is hanging outside the window. I have been having trouble sleeping lately (can't imagine why) and find myself watching early morning PBS for kids. *Mr. Rogers' Neighborhood* is going to come on soon. Right now, I'm learning where plants come from and all about the different colors in our world. It's comforting.

I've been spending a lot of time with Marley and Catie lately, and I just wanted to share a few tidbits. First of all, it is a consistent pleasure for me to be with them. I look forward to seeing Marley fly down the hill toward me in his manual wheelchair after a morning at the high school; and Catie walking up with her violin, having started her first year of middle school. It sounds a little funny, but getting to be the one who picks them up makes me feel cool.

So Marley is in his wheelchair most of the time and gets tired in the afternoon, but this whole radiation thing seems strangely normal—which I think Jennifer mentioned too. There is a steadiness, a solidity in Marley, and in the routine, that is a bit baffling. I suggested to Marley the other day that we skip his normal appointment and find an alternative source of radioactivity…a nuclear waste dump perhaps. I think he enjoyed that idea. Anything but the big sterile room with the swiveling monster machine.

Then again, any large machinery is pretty cool. (I have never talked about cars more in my life! I'm discovering my 16-year-old male side that thinks spiral hubcabs are the bomb…and, oh man, check out that cherry Mustang!)

The sky is getting pink now, and the Teletubbies are on. Po

and Tinky Winky think Dipsea's hat is too big!

Catie is supremely excited about school and feeds on the social dynamics of her class. So much energy! Our latest thing to do after school is to eat sticky rice with teriyaki sauce outside at a busy intersection in Ashland and watch other kids hang out.

The other day, just after the Trade Towers and the Pentagon were hit, I met Marley at school and the first thing he said was that he hopes we don't just go bombing people without knowing who did it. I think my jaw dropped open for a moment before I recovered and said, "Yah, me too." Of course we went on to discuss the appropriate uses of M-16s, but hey, the love is there. Really, it is. Everywhere. In all of us.

Take good, sweet,
honest care,
Selene

"Bring it on!"

"Artillerymen believe the world consists of two types of people: other artillerymen and targets."

—military saying

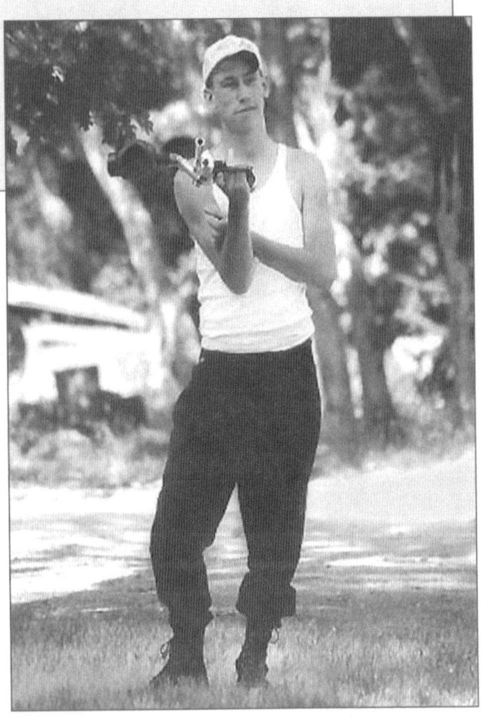

Marley flipping Jay off because Jay asked Mars not to shoot the deer with his paintball gun before Jay got to shoot them with his camera.
Photo: Jay Newman

Monday, September 17, 2001
Subject: "FOOD FIGHT!"

Howdy Gang!

We got a new dog yesterday! This was a big step for me since Sage, my beloved 16-year-old dog, died just before Mars got sick. Sage was the world's best dog, so this new family member has some big paws to fill. Zipper is very sweet, eager to please, and willing to learn, although her first day with us probably made her question the sanity of her new owners.

Yesterday, we had our first annual food fight! Jennifer S. was one of the 20 brave people who participated. Today, she sent me a copy of an e-mail she wrote to her friends describing the adventure. I thought I'd pass this wonderful story along to you.

Next year, you've all gotta join us!

Love you,
Jennifer

****

• From: Jennifer S.

Friends,

I went to a huge, crazy food fight today out at the lake. It was in honor of a 16-year-old friend named Marley, who is unique in many ways, including the fact that he is currently battling a mean case of cancer. He has lost a lung, a knee, and a rib in the last year and a half and goes between a wheelchair and a cane. We were hiking buddies before the diagnosis, and it's been hard watching him lose his strong teenage physical energy, especially because it's still there emotionally and spiritually.

Anyway, we had a riot at the food fight, which consisted of all varieties of armaments—huge vats of buttered noodles, cooked rice, boxes of too-ripe tomatoes, plums, strawberries, and a couple of crates of way overripe cut up melons. There was potato salad, mashed potatoes, chocolate pudding spooned into crusts, lots and lots of squirty whipped cream, and some really really gross creamed corn! Blech! CREAMED CORN! It was SO disgusting!

I arrived armed with industrial-sized squirt bottles of ketchup and yellow mustard, which I highly recommend as very effective weapons to anyone attending a food fight. As this was my first time, I didn't know what to expect and was quite impressed by the number of times food fight food can be reused, especially when you hold the bulk of the battle on tarps. The food just dropped and mixed in with all the other slop and got even GROSSER! I rubbed a handful of crushed-up tomatoes into this woman's hairy armpit and slathered a fat mom's belly with chocolate pudding. Then I stuffed the back of Marley's shorts with a tortilla brimming with noodles, mashed potatoes, and a big helping of creamy corn and gave the whole package a good shmushing.

After we were all sticky and coated and exhausted, we jumped in the lake, which turned out to be lined with soft silty mud and before you could say "this is something out of a bad summer camp movie," we were covered with this slimy mud. Eeewww. Because it was 96 degrees, even after having gone for a final rinse-swim, the fine layer of silt was left everywhere—baked right on. One of my ponytails was caked to my head with—well, as a matter of fact, with CAKE—and the other one was plastered hard with ketchup. It was SO MUCH FUN.

Jennifer S.

"My philosophy? Life is this beautiful buffet, but you get just one trip through the line, and only one plate. And there's no room on my plate for the green Jell-O."

—Daniel Liebert

THE BEDTIME RITUAL

A Land of Dreams

Globally, locally, and in my own home, life seemed to no longer make any sense. Everybody seemed to feel they were caught between a rock and a hard place with nowhere to move. Fortunately for me, there was always bedtime. This sweet-and-sour event happened every night for the two weeks of every month that I had the kids. It was the most important event in my life during these turbulent times. Our ritual rarely fluctuated, becoming something we could all count on.

Both kids brushed their teeth; then I followed Catie up the ladder to the loft. Lit by flickering homemade candles, we crawled on our knees ten feet to her bed. We had to be sure to keep our heads in the center of the peaked roof, to avoid smashing our foreheads on the thin round logs spaced every four feet. As I folded back her down blanket and rose-patterned flannel sheets, I said a silent prayer to the spirits of old cabins, the ones built with love. I pleaded, "Please keep my little home from leaking or falling down. If my house falls apart now, I'm pretty sure I will too."

I thanked the spirits for the strength of those skinny poles that held their load of plywood, tar paper, and green flecked shingles. (Who needs insulation, anyway?) The poles were cut and peeled right on this land, forty years before, by the guy who built the original cabin. Every night that I tucked Catie and Marley into their beds, I felt guilty I hadn't yet found the time or energy to follow through on the plans for an extension on the cabin. My contractor friend, Rhys, had agreed to help me, but available time was extremely limited. Catie really needed a room she could stand up in and Marley deserved more space—what would happen if he became wheelchair-bound before construction started? My mind reeled with how I could work harder to make our lives easier as Catie hopped into bed.

"Time keeps on slipping, slipping, slipping into the future."

—Steve Miller Band

I snuggled next to Catie, stroking the hair off her super soft, high forehead. "How you doin', little one?" I rarely got a straight answer out of her. It didn't seem to matter. She mostly kept her feelings tucked inside her like a jack-in-the-box. I learned that trying to pry her feelings out was a stupid thing to do. When they came out, it would be on her timetable and it would almost always come in a flood, requiring time to mop up the tears and more time to patch her little broken heart together. Time was something we never had a lot of—not with Marley around.

Marley was below us, in his little room, waiting his turn to be tucked in. It never failed; just as Catie and I settled in and found that special moment of privacy, we would be interrupted by Marley. "Moaaaam!"

I'd call down, "Just wait a minute, Marley, I'll be right there."

Patience was not a word in his vocabulary and Catie knew it. She also knew how the threads of his life were wearing dangerously thin, even though he still acted "normal" enough. I'd stroke her hair more, knowing that she was hurting inside just like me. We both knew each other's thoughts like they were our own. Words just weren't enough. There were so many contradictory feelings, neither of us had the courage to begin voicing them. It seemed like if we did, we'd make that mysterious lifeline of Marley's even thinner by making our fears real. And God forbid we should ever stoop so low as to complain about his complaining. Every time we did, we ended up feeling like crap and we worried our last words to or about him would be ones of selfish cruelty. Nevertheless, resentment still lurked in the dark corners of our minds with guilt, glorious guilt, hiding just behind the resentment.

Marley would moan again, "Moaaaam!"

Catie and I would roll our eyes up to the heavens, in a silent conspiracy, asking for strength and patience.

"Hush, Marley, let me say good night to Catie."

Knowing her turn was up and that I needed to go to Marley's side, she'd just say, "I love you, Mom" and she'd open her arms to me, waiting for her hug and kiss. I knew she was sacrificing her rightful time with me because Marley needed me more.

As I blew out each yellow flame, I would say, with all of my heart, "I love you so very much. Sleep loose, Sweetie."

Then the game would commence, just like it did the night before and would the night after for years to come. It was like we had memorized our scripts.

ACT I

In the darkness, I could feel her smile as she said, "But, I love you more!"

"I don't think so, Catie."

"I know so, Mom."

"Sweet Love, I'm older so I have more love to give."

"Whose rules are those? Give it up. I love you more and you know it."

"Go to sleep now. I'm really glad you love me." My head would disappear down the hole in the floor of the loft. Just as my foot would touch the carpet below, she'd get in one last volley.

"Mom?"

"Yeah, Love?"

She'd pause, holding my attention for just a few precious seconds, "I love you more."

I'd smile and respond, just like always, with my best imitation of a stern sounding voice, "I don't think so! Now go to sleep!"

I'd turn my attention to Marley, as he'd call out to me, sounding something like a cow giving birth, "Moaaaaam!"

"Hang on, Mars, I'm gonna go get your pills."

"Howry up!" He demanded.

I headed into the kitchen and loaded up a little silver cup designed for side orders of sauces, that I had "borrowed" from my favorite restaurant. The familiar chiming sound of twelve or so pills filling the cup was a comforting ritual. I was actually *doing* something that might help Marley. I sometimes questioned if these vitamins and herbal remedies would have a dramatic effect, but at least I knew they wouldn't hurt.

"Moaaaam!" The cow was giving birth to twins.

"I'm coming, Marley…just have to get some water."

Into the water glass, I squirted some of the clear liquid aloe that the kids and I called "wetter water." I kept his prescription drugs separate from the other pills, because he was in control of his pain medication. He didn't care about the cupful of colorful caps and tabs; he trusted that I was giving him good stuff. I think he thought it was sweet that I would spend the time to research new pills and give them to him religiously. As far as alternative medicines went, he'd take anything as long as it came in pill form. As long as my choices met this requisite, he wouldn't say "no" to something that just might be helping. Hell, something was working! He was still alive.

He always relaxed when I walked into his room. He loved the bedtime ritual. He tipped the silver cup to his open mouth, taking all the pills at once. I had to concentrate on not gagging as he leisurely took the glass of water from my hand. I hate pills. I swallow them one at a time followed by large gulps of water. It would have taken me fifteen minutes to down what he took in one gulp. Then I'd open my other hand, exposing the "big boys" that took the pain away.

A Pain in the Ass

I would sit carefully next to him on his bed so as not to bump or jar his hip. From my outstretched palm, he reverently plucked his painkillers. I knew by which ones he chose what his pain level was. His long arm would extend toward me until he found my hand curled in my lap. My smallness was immediately apparent, as his long-fingered paws made mine disappear. He was so incredibly tender with his lover-like touches.

His scarred, battered fingers slowly rubbed my wrist ever so gently and methodically while he whispered, "Ma, my body's not coopawrating wif me enymawr. It's jus' fallin' apawt on me. I feel like I'm an owld man."

What does a mom say to that? I came up with something lame like, "Damn, I'm so sorry you're hurting, honey. I wish I could make it all better. Is there anything I can do?"

I'd reach for the tube of Rescue Remedy cream before he

could respond, but he did anyway, "Yeah, give my hip some love, will ya?"

As I massaged his long lanky body, with bones protruding everywhere, I realized how healthy he always looked when he was moving around. Maybe it was the long johns he wore that made him look a little more padded. Maybe it was the bright T-shirts that caught my eye or the thick camouflage flannel shirt he wore unbuttoned that flapped in the wind. Maybe it was the fact he just radiated Life. But whenever I saw his bare body, I was always taken aback by how thin he had become.

He loved being loved and touched. He wasn't shy about his body. Not at all. On the contrary, when he was younger, we had to teach him that in our world, he had to concentrate on wearing clothes so as not to give other people the wrong impression. He learned the rules, but I don't think he ever really understood what the issue was.

"Ow! Not so hard."

"Oops, sorry, I was barely pressing."

"Well do it lighta. Okay?"

"How's this?"

"Tanks, Ma. Much betta."

Whenever I stopped, he'd moan, knowing I was going to go away.

He asked, "Can I just cwawl back inside you, Mommy? I'd be safa in there." He would look at me with puppy dog eyes and protrude his lower lip in a masterful pout.

If I'd been true to how that felt to my Woman Self, the dam would have burst and a river of salty tears would have flooded Ashland. I was jealous of all the people tucking their healthy kids into bed, oblivious of how close death is to us all.

I smiled and just looked at him softly, imagining I was wrapping my 6'2" baby boy in my soul's arms. I cocked my head and replied, "Sweet Pea, if you crawled back inside me, there wouldn't be a me left to keep you safe!"

One side of his thin, wide mouth almost touched his ear in a sly grin as he curled toward me to put his head in my lap. He'd let out a deep sigh that seemed to fill the room with a private and hopeless grief. In silence, all I could do was to stroke his curly hair back and rub his big ears. I watched the glow of Marley's light slowly dim as the 12-volt battery drained itself, reflecting how I felt inside—my life-light slowly dimming.

I did my best to pour enormous amounts of invisible love throughout his being, wondering how many more times we would be able to do this bedtime ritual. "Good night, darlin'."

Then, to keep me there longer, he would ask, "Will you wead to me tonight?"

"No books tonight. It's late."

In a mocking voice, pretending to be snide and huffy, he'd whine, "You book Nazi!"

I'd roll my eyes as I flicked off his light and say, "Lights out."

Act II

"Night, Ma."

"I love you, Marley."

"I love you too, Ma."

Some nights, when the house was filled with feelings thick enough to cut, dear Catie would listen to Marley and me talk. The actual distance from her bed in the loft to Marley's bed was a mere ten feet, separated only by the board and bat that used to be the exterior wall of the original cabin. The wall separating the two bedrooms, covered with a tapestry on both sides, didn't exactly act as a sound barrier.

As I walked into the candle-lit living room beneath Catie's loft, she'd call down, "Good night, Mom."

"Catie, you should be asleep by now. Good night, Lovey."

This was Marley's cue to keep the process alive. "Good night, Catie Batie."

"Good night, Marley."

Whenever Rhys had dinner with us, he'd spend the night and join our bedtime ritual. "Good night, Catie."

"Good night Rhys."

"Sleep well, Marley."

"Yeah right! Like that's possable! 'Night Weesee Peecee."

Mars would try to keep the game going with one last try, "'Night, Ma. I love you."

"Geeze! Good night you two. Now, go…to…sleep!"

It was something out of a TV show from my childhood. I could just see the camera coming in for a closeup of the open windows of the Walton's house bathed by moonlight. And John Boy would say good night to grandpa and grandpa would say good night to Mary Ellen, who would then say good night to whoever was in the next bedroom and so on.

The Grand Finale

Ahhhhh. When the day was done, I could take off my mom hat. On the nights Rhys stayed with us, he and I would talk, curled up together by the wood stove or, if it was warm enough, on the couch outside. He would hold me tight and let me babble. But on most nights, I would be alone after the bedtime ritual was done. I'd concentrate on my quiet and soothing ritual of hand-dipping candles. As soon as I crawled into bed, my beloved cat Salsa would settle herself across my neck, or with her body tucked close to the curl of my body and her nose resting on my ear. If I wanted to cry, now would be the time. I could bury my face in her fur and create mind scenes of what life would be like after Marley died.

I'd imagine what it would feel like to be cleaning and find his Legos or ones of his knives tucked into a corner. I wondered what it would be like to only tuck Catie in bed every night. Would we still play the good night game? Most of the time, there were no tears, just a sense that I was preparing myself for a future I could not fathom. Logically I knew he couldn't stay alive too much longer but…it was Marley, after all. I had to take that into consideration.

Then I'd ponder the opposite extreme. Shit! What if he stayed alive? That was enough to make me want to cry too. He couldn't read. He couldn't write. Some of his bones simply didn't exist anymore. He would always be in pain. Could he defy the odds and actually regenerate bone tissue? Maybe…Who knows?

Even if he did, the kid wasn't likely to be able to live without assistance. On the other hand, he would most likely find a woman who would be hopelessly devoted to his brand of love. Real Love. Anything was possible.

Why bother thinking about any of this? It always seemed impossible to cover all the bases, but I had to help Marley (and Catie) be prepared for everything. Planning for everything seemed next to insanity, but I had no choice. The interior of my brain swirled around in technicolor, and I envisioned lovely padded walls with nothing to look at or nothing to do. The comforting depth of darkness would finally carry me off to a world of dreamy adventures where I could breathe under water and watch the waves curl above me. No pain…That's what I always told Marley…"Sleep. When you're asleep you feel no pain."

Tomorrow would be a new day. I never knew if that was a good thing or not.

"We must pass
through solitude and difficulty,
isolation and silence
to find that enchanted place
where we can dance our clumsy dance
and sing our sorrowful song.
But in that dance, and in that song,
the most ancient rites of our conscience
fulfill themselves in the awareness
of being human."

—Pablo Neruda,
Toward the Splendid City

Chapter Eleven: Losing Patience

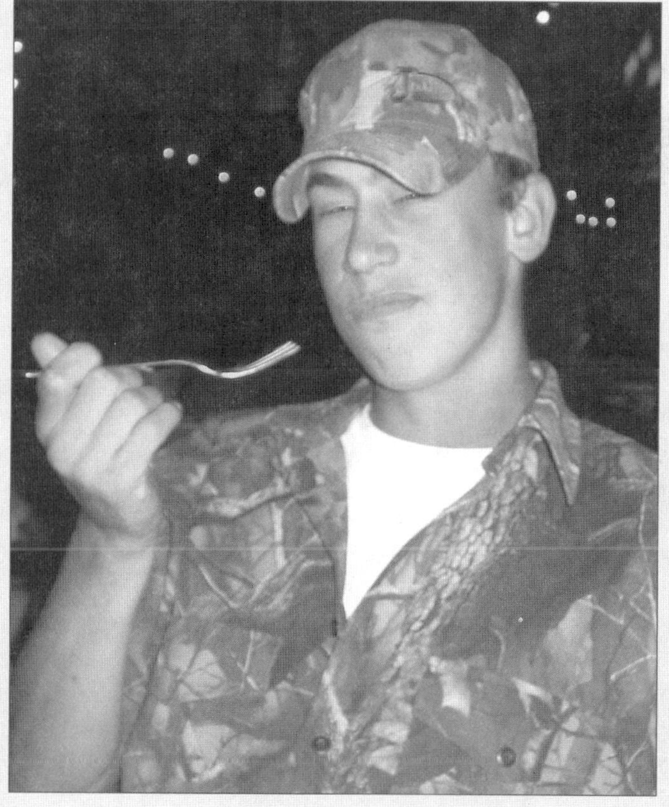

"Bite Me, Bambi!"

Photo: Mandy Little

LIVING WITH CANCER

A Different View

The medical profession doesn't try to "cure" heart disease or diabetes, they try to manage the illness so the patient can live a longer life. They give small doses of drugs that help control the disease. I'm not sure why they deal with cancer any differently, but they do. For some reason, we are still trying to cure cancer rather than finding ways of living with the disease.

I'm kind of glad that chemotherapy didn't work for Marley. I think he stayed alive so long because we had no other option than to treat his disease as if it were an ongoing chronic illness. Because there was no "cure," we were forced to take a long-term view, and that helped us make better decisions about the pace, duration, and invasiveness of treatments. Our objective was to allow Marley to live better and longer.

Marley's friend Ben would come visit me at the office every week to ask if Marley had been cured yet. I tried to explain that cancer is something Marley was just going to have to deal with one step at a time. Ben never did quite understand this, and he always walked away disappointed. There were a few things that Drew said that made me wonder if he, too, had the image that this was all just going to go away. He'd say, "If the tumors would just stop forming so fast, then Mars would have a chance to heal up." For him, apparently, there was some hope that Marley would outgrow the cancer. I worried about Drew not being able to face the odds that Marley was going to die from cancer, but never said anything because I was afraid he'd get mad at me for not trying hard enough to find a way to stop the cancer. I secretly hoped Drew's view was more accurate than mine. I wanted Marley to grow old too.

"One day everything will be well, that is our hope. Everything's fine today: that is our illusion."

—Voltaire

Monday, September 24, 2001
Subject: "SOCIETY'S BLINDNESS"

Hello all,
The recent ruin of the two Towers has made life's clear lines blurry with confusion. For the past two weeks, work has been next to impossible, but the deadlines live on. The kids are gone and the BRI office feels more like home than home. Being with people is a comfort, yet I'd rather be solitary and deep. So I took the weekend off to add streams of tears to rivers of grief.

If you want to know more about how my life feels, the video "*Wit*," starring Emma Thompson, is required viewing. (Have lots of tissue on hand.) After watching this video, all I could do was bathe in the sun and write poetry.

Towers of Love

I wonder about the seconds before their choice to leap.
I worry about the masses who still seem to sleep.
As my son plods on through life...

What is it that we've done, that makes so many hate?
On our house of cards, we must concentrate.
As my son plods on through life...

Will we see that an eye for an eye will leave us blind?
As Death hovers close, the arms of Love is all I find.
As my son plods on through life...

I know, like cancer, forgiveness spreads all-mighty fast.
Help make our children's future be different than our past.
As my son plods on through life...

So even though life feels so insanely insecure and hopelessly absurd, I have faith there's a reason, a method to this madness.

Stay safe,
Jennifer

MISUNDERSTANDINGS

It's Nature's Way

One common question of the terminally ill that Marley rarely asked was, "Why is this happening to me?" The few times he did ask, I never had a good answer. Sometimes it's hard for parents to confess they don't have a clue. I usually came up with some pretty outstanding explanations, but I had to admit that I *was* clueless. I don't believe God or the All-That-Is just makes random picks from the herds of creatures on Earth. I'm more comfortable thinking we co-create our lives with the All, on a soul level, before we enter our baby bodies. When we're done fulfilling our contracts, then we can go Home.

Those are my beliefs. They are constantly forming and reforming. Having an answer and believing I know the answer are two very different things. Marley didn't need my beliefs, he needed his own, so I did my best to keep my beliefs to myself. "Beats me!" is all I could ever seem to muster. In response, I would add something uplifting like, "All I do know, Marley, is that you're doing an amazing job of playing a great game with the crappy cards you've been dealt." That would satisfy him.

What was remarkable to me was how little he felt sorry for himself. The Marley Man somehow took the pits along with the fruit without question. Maybe it's because he spent time at both of his homes observing nature's way. Marley saw how coyotes would stalk a birthing cow, lying in the pasture, waiting to attack the calf just as it was midway born. Marley had no problem helping Drew shoot at the coyotes to protect their cows, but he never questioned that the coyotes were just doing their job. If the coyotes escaped, they would just run away and do their best to find more prey. If the cow survived, she didn't seem to grieve, she'd eat more grass and try to get pregnant again. Life goes on.

Marley watched a variety of creatures being born. He also watched them die. When Sage, our canine companion, died, we all grieved. As sad as the event was, Marley knew it was her time to go—she was old. He knew that was simply the cycle of life. He experienced it every season with the plant kingdom. We all do. Some of us just forget, or maybe we think humans are immune to the ways of nature. Marley knew he was going to die—he just didn't focus on it. Like the rest of us, he didn't know when or how. None of us do, even if we have cancer. When we get right down to it, life is pretty mysterious. That's nature's way!

"God does not play dice with the universe."

—Albert Einstein

"God not only plays dice, He also sometimes throws the dice where they cannot be seen."

—Stephen William Hawking

Mixed Messages

I personally think TV, microwaves, cell phones, computers, and credit cards are the downfall of our civilization. But who am I to talk? I was a walking contradiction. I was working on a computer ten hours a day. I was spending way too much time in too many hospitals, and I got a cell phone so I could work during our travels. When we went to Maui, I had to break down and get a credit card just to rent a car. At work, I was surrounded by fact junkies, while I don't believe 90 percent of what's reported. And yes, I admit, I sometimes used the microwave at the office. The icing on the cake was that I worked for a corporation! Away from home, I was knee-deep in everything I detest; nevertheless, I managed to keep my personal sanctuary in the woods void of most technological innovations.

Drew grew up on Long Island, but moved out west and became a tofu-eating hippy. Then one day, two escaped horses roamed on to our property. He caught one, rode it around the yard and decided to cut his hair and become a cowboy! So maybe Marley inherited our ability to dish out mixed messages.

Marley didn't read, so computers were not important tools for him except for playing games on. Marley was possibly the most extroverted, social critter I have ever met, but he hated talking on the phone. His sense of fashion was mind-boggling. He loved '70's-style fancy silk shirts because he loved the way they felt against his body in the wind. He wore T-shirts slashed to ribbons because they pissed people off. One day he'd wear a stained T-shirt, ripped jeans, tennis shoes completely wrapped in duct tape, and a ball cap stained with sweat. The next day, he'd wear a white cotton shirt, leather vest, dress jeans, cowboy boots, and one of his many cowboy hats. Marley was a cowboy through and through (except when he wasn't).

He cared about animals, emergencies, bikes, and ATVs. He didn't care much about other cultures, political rules, or new trends, and yet, his preferred bedtime reading was *National Geographic* (with the exception of *4-Wheeler* magazine). He also knew which politicians were trustworthy and which weren't, but didn't much care to discuss why.

It was never planned that both of the homes that the kids lived in wouldn't subscribe to television, newspapers, or listening to radio news. Other than a lack of reception in the Colestin Valley, I don't know what Drew and Cindy's story was, but I chose not to have electricity. Marley would watch TV when he was at the office. Lots of TV. His program choices were Country Music Television (CMTV) and anything on the Discovery Channel that focused on surgeries, emergencies, or disasters. He would also watch national news.

Crash and Burn

On September 11th and the weeks following, Marley watched CNN nonstop. He took it all in. It wasn't the act of terror he was fascinated with, it was putting himself in the shoes of the emergency staff and the people in the buildings. He wanted to be there, digging through the rubble and stitching people up. It was a real-life disaster happening before his very eyes. He lived for that kind of excitement. If he had been there, his long arms would have been wrapped around the fearful and the ones grieving their loss. His love would have soothed those in need (especially the babies). I never heard him talk about the injustice or how terrible it was that so many died. To him it was the same as if a tsunami wiped out a village.

Somehow, he saw the 9/11 disaster as nature's way. He knew more about what was happening in the world than I did. His views helped Catie, Selene, and me feel calm as we did our best to understand what seemed incomprehensible. I'm not sure how he did it, but Marley made life make sense. There was a wisdom in Marley that I could feel in his touch and see in his eyes. He was telling me that everything would be alright, and I felt I had no choice but to believe him.

***"Life is thickly sown with thorns,
and I know no other remedy than
to pass quickly through them.
The longer we dwell on our misfortunes,
the greater is their power to harm us."***

—Voltaire

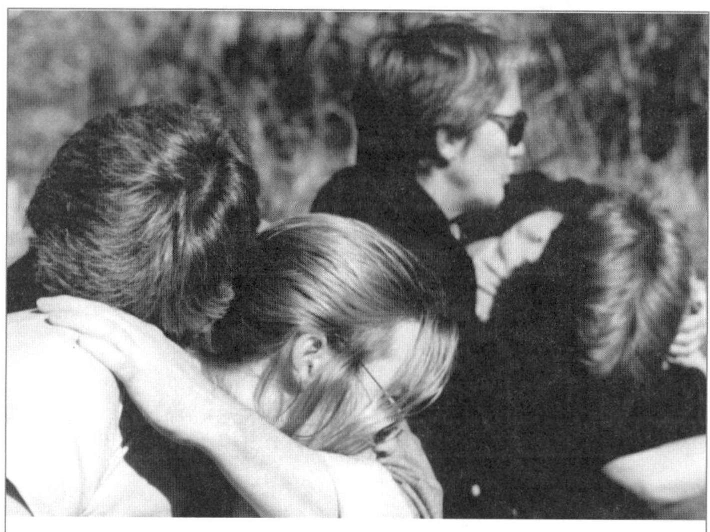

"Holding On"
Joseph, Peter, Julia, and Rawley Gunnels

Tuesday, January 1, 2002
Subject: "ANOTHER YEAR—ALIVE & KICKIN'!"

Howdy Gang,

Happy 2002! It's New Year's Day. Marley, Catie, and I decided to celebrate by getting a hotel room in Ashland so we could watch TV, swim, and soak in the hot tub. It was a fun way to spend New Year's Eve.

We sat on our two queen sized beds and recapped 2001. As we listed memorable events, we realized our calendar was focused on the different tumors; even our Maui trip was remembered by Marley's fall in the bathroom. Oh well…no one can say our lives are boring! 2001: Three tumors (knee, shoulder and hip), two surgeries, and three rounds of radiation—the same as in the year 2000. I hope it's not a pattern.

Marley has managed to remain in school since fall. His favorite class is shop. His teachers all love him, and his strength is generating thought-provoking discussions. Needless to say, Marley has a unique perspective on life and, because writing and reading are not skills he can lean on, conversation is the technique he uses most.

He uses his manual wheelchair when at school, but he leaves it there and uses his cane when he needs support at home. Most grocery stores these days provide wheelchairs or motorized carts so he can shop with Catie and me. He is tired most of the time, yet is most happy rigging elaborate ways of climbing trees without having to use his legs much. He set up a Cirque de Soleil-type rigging high in an old oak for Catie. It's a sight to see: 25-foot ribbons of cloth that she wraps around her body as she practices her aerial dance techniques. He says when he's doing that kind of project, he forgets about the pain. When the snows came, his idea of a good time was to put chains on the car just to take them off again. (Strange child.) Come to think of it, maybe lying on the snow numbs the pain in his leg.

Catie is tall and beautiful. It's scary how fast they are growing up. I feel something special when both children stand on either side of me, resting their elbows on the top of my head! Catie's first report card as a middle school student was perfect, a 4.0 GPA. She's every teacher's dream. She loves school. Her idea of fun is to do extra-credit projects with elaborate detail. (Another strange child.) And to think they both came from the same set of parents!

My goal for this year was to be able to manage my crazy work load, yet have more time for my kids—an important thing to focus on when you start hearing, "You love your job more than me." I'm proud to say I think I finally accomplished my goal. Okay, so I don't have any friends anymore, but I have a deep connection with ME which gives me unlimited energy for working hard. The workload for 2002 will more than double at work and at home. If Marley's health status twists, I'll simply roll up my sleeves a little higher. I'm ready for whatever Great Spirit dishes out. (Knock on wood.) I'm beginning to think of life as an Olympic sport with two choices: jumping for joy as if I'm winning a medal or wallowing in the agony of defeat.

I hope you know that I love you all and lean heavily on your support and prayers. I am most thankful and ever mindful that you are there. I also hope you understand that you are part of a young man's life that will have ripple effects on the way we all live in the future. I don't know the details yet, but I have a strong sense that this is true. Keep the faith and stay true to that Still Small Voice Within. Together we will rock the world! I'm proud to be sharing the planet with you.

May all your wishes for 2002 come true,
Jennifer

TALK ABOUT DYING

In Other Words

Death is probably the most uncomfortable topic I've encountered in our society. If I were to make a list of all the subjects that are taboo, I bet I'd find they all lead to the same place—our fear of death. We all are surrounded by death constantly, yet we do our best to sidestep the conversation.

When I'd bump into people around town and they'd ask me how Marley was doing, it was like they were walking on eggshells. I hated it. They wanted to keep their verbiage indirect, impersonal, discreet, and covert. I never could figure out if this was for my benefit or if it was so they could walk away from me and not feel the brush of death.

All I know is when my death is near, I would appreciate it if the people around me talk about it without mincing their words and hiding their feelings. Can you image how healthy it would be if Marley's eight doctors, each in their own way, had found a way to hold him and just say, "Damn. I'm really sorry there's nothing we can do that we haven't tried. You're a good kid, I'm glad to be your doctor." What a concept! It's not the doctors' fault Marley was dying. Technology, or lack thereof, was not the cause. Nobody failed, including Marley. I kept telling myself, "Shit just happens."

Word Play

When we die, we:

are dead as a doornail
take the big sleep
kick the bucket
cease to live
depart
rest
lose our life
pay nature's debt
take our last breath
go the way of all flesh
launch into eternity
hand in our chips
meet the end
perish
pass away
bite the dust
bite the big one
drop into the grave
give up the ghost
join the majority
drop dead
expire
end our days
meet our maker
lay down our life
are six feet under
end our earthly career
have bought the farm
yield our breath
breathe our last
drop off
pop off
are no more

A Straight Shooter

Whenever Marley asked to see Diane, our ever-loving local oncologist, we knew we were facing stormy times. Whenever I made a new appointment, my stomach always felt queasy with fear and I knew it was a good time to pray hard. At least I knew she would shoot straight with us, no matter what.

We were lucky to have found Diane. She was a pediatric oncologist, serving kids with cancer. Her heart-wrenching specialty was balanced by also being a general practitioner: taking care of little kids with bruises, breaks, and runny noses. An appointment with Diane was like visiting Grandma. She always wore a comfortable dress and a bright apron. In the front pockets of the apron, a prescription pad and a stethoscope were hidden where a spoon or a hot pad should have poked out.

Her tiny examining rooms never had enough space to accommodate one oversized kid and three parents. But these tiny rooms were the only ones I've seen that had fun stuff to look at on the walls and piles of children's books stacked on a special shelf under the exam table. Diane would breeze into the room and sit next to Mars on the table. She, too, knew if Marley was visiting her, another storm was brewing.

She had a wonderful way of revealing that she was human. From the start, she knew that we knew she had never encountered a patient with squamous lung cancer, so she didn't have to pretend. We were in this together. She was the one with the prescription pad and the one that could sit in with the other doctors from all the hospitals to discuss our case. She was our advocate, making sure everyone was well-informed and was on the same page. We trusted her to represent us, and treat us like the intelligent parents of a unique child with a terminal disease.

The start of almost every appointment began the same way. Drew, Cindy, and I would be squashed together along one wall. She would turn her attention to Marley.

"Hello, my boy, what's up? How are you feeling these days?"

An Eeyore-like moan would fill the room, accompanied by an exaggerated exhale. He'd groan, "Shitty."

She'd respond sarcastically to Marley, "Well, I didn't think you were visiting me just for fun!"

She'd cock her her head toward the three of us, with an expression that relayed, "I'm so sorry. Are you ready for another round?" We'd quietly nod in resignation. Then she'd ask, "So, my boy, where does it hurt?"

"Things are going to get worse before they get worse."

—Lily Tomlin

Patient Love

It must be really tough for doctors to know their patients are going to die and there's not a damned thing they can do about it.

It took Marley's radiation oncologists about six tumors for them to stop saying things aimed at Drew, Cindy, and me; like: "He must be really careful not to do activities that could put his now brittle bones at further risk."

We'd point to Marley and respond, as if we were defending ourselves, "You've gotta be kidding?"

There's Marley; sitting cockeyed in the chair with one elbow slung over the chair's back, the other arm stretched out on the window sill. His long fingers flicking the always closed blinds that concealed the view of the concrete wall of the next building. His legs would be stretched out, long and lazy, but his foot would be keeping the beat to music that only he could hear. He'd probably be wearing camo pants and a T-shirt that read "Jump hard. Die young." His body language said, loud and clear, "Whatever! Do what you have to and get me out of here fast!"

The doctors also finally stopped considering the fact that we were reaching the limit of how much radiation his body could withstand. Until this point, they kept warning us that the total accumulated radiation quota was being reached. (Like we had any control over how many tumors grew.)

"Blah, blah, blah." There were no limits. We all knew that. Their medical journals said not to give more than this amount of radiation in this amount of time. The reality was, we didn't have a choice and they didn't have a clue. We were in no-man's-land.

In the very beginning, they warned us that developing a secondary cancer caused by too much radiation was the major risk. That didn't seem to be an issue, because it usually takes five to ten years for most cancers to manifest. But that was when we all thought Marley's chances of surviving the first year were limited. Now in his third year, I could see the doctors starting to sweat, because he simply wasn't getting enough time between tumors and treatments to heal.

These poor doctors had lost their carefully maintained reserve toward our family. I even sensed a little bit of respect and honor leaking out of the cracks behind closed doors. But what doctor wants to start loving someone who's just going to die?

It seems we are all trained to not be vulnerable with someone who might leave us. Imagine how different relationships could be if we entered them acknowledging that separation will occur. Imagine being able to say, "I love you more now, because I know you will be leaving me and I want to savor every moment." Marley taught me that.

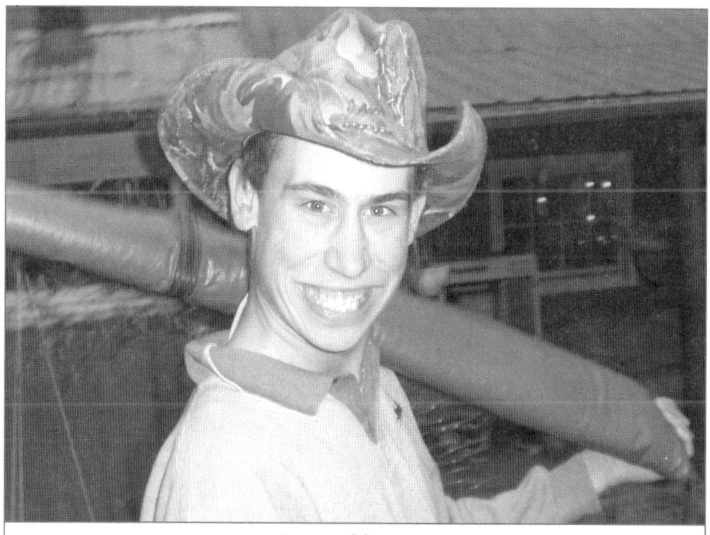

A crazed hunter!

Photo: Reagan Burrell

Monday, February 25, 2002
Subject: "STICKING OUR NECK OUT"

Dear Marley Network,

Life never ceases to amaze me. The weeks flip past like waves crashing on the shoreline. Catie excels in school and has fallen in love with skiing. Marley packs his *Cabela* catalog (hunting accessories) around with him everywhere. He loves playing his virtual driving games and is finally riding his bike again. What other kid goes from a riding in a wheelchair one minute to riding on a BMX bike the next? I actually caught him jumping his wheelchair off a ramp at school while he was waiting for me one day. I barked at him but, to tell you the truth, I really don't know if I was worried about his body or the wheelchair!

Just a note to let you know Marley has a new lump on his neck right near the Adam's apple. There are some things we know and many facts we don't yet have. I will be sure to send you solid info when available.

What we *do* know
Only the left side of the thyroid is affected. Marley looks and feels great! There's no pain or discomfort associated with the lump. We discovered it at Diane's office due to the shadows cast by the overhead fluorescent lights. (A lucky accident.) That same day, it was confirmed with an MRI.

What we *think* we know
This lump is cancerous. This is not, in itself, life threatening.

What we *don't* know
If this tumor is *on* the thyroid, it's our old friend, squamous cancer. If it's *in* the thyroid, it's probably a new type of cancer. To find this out, we'll be doing a very simple procedure called a *small needle biopsy*. We'll do this within the next ten days. We'll

also be getting an MRI of his brain to compare to last year's and a CAT scan from jaw to pelvis to learn if anything else is going on in his body.

Conclusion

When we put all the pieces together in a week or two, we'll be able to know what we're dealing with and what our options are. In the meantime, I ask you not to worry and not to jump to conclusions. It's Marley we're talking about, so none of the normal rules seem to apply. I also ask that you simply pray for clarity and Right Action. Know that I will contact you when we know more. Not to worry....

We love you all,
Jennifer

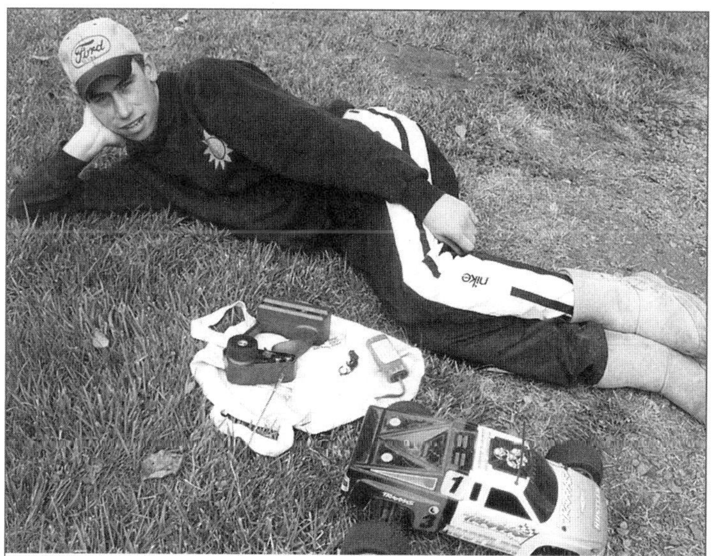

Mars with his favorite remote controlled race car.

Photo: Reagan Burrell

FRUSTRATION

Tipping Over the Edge

In the very beginning, my oldest brother, Tip, had sent me some herbal pills designed to lessen the impact of the American Medical Association's cancer cures. He suggested that I contact a doctor in Maryland who supposedly had the "cure for cancer." This method of preventing and curing many ailments was based on radical dietary changes, designed to cleanse existing toxins and build the immune system's strength. It was a great suggestion.

Two years had passed since Tip's gentle suggestion, and Marley's condition was getting worse. In the meantime, one of Tip's dear friends had been diagnosed and died from brain cancer. Tip hit the wall—his patience had worn thin and he could keep quiet no longer.

> Tuesday, February 26, 2002
> Subject: "CURES"
>
> • From: Tip
>
> Jennifer
>
> I have become quite exasperated with friends who have chosen to die from cancer when it is so unnecessary, so curable.
>
> Now you are anguishing about Marley's future. You've got two options. 1) Do nothing and let the AMA doctors take all your money as they wring their hands and suggest a good undertaker, or, 2) Seek out the prevention and the cure—it's so simple, easy, and cheap.
>
> If Marley croaks from cancer, I'll know you didn't seek the alternative truth.
>
> Tip

After reading his e-mail, I sat at my desk with my jaw on my keyboard. As I responded, I realized how much pain my brother was in, and how defensive I felt.

Tuesday, February 26, 2002
Subject: RE: "CURES"

Dearest Tip,

I can't make Marley do, think, or feel *anything*. I can give him pills, but I can't make him swallow them. I can measure a teaspoon of the miraculous Noni Juice, but can't pinch his nose closed until he swallows it. I can make an appointment for him with a world-renowned instant-touch healer, but it won't do a bit of good unless he wants it to. Do you understand that?

Just remember, for some, choosing to do what it takes to prevent dis-ease is hard enough, and to cure disease that's already manifest seems more difficult still. Everyone learns at their own speed. It's been my toughest lesson: to allow people to suffer if that's what they choose, and to love them still.

I agree with you, my frustration level is at an all-time high. How can he just roll over and die? I'm offering alternative solutions that are amazing and simple—reams of research have been done, contacts made, and products purchased. Many of these solutions don't seem to interest him. He's doing this illness differently than you and I might, but I find I have to respect his way. He's an amazing human with his own agenda and style.

For the record, I've contacted your doctor. I was told their products may be too specific for Marley's illness and are designed for adults, not young people.

I'm so thankful you're in my life. Between you and me, sometimes I'd like to shoot the boy and put the rest of us out of our misery. And then I hear that little voice saying, "Maybe this isn't about whether he lives or dies at all." So I keep learning. And I keep loving.

Thanks for being there.
Thanks for caring,
Jennifer

Tuesday, February 26, 2002
Subject: "TIP'S FRUSTRATION"

Dear Network,

My brother, Tip, has been having a very hard time understanding why this is happening to Marley. He has expressed frustration about our inability to find a cure. In the following e-mail he focused on finding the cause. As I responded to him, I thought some of you might be asking similar questions, so I'm including you in our conversation.

~~~~~~

J

Man, I'd look around your place—there's gotta be a toxic waste dump somewhere close by!

T

~~~~~~

Dear Tip,

Both Drew and I live way out in the country, up in the mountains where the air is clean, the stars are bright, the water is good, no cattle are above us, etc. At your suggestion, I did check on the radon levels for this region and they are very low. The only other thing I can come up with is the railroad tracks, which pass by both houses about three "blocks" away. I have no clue of where else to even explore the cause of Marley's cancer, which most likely began when he was five years old.

If you're reacting to the possibility of secondary cancer, that would be due to the "solution,"—using radiation. We were warned that this could happen but were also told not to worry about this for quite some time. Everyone agreed it was worth the risks because of the limited survival rate for this level of lung cancer.

Jennifer

I DID IT MY WAY

In Your Face Honesty

Tip had just recently lost a dear friend to brain cancer. He had had it with this disease and the fact that war wasn't being waged against the dying process. Not only did he want me to fight harder, he wanted me to find a cause. He was one of the few that openly challenged what was happening to us, and how we were choosing to react. At first, I was stunned. Then I started to understand that Tip was righteously angry that two people in his clan were being carried away "before their time."

In the very beginning, Tip sent me herbal products designed to reverse the effects of this disease and a book describing the diet changes required. I researched the herbs and indeed, they all were beneficial for various stages of battling cancer, including the ones associated with healing from chemo. Because they were in pill form, Marley would take them, but a permanent change in diet was not an option for Mars.

It seemed, as far as Tip was concerned, that Marley's lack of desire to battle his cancer was a lack in my parenting skills. I found myself in the position of defending Marley's self-imposed limits, stating I had no control over my son's choices. My biggest lesson was how to support someone else's decisions even if it meant I was most likely going to lose them.

I keep asking myself how I would play the game if I were dealt Marley's hand. My response has become my rating system for how much I want to live. I found that it is not so much that I adore living, it is that I want to do my best at living the best I can while on planet Earth. I hope I am never faced with this challenge. If I am, I pray my desire to survive is great, and that I have the courage to make great life changes. But the truth is, I don't know.

> ***"Our lives improve only when we take chances — and the first and most difficult risk we can take is to be honest with ourselves."***
>
> **—Walter Anderson**

Friday, March 8, 2002
Subject: "TWO NEW TUMORS"

Hiya Gang,

Here's an update on the results from the three tests:

1) The biopsy of the tumor in the thyroid area shows our friend squamous carcinoma has metastasized again. An MRI shows that it seems to be not just ON the thyroid, but possibly WITHIN the thyroid as well. The good news is that it's not obstructing the airway. The bad news is, the nerve to the voice box is in this area too. Under normal circumstances, both surgery and radiation would be the standard operating procedure BUT...

2) The CAT scan (from jaw to hips) shows that he also has a new growth in an old place; his *iliac* (the big, wide, flat area of the wing-shaped bone of the hip). Surgery is not an option, as we discovered with both his hip and his shoulder previously. Radiating a second time is our only option.

Because we have two tumors to deal with, we are leaning away from surgery to the neck. It's too much for his body to deal with, especially without high odds they could get all of the tumor via surgery. They say it's hard to know what they're dealing with until they actually get in there. Hmmmm. I don't think we'll take that option!

3) And finally, the MRI of his brain shows no cancer!

On Monday night, I was trying to wrap my head around the travels of squamous as I slipped into a lovely state of "here we go again"–type depression. I counted the feet of incisions and the hours of radiation, and then I drew an outline of a body and started putting Xs on the spots where this cancer has made appearances. I was trying to make sense of the different body systems affected, sides of the body, timing,...anything. The result? Nothing.

Check it out: (3/2000 – 3/2002)

<u>2000</u>
Left - **Lung** – surgically removed and radiated

Left - 6 **Lymph Nodes** (mediastinum) – removed and radiated

Left - **Arm – Subcutaneous** marble-like tumor – removed and radiated

<u>2001</u>
Right - **Knee – Bone** – removed, replaced, and radiated

Right - **Shoulder – Bone** – radiated

Right - **Hip (iliac) – Bone** – radiated

Right - **Shoulder – Bone** (2X) – radiated again

<u>2002</u>
Right - **Hip (iliac) – Bone** (2X) – to be radiated again

Left - **Thyroid** – Treatment Undecided

Wow! And the kid keeps going and going and going! He looks good; you'd be amazed. He continues to go to school. He uses his wheelchair, cane, or nothing—depending on the situation. He's 6'2" with a knee that doesn't fold well and a hip that hurts badly, so he now avoids little cars, bleachers, walking long distances, and movie theaters. But, other than that....

I have the weekend ahead while the kids are with Drew and Cindy. So, after a week of working very long hours, I'm going to go kick back, chop a few trees down, split a little firewood, and read my novel!

One more doctor appointment on Monday and we'll know exactly what we're doing. I'll keep you posted.

Have a great weekend,
Jennifer

WHO'S IN CHARGE?

Lymphing Along

To date, the cancer had affected the respiratory system, the skeletal system, the muscular system, and the lymphatic system. Having just six small lymph nodes test positive was more worrisome than all the other tumors. According to Frederic Martini's *Fundamentals of Anatomy and Physiology*, "the lymphatics are found in all portions of our bodies except the central nervous system, and the lymphatic capillaries offer little resistance to the passage of cancer cells. As a result, metastasizing cancer cells often spread along the lymphatic. Under these circumstances, the lymph nodes serve as way stations for migrating cancer cells." As with my father's cancer, I knew that at any time the cancer could pop up anywhere using the lymphatic system as a means of travel.

The Endocrine System

This new tumor involved the endocrine system, and marked a whole new chapter in Marley's cancer charts. The biopsy of the new tumor told us that it existed, but not how extensive it was. The CAT scan could not differentiate between his thyroid gland and the growth. We knew the tumor was growing *on* the gland, but had the cancer cells actually infiltrated the thyroid itself? If they hadn't, surgery would be an option. If the tumor had invaded, we'd either have to remove both tumor and gland or just nuke the tumor and hope for the best.

In order to make a decision about this new tumor, we had to learn what the thyroid does. In order to do that we had to learn about the endocrine system. The endocrine system includes two small glands in the brain (pituitary and hypothalamus), three glands in the rest of the body (thyroid, adrenals, and testes/ovaries), and two organs (pancreas and kidneys). Although this system involves few organs, it controls every part of our body. This is our body's chemical laboratory, producing and storing critical hormones that control every other system of operation.

The endocrine system supplies hormones to the lymphatic

system, keeping our immune functions firing. It rules our heart rate, kidney functions, body fluids, electrolyte balance, muscle growth, and stimulates our respiratory activity. Without the hormones controlled by the endocrine system, no sperm would find its target because no egg would be there to receive it. Babies would not be pushed from the womb, and no milk would be produced.

The books warned that a malfunction of the endocrine system would also effect the regulation of calcium levels needed by our bones. The thyroid gland is directly responsible for the secretion of calcitonin, which reduces the concentration of calcium in the blood. Too much calcium in the bloodstream can be fatal. (At the time, we had no idea how important this tidbit of information was going to be…neither, apparently, did the doctors.)

Learning about the endocrine system made us more aware of how advanced Marley's cancer was. The thyroid gland has two lobes, one on each side of the Adam's apple. They join across the windpipe, just below the voice box. Because of the growing size of the tumor on Marley's thyroid gland, within a week, breathing became more difficult when he turned his head from side to side. (An enlarged thyroid can actually cut off the air supply through the windpipe.) Because Marley's tumors had always grown quickly, there was no time to waste—a specialist was definitely needed.

Define "Special"

We were referred to an ear-nose-throat surgeon who was top in his field. The only problem: He was on vacation, leaving the care of his clients to his son. Okay—like father, like son—right? Wrong! We showed up for our initial appointment and were greeted by a man in his early thirties. He wiped his sweaty palm off on his pants as he told us this operation would be a no-brainer. We had done our research. We knew the two nerves to the vocal cords ran alongside the thyroid. We also knew how important this little gland was. This was not a good time to be cocky.

He said the only choice we had was to remove the tumor surgically and he wouldn't know how radical the *thyroidectomy* would have to be until he got in there. His attitude of "it's no big deal" made Drew, Cindy, Marley, and me almost run out of his office. Instead, we walked. We stood in the parking lot, kicking the tires on Drew's truck. Cindy calmly asked, "So, how'd you like this guy?" Within seconds, we were all frothing at the mouth, babbling about what an idiot this "kid" was.

On Firing a Specialist

We reported back to our oncologist and said we didn't want this guy to touch Marley. We had learned from our experience with the Portland surgeon who did Marley's knee replacement. If we had bad feelings about a doctor, we would trust our gut instinct. We bravely rejected this surgeon's help, but time was running out. Instead of starting the interview process again, we opted to rely solely on the skill of our radiation oncologist.

Our justification was that, even if we did find a surgeon that we liked and trusted, we believed this particular operation was too dicey to take a chance on. If the surgeon screwed up, the risk was irrevocable damage to the vocal cords. The irony of facing the possibility that Marley would lose the ability to speak was simply too much, considering it took him so long to talk in the first place. Besides, his hip had to be radiated ASAP and putting Marley through surgery and radiation at the same time seemed just a bit cruel.

Little did we know we had just burned a bridge. Apparently, when you consult a specialist who is a part of an office of like professionals, it is deemed unethical for another doctor of that same office to take your case. Had we known this, we might have simply done phone interviews with the other ear-nose-throat specialists in that office *before* we made our initial appointment. After the fact, we received rave reviews about a woman who also worked in that office. We learned this little rule the hard way.

"What you risk
reveals what you value."

—Jeanette Winterson

Thursday, March 14, 2002
Subject: "DECISION MADE!"

Beloved Marley People,

Looks like we're going to do just the radiation—no surgery! We begin radiating both the hip and the throat on Monday. Should last for a month or so (5 days/week).

The risks are relatively low, and the outcome should be just as effective as the surgery probably would be.

Looking forward to being with Marley and Catie for the next two weeks, which includes Spring break. (They come back tomorrow.)

Not much else to share, except I love you all.
Jennifer

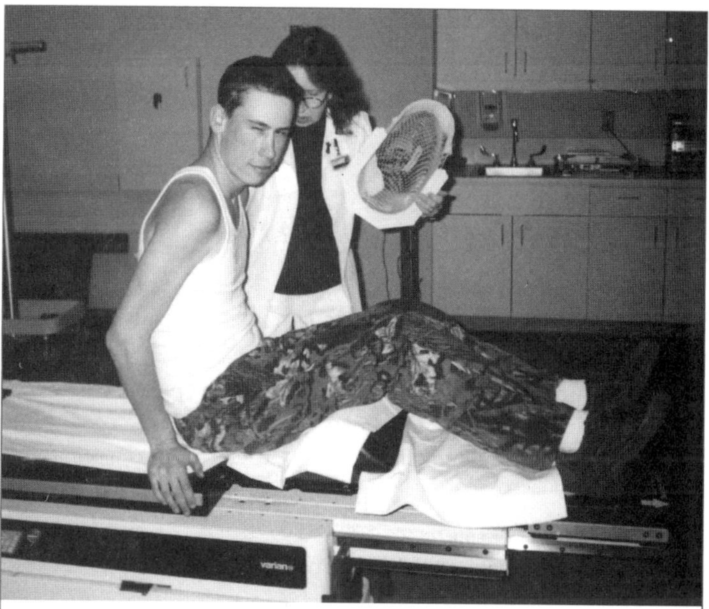

Marley obviously enthused by another round of radiation!

Wednesday, April 3, 2002
Subject: "YET ANOTHER TUMOR—
GIVE ME A BREAK!"

Howdy Folks!

Spring has sprung. Yahoo!

Marley is in his third and final week of radiation for the tumor in his hip and the one on the left side of the thyroid. Just a few days before the end of this round, another tumor was discovered. This time just to the right of the first thyroid tumor. Geeze Louise! It feels like a marble on his Adam's apple.

Marley told me about this one on April 1st. I thought for sure he was trying to pull my leg. No such luck. It sure would have been nice if it *were* an April Fool's joke. Oh well.

He feels relatively good. He's always tired, but there's no pain in his neck area. The doctors aren't even going to biopsy this one, just nuke it. How can a new tumor develop while he's being radiated in almost the same spot? "Almost" is the key word. The laser line for the first one is very specific to avoid doing more damage than needed. Who would have guessed? It sure didn't show up in the pictures taken just a month ago.

Never a dull moment in the wonderful world of Marley Jacob Pratt! All we can do is just take it one step at a time.

Take care of yourselves—and I encourage you to enjoy the world's wonders...they're everywhere!

Smelling the flowers,
Jennifer

P.S. Marley's voice has begun to change due to the radiation, and his neck has an oval tan line around his Adam's apple. Now Marley proudly calls himself a "red neck."

SUICIDE WATCH

Troubles at School

Marley was losing his appetite for school. About the only things that kept him going were his job in the lunchroom and his two elective classes, carpentry and shop. The only problem was that he was having increased difficulty leaving his wheelchair and standing up for long periods of time. All three of his favorite classes required him to be upright, and there was no easy solution.

We talked at length about asking the school to get mats for the kitchen floor so it wouldn't be so slick, and we talked about rearranging the layout of the shop classes so he could get his wheelchair in there. He said, "It's no use, Ma, they don't care and neither do I. I don' have the enagy to do any o' that stuff anyway." It was a good thing summer was just around the corner—school was almost over.

I received an e-mail from Marley's special-ed teacher, Holly, who also had been his main advocate at the high school during his first two years. I could tell she was really worried about Marley.

Thursday, April 18, 2002
Subject: "TROUBLES AT SCHOOL"

• From: Holly

Dear Jennifer,

Here at school Marley really seems to get tired easily. He actively participates in any discussion we have in Social Studies and English, and always has opinions and analogies to offer, but can't focus for long, complains of headaches and fatigue; and later he'll say he hates the class. Last week, when I had a sub, he spent an entire class sitting outside in the sun while the class made tacos. She checked in with him frequently, but reported that he just seemed very depressed and listless. Bonnie (cafeteria manager) told me today that Marley has

> become very distracted and is unable to remember the steps to putting together a sandwich in his job. I suspect that's why he wants to quit.
>
> Today I set up a meeting for him with Demaris so he could just talk, and he was really glad to do that. Demaris is able to see him during third period beginning Monday, and continuing as long as needed. We are also working on something for fourth period where he can practice public speaking with Shianna—I'll let you know if that comes through.
>
> You should also know that on the day he sat out during the cooking class, he told Beth (the nurse) that if he still felt this bad in two weeks he was going to take a gun and kill himself.
>
> I returned to school this week after my illness, and he has seemed more positive. I have been trying to monitor his moods and attitude carefully, and today he seems more agitated and uneasy, and I wanted to be sure you had been told about that comment to Beth.
>
> We're willing to do whatever we can to set up Marley's days so that he enjoys them. Hopefully, with some creativity, we can get something in place quickly.
>
> Holly

No matter what Marley said, the fact was the folks at the high school really did care, but change never happened fast in that setting. Marley had a love-hate relationship with Holly, but I knew she had always bent over backwards trying to get him what he needed to stay involved. The only problem was follow-through and cooperation with other teachers. Generally, one out of every four great ideas actually happened.

Getting Demaris' help was one of Holly's most brilliant solutions. Demaris was a "transition counselor." I was never sure what that meant exactly, but I was glad she always had time for Marley—he adored her.

Friday, April 19, 2002
Subject: "RE: TROUBLES AT SCHOOL"

• To: Holly, Ashland High

Thanks Holly,

I really appreciate your letter, and hope this reply can help give perspective.

Medical Update:
Marley is no longer being radiated for his hip and the #1 neck tumor. He is only being radiated for #2 neck tumor that will last until Tuesday or Wednesday. The effects of the radiation will be felt for another two to three weeks after that. (We're expecting a sore throat and more fatigue.) We're checking into the increasing pain in his thigh and hip. I'll keep you posted.

I have found Marley's discomfort is felt more when A) he's not being active, B) he disagrees with the activity, or C) he's bored. Marley gets headaches at school and not at home. Hmmmm. Please remember, the official report states Marley is "mildly mentally retarded between 9 A.M. and 3 P.M." See a pattern?

Depressed and Listless
One major reason Marley may be depressed is because he's battling a vicious and unrelenting case of lung cancer. He is depressed because he has nothing to look forward to at school. He can't quite figure out why he's there for seven hours each weekday, when he could be behind a roto-tiller creating his very own garden, or mowing the lawn with the tractor he just spent ten hours putting together using the instruction book!

Kitchen Job
Marley felt that he shouldn't be doing the kitchen job because he's "not all together." I agreed that at that job he needs to be

focused to remain safe. It's also tough for him to stand for long periods and he worries about slipping because there are no floor mats. Yes, let's get Marley out of the kitchen, for everyone's sake!

Regarding Suicide:
Marley's brand of sarcasm and communicating his feelings is a bit rough around the edges. He's been successful in letting us know he's seriously not happy, and we've been put on notice to listen. In his position, I must admit, oncoming Mack trucks and busy railroad tracks would start to look pretty good.

For the record, in November, he said he'd be happy to live for another 20 months. (With his understanding and use of numbers, it's difficult to know if he's thinking about two days or two years.) He's also said he hopes he dies from something other than the cancer, ie: rattlesnake, bike wreck, falling off cliffs, etc. Scares me, but I have to respect it. All we can do is try and make it possible for his life to be a little more interesting and worth living for. The rest is up to him.

The Future
Beth, Demaris, Shianna, Drew, Cindy, you, and I, and anyone else who is involved with Marley, should know we have a frustrated earth dweller on board. He has made his feeling known (duh!) yet feels relatively powerless to change the events that govern his life. Is there anything else we can do? *That* is the question. Let's continue to be inventive.

Marley has made many of us question the standard operating procedure of living. Thank God. Someone has to do it. May we all learn well!

Many thanks,
Jennifer

Chapter Twelve:
HOPE

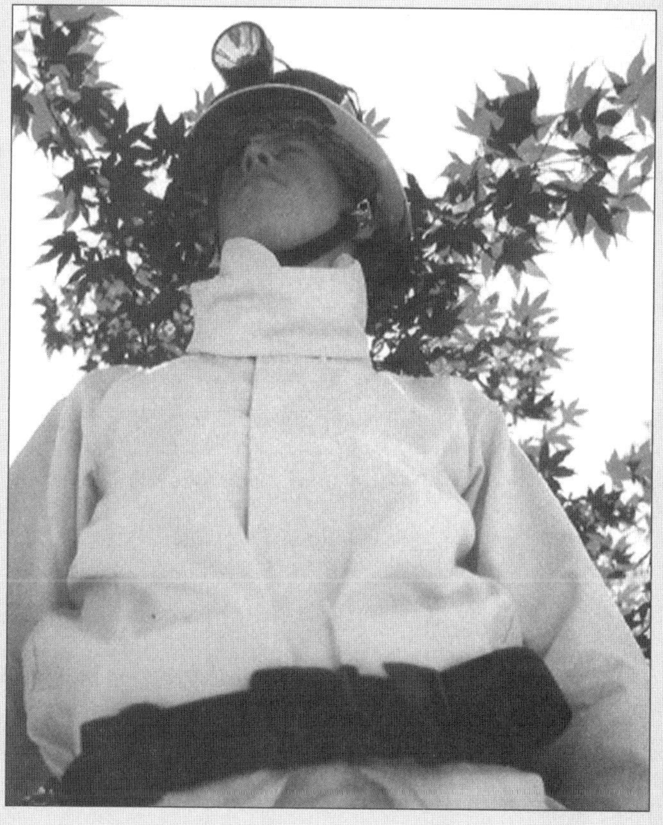

Firefighter Marley

Photo: Jay Newman

RADIATION

Total Recharge

Springtime is an extraordinary time of year. Somehow it didn't matter how intense my life felt when I was outside soaking up the sun's radiating energy. I could literally feel the rays healing me, recharging my batteries. Even though my current life story looked pretty grim, it didn't feel so bad. I had time off when the kids were with Drew and Cindy. I knew they were in good hands, and they loved being with Vanessa and Laura. I had two weeks to take care of myself so I would have the energy to take care of Marley and Catie when they returned for my two-week shift. It was a good deal.

The spring of 2002 was incredible; the blues seemed bluer and the whites seemed whiter than normal. Maybe edging closer and closer to death's door made me start to appreciate everything a little more. I was actually feeling more alive and full of love than I had ever felt before. Physically, I was strong. Emotionally, I felt calm and ready for anything. Mentally, all systems were firing at 100 percent capacity. And spiritually, I felt like I was standing with my arms open wide in the middle of a beam of radiating love. It sounds corny but I felt high, like my life was totally on target.

"Since my house burned down,
I now own a better view of the rising moon."

—Masahide

The weather was superb, and I spent as much time as possible at home working as hard as a body can. I adored working up at my place, surrounded by the music my wind chimes made. It was my style of therapy. I listened to books on tape as I unearthed boulders to build retaining walls, shoveled dirt to prepare new garden spaces, moved log piles, and split more wood for next year. I built a brick wall around the firepit, because I knew the crew would be gathering again now that the snows had melted. For most of May, I was burnt to a crisp and as sore as I'd been in years.

Evolution

I also spent my time just sitting outside in awe of the beauty of nature. I declared that a part of my goal was to imitate my beloved cat Salsa and my dog Zipper. They seemed to know so much about doing nothing. I pondered why we don't act more like our fellow animals and questioned if we really are an evolved species.

Like the flowers, Catie was blossoming. She was high on skiing, feeling that she'd definitely found a calling. It was pure joy to witness her loving something so much. She worked her beautiful, strong, tall body hard and came home exhausted but elated. Finding rides up to Mount Ashland consumed her free time—the ski season was ending, and she didn't want to miss any opportunity to speed down the slopes. Meanwhile, she was also jazzed about school and continued to get straight A's. I think she too was riding high on a mysterious wave of energy.

It was like all three of us, in our own ways, were gobbling up life and savoring every last morsel. Marley was staying as busy as humanly possible, ignoring the pain he felt. At Drew's house, he had taken it upon himself to build a bridge over a 15-foot-deep ravine. Using the Mule, he somehow managed to get two 30-foot long, 12-inch wide pieces of steel across the span of the ravine. No one was aware of what he was doing until he was done. Drew was amazed, because those planks of steel were extremely heavy, and he couldn't explain how Marley had done this without having them fall into the ravine. If they had, Drew reported, they would have had to hire a crane to come lift them out.

At my house, Marley spent countless hours finding new ways to use the endless yards of climbing rope that Sunny gave him on every birthday. One morning I woke up to find that Marley had spent hours carefully tying a grove of oak trees together. I couldn't figure out why he had done this, and I thought it was an eyesore.

I blurted, "Jesus, Marley! What possessed you to tie the trees up?" He didn't bother talking, he just smiled at me and proceeded to use the web of rope to climb to the tree tops. I nodded, impressed, and said, "Cool!" as I walked back in the house.

"Everything that is really great and inspiring is created by the individual who can labor in freedom."

—Albert Einstein

While Marley had been fighting battle after battle with cancer, he was also growing up. The evolution from boy to man was striking. It wasn't just that he was taller, it was the way his jaw, cheekbones, and forehead were more defined. His shoulders were broader and the muscles were much larger. His upper body had definitely become very buff from using the wheelchair while at school— although his left leg looked like a tree trunk, while his right one was growing thinner and thinner from under-use. Even though the cancer was chewing through his body, attacking one part at a time (sometimes two), Marley was looking good.

To add to his manly persona, Marley's voice had radically changed. We discovered that radiating the tumor on his thyroid gland, just below the surface of the skin, was a tricky business. The beam had to be aimed just right so the nerves and blood-flow to his brain wouldn't be fried too. The radiation oncologists had to come at it from the rear, just below his ear, so they wouldn't nuke his vocal cords too much. Even so, his voice began to remind me of a cartoon character, or like a middle-aged lumberjack who smoked too much.

As the effects of the radiation lessened, his voice became no longer comedic, but instead very adult. The shift was subtle and slow. His transformation wasn't just physical—everything about Marley had changed. The way he expressed himself and treated others was less self absorbed. I realized that I still thought of him as the fifteen-year-old who got sick, so I started observing him more. As his strength began to return, I would stand back and watch him with wonder as I realized Marley had become a man.

***"Change is inevitable.
No one would argue about something so obvious.
Yet we're always surprised when it happens."***

—Gloria Karpinski

Friday, June 21, 2002
Subject: "HAPPY BUT TIRED"

My Dearest Marley Network,

It's late and at the end of a very long week. I've wanted to write for over two months but, when I have both work and the kids to tend to, spending a couple of extra hours at the office is not in the cards. I passed the kids off to their dad this afternoon, soooo... here I am with you.

THANK YOU

I wish I could communicate how close you feel—it's like you're with us daily—even those of you we don't know. Marley's rock fountain is just outside my window here at work, reminding me of your love. There is electricity here for the fountain's pump, and this is where we seem to always be. I've noticed the folks who walk by the office are also touched by the very unusual fountain outside this beautiful old red schoolhouse. Your love and healing are felt by many.

UPDATE

Since the last round of cancer (a second tumor in the hip and two new ones on his thyroid), we've just been cruising. Marley's voice got very deep and raspy but is sounding more normal now. The skin on his neck was very burnt by the radiation. It bubbled and peeled. Two months later, it just looks very tan in one patch. Apparently this effect may remain for years.

His energy level is generally very low. Nine times out of ten, if you ask him, "How are you?" He'll respond with one, long, drawn out word, "Tired!" But he's still like the Energizer Bunny. If you tell him his buddies Luke and Lucas are waiting for him to show up with his Mule, he's off like lightning for ten hours of exploring the back country of the Colestin Valley. He pays for it later but he doesn't care. When he's doing things BIG, he seems to forget about the pain and lack of energy.

FIRE!

Catie has joined Marley as a member of the Colestin Volunteer Fire Department. Twice a month, they go to training sessions in preparation for what looks like a very dry summer. Marley was just fitted for his official firefighter's outfit. Since Marley was a wee one, he's wanted to be either a firefighter or an EMT (Emergency Medical Technician). Catie wants to be a doctor. So somehow it makes sense that they're getting some very serious training, very young.

SCHOOL

Marley's finally in the best possible scenario for next year—an alternative school called The Wilderness Charter School. There he'll spend half the day learning the basics in creative ways. The rest of the day will be spent at the high school doing electives: auto shop, woodworking, and photography. The kitchen staff has asked for him back next year if he's able. We're all thrilled. Maybe it'll be a reason to get up and suffer through his arthritic first hours of each day.

CURRENT STATUS

Marley's a 6'2", 165-pound 17-year-old. Catie's a 5'5", 114-pound 12-year-old. I look up to them both from my 5'2" perspective, feeling older and older. What really threw me was when Marley beat me arm wrestling last week. Something giant shifted for me. I no longer feel like I'm in control (like I ever was). We joined the YMCA. Marley can swim and try to build up the strength in his knee and enjoy the hot tub's healing. Catie can play and be social. And I can work on my arm wrestling muscles.

In a nutshell, Marley's knee continues to be very painful and he has very low energy. With your help and the help of alternative therapists we're currently seeing, Marley is trying to tell the cancer it is not wanted. Sometimes it feels like we're staying just ahead of the cell growth, buying him enough time so his body can heal a bit before the next wave hits.

THE FUTURE

Unknown! Changes on all levels are brewing. Visiting family and traveling seem to be what matters most to both the kids. Marley talks of wanting to travel around the country visiting family in a big motor home. (Unrealistic but fun!) Marley wants to play hard and dream big (forget the little steps). He's been talking about his Western Rest Home idea. He's very serious about this rest home, designed for the kind of folk who would quickly curl up and die if put in a traditional rest home. I wish I had an extra million dollars and a few extra hours each day to make his vision a reality.

Anyway, I'm fried. I have the weekend before me to plan how best to juggle maintaining current real-world needs while creating our fantasy world.

I love you all,
Jennifer

P.S.

• Congratulations to Catie for perfect grades in her first year of middle school.

• Mabel Fenstemmer (whoever you are), we think you rock! Your care package of gems was well received, but our thank you gift was returned. Are you a part of Marley's Network, or are you a mysterious angel?

• Marley's website is being overhauled by our beloved friend Debbie. Will keep you posted on its progress.

FIGHTING FIRE WITH FIRE

Prepared for the Worst

Luke, Marley, Catie, Lucas, and Lucas' younger sister Andrea all joined the Colestin Valley Volunteer Fire Department. This was a very smart thing that Steve, the fire chief, encouraged. Other than Laura and Vanessa, this group consisted of the Valley's entire population of teenagers. Three of these teenagers (the Coyotes) spent most of their waking hours on gasoline-powered vehicles, roaming the nearby mountain ridges. Steve's decision was likely to save that dry little valley from being torched by careless teenagers! He was educating them and putting them in charge of protecting the region. Their job was to cruise around (which they were doing anyway) and act as roving lookout scouts.

Marley took his job very seriously. He was bound and determined to be the first one at the scene, any scene. Just in case, he always had what he considered a proper emergency rescue kit on hand. This meant a lot of rope, pitons, water, bandages and, of course, duct tape. He even had a miniature first aid kit strapped to his wheelchair at school and another on his backpack.

On the day that Lucas, Luke, and Marley were going to Dreadford to be outfitted for their official bright yellow firefighter suits, they stopped by my office on the way to Luke's mom's office to pick up one of Marley's bikes. Ten minutes later, I got a call from Marley asking me if I could drive him to Dreadford because Luke had to go to the hospital.

"Say what?" I exclaimed, "What happened?

Marley described how he was having trouble holding his cane while trying to steer his bike while Lucas was pushing him. Luke took the cane for Marley and, while jogging next to the bike, he managed to stick the end of the cane between his feet and he tripped! Apparently Big Luke hit the pavement hard and broke his collar bone. I had to laugh. Poor Luke. It was going to be hard for him to get sympathy with Marley around. Luke couldn't get away with much complaining, so it didn't take long before they had their fire suits and were ready for action.

A few weeks later, Marley was driving his Mule on the back country roads in the Colestin and saw a plume of thick black smoke coming from the Hilt Store. He hit the gas and was determined to save the day, but by the time he got there, the fire chief and his team had already put the fire out. A Volkswagen bus had caught on fire about 25 feet away from the two gas station pumps. Because Marley was there and had come prepared with his new fire suit, the chief let Marley lend a hand in the clean-up. Marley was most enthused about his role and thrilled that his fire suit was forever streaked with black soot stains and smelled like smoke, the way it was supposed to.

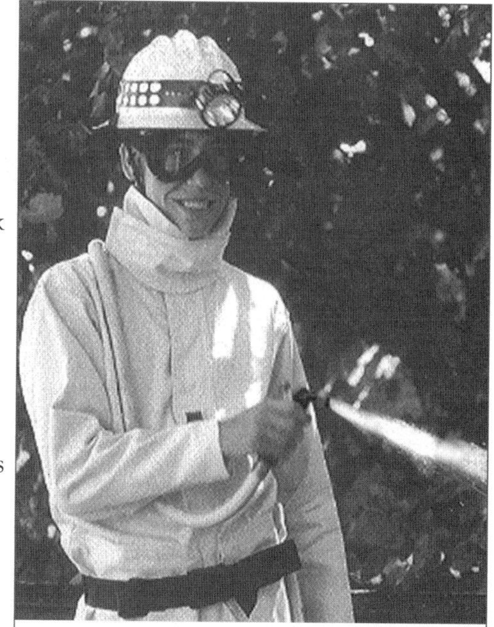

"Prepared for Action!"
Marley in his new fire suit.
Photo: Jay Newman

Throughout the rest of the fire season, Marley took every opportunity to protect the valley. Drew said he was out the door and on his Mule at the break of day, and most days didn't come home until dinner time. Drew complained because Marley was never around to help with the chores, mainly moving the long irrigation pipes in the hay fields. I asked Marley what he did all day and he said, "Mostly I go up high and just watch."

I asked, "What are you looking for?"

He looked at me like I was a little slow and told me, "From up thar you can see smoke."

Okay, so I did feel a little dumb but I kept on pressing for conversation—a little glimpse into Marley's world. "When there's no smoke, what do you do all day?"

I knew by his shrug I wasn't going to get a whole lot out of him, so I gave up trying. Then a few minutes later, he said, "Ya know, Ma, it's nice jus' sittin' up thar and watchin' the clouds go by. Jus' sit. That's what I do."

I never seem to let things go, so I had to pry just a little more. "Do you think about having cancer and what's happening to your body? Do you ever get scared or feel alone?"

It was a nice try, but he looked at me and simply said, "Nah." Conversation done.

As an ex-wilderness quest guide, I was pleased that he was spending solitary time. I knew the balance of nature always has a special way of healing wounds and inspiring growth.

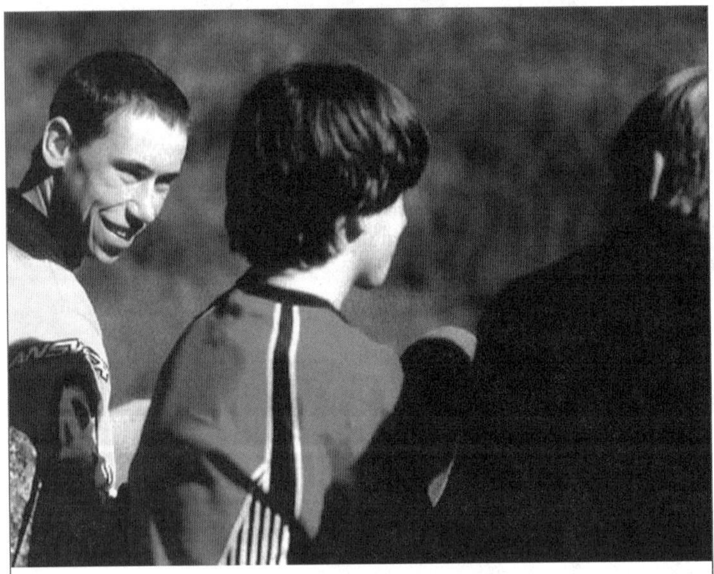

The Coyotes: Marley, Lucas, and Luke hanging out on a ridge top.
Photo: Jay Newman

THE OREGON COUNTRY FAIR REVISITED

You Only Live Once!

Last year, Marley, Catie, Jay, Jeff, my best buddy Andrea, and I piled in the Suburban and ventured to the Oregon Country Fair, four hours north. We'd had a great time and, this year, everybody wanted to repeat the event. Andrea was on the East coast, so she couldn't join us, but Selene was in town and wanted to come. When Selene was little, she used to spend the summers with us, and I'd take her to the Country Fair. She knew what she was getting into and was excited and raring to go.

I was a little more concerned this year, because Marley was increasingly dependent on his wheelchair and on his painkillers. I knew he would be constantly surrounded by one or all of our crew, but going to the Country Fair was still a hard journey. Both his shoulder and his pelvic bone were rapidly disintegrating, and he'd have to tax both to the limit during the weekend. But he knew what he was up against and still desperately wanted to go. What the hell! We all deserved to play as hard as we could, especially Marley—it had been another tough year and, like he kept saying, "Ya only live once!"

"You only live once—
but if you work it right, once is enough."

—Joe E. Lewis

Circus of the Sun Dragon

During this little vacation, Selene's personal goal was to show Marley a *really* good time. She had convinced me that we should drive up to Portland, before going to the Country fair, to see Cirque du Soleil perform *Dralion*. I had seen this amazing troupe perform on video, but never live. Both kids really wanted to go, so I agreed. I just kept my fingers crossed that we would all survive the weekend.

On Thursday morning, we left Ashland and drove six hours to Portland to experience the most bizarre "circus" act I could ever imagine. The videos I had seen of their various shows were outrageously entertaining, but seeing it up close and personal was a different story. Women slithered down 30-foot long ribbons of material while boys danced on top of giant rolling balls. But when the silver-painted juggler in a G-string tossed balls ten feet up to a hanging trapeze artist, using the nape of his neck, I thought I was going to explode! As my sister Constant used to say, "I was having containment difficulties."

I was blown away by the absolutely perfect execution of extreme feats. I felt like a little kid. I sat spellbound with tears of joy streaking my face. Catie looked at me in horror when she saw that I was crying. I had to explain that I was just too happy to contain my emotions. Marley, on the other hand, was having comfort difficulties sitting on the wooden bleachers. He had poked fun at me for insisting on bringing a pillow for him to sit on, but ended up thanking me profusely for the extra padding.

We were all floating three feet off the ground when we piled back into Indy and drove two hours south to the Country Fair, just west of Eugene. It was about 10 P.M. when we met Jeff, his new girlfriend Annie, Jay, Eric, and Eric's sister Liz, at the campground. Catie, Marley, Selene, and I spent the next few hours excitedly trying to describe what we had just seen, all talking at the same time. It was a great energy to have in preparation for the next two days.

The Main Event

The following morning, we spent hours putting on glitter, cool clothes, and creating weird hairdos. It was Marley's second year of being at the Country Fair in a wheelchair, so he knew how to prepare. He took off the footrests and armrests and was ready to roll. Once again, he did a remarkable job of negotiating through intense crowds over rough terrain.

Jay's love for Marley was a wondrous thing to witness that weekend. He was never very far away from Mars, and he was willing to wrestle with Marley endlessly whenever the frustration or pain levels began to rise. This year, Marley didn't do much exploring. Instead, he spent most of the time on our big blanket at the main stage, listening to one great band after another and being visited by other friends who were also at the fair. Whenever he did explore, I knew he'd be watching the flint knappers, or the

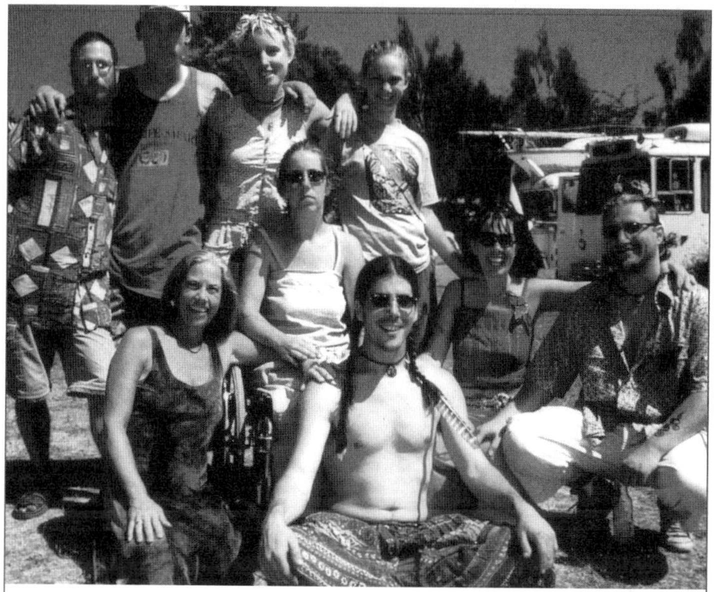

Jay, Marley, Selene, Catie, Jennifer, Liz (in the wheelchair), Eric, Annie, and Jeff at the Oregon Country Fair, 2002

Photo: Jay Newman

fire makers, or he would be learning how to make giant fish nets.

We had a phenomenal time that weekend. Marley was so cool and was such an instrumental part of pushing us all to have extreme amounts of fun. We had come armed with glow sticks: long tubing filled with phosphorescent chemicals that glow in the dark. Marley kept inventing new ways of connecting them to ropes for a unique light show. Our attitudes and Marley's creativity rubbed off on all the nearby campers. It turned out to be the best campground party that I've witnessed in all the years I've been going there. It felt like everyone there became one family. Usually everyone is friendly, but this year was special. Our camp became the hub of action and Marley was loving it.

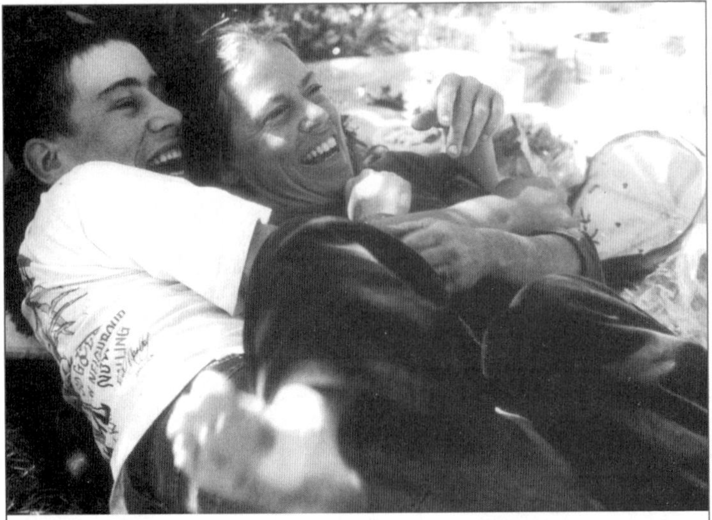

Marley and Jennifer playing at the Country Fair
Photo: Jay Newman

Accidents Do Happen

We decided to return taking the long road home, traveling west to the Pacific Coast Highway. When we stopped to have a fresh seafood dinner, Marley was so happy to be back on smooth pavement that he did one trick after another in his wheelchair. After dinner, he did one last flying leap off a very high curb and the wheelchair buckled under the stress, snapping the metal supports.

The wheelchair was transported on a bike rack attached to the back of the Suburban. The following day, I made a grave error in judgement and backed into a light pole hidden in my only blind spot. The four-inch diameter pole bent Marley's wheelchair in half. I had to laugh, thinking to myself that gods were making it so my auto insurance would probably cover the already broken wheelchair. Yes indeed, the following week everything was back to normal and Marley had a new wheelchair.

"Problems are only opportunities in work clothes."

—-Henry Kaiser

Thursday, August 1, 2002
Subject: "THIRD NECK TUMOR"

Hiya folks,

Timing Is Everything!

Wish I had more spunk to write a fun letter. But today we finished our first *Uncle John's Bathroom Reader For Kids*! In one of our traditional deadline crunches, I have managed to work way too much. I'm not sure I'm proud, just amazed that my last day off was Sunday, July 21, and since then I've clocked in 119 hours. Sure wish I was being paid overtime! I'm tired but completely satisfied—it feels really good to work with a well-trained team of really cool people, successfully creating a product that will sell very well and make people happy. Enough… it's done! Sure feels good to say that. Best yet, tomorrow the kids begin their two weeks with me! I can focus on relaxing and loving up my children before the next deadline for our annual 500-page *Bathroom Reader* is due (Sept. 30th).

As always, Marley's timing is impeccable. He's picked the perfect two weeks to require my attention. Yup, he's got another tumor. This one is in a lymph node on the left side of his neck, just below the curve of the jaw line. If you took my hand (it's small) and cupped it against your neck, that's how big it is. Kinda makes him look like a football player with a thick neck.

Takes a licking and keeps on ticking!

I saw him today at the radiologist's and he looked great. He was full of sarcastic smiles and big, warm, loving hugs. Cool kid. I really like him. He has a flashy gold cane decorated with duct tape that he uses most of the time (his knee really hurts). Somehow it all works with his "look." He's a tall, tan, lanky cowboy that looks like he got bucked off a mean horse.

Don't know what procedure we'll choose. There are definite

pros and cons to consider regarding radiation. There's been a lot of radiation aimed at his poor neck recently. We need more info about the possibility of surgery. Drew, Cindy, and I are cautious about the skill level of the doctors here in the little old Rogue Valley, but we still need to investigate. While the info is gathered, I plan to have some fun with Marley. That's what counts.

Well, the manuscript has finished printing out and I get to go home and look it over again tonight. (I'm a glutton for punishment.) But first I'm going to type a poem written by Marley that I found on the living room floor this morning.

– Marley –

Ornery, driven, outdoorsy, tough

Brother of Vanessa, Laura, Catie

Lover of fire fighting, the Colestin Valley, four-wheeling

Who feels happy at mud holes, sad with cancer, lost at not knowing where I am going in life.

Who needs love, four-wheeling, and chaos

Who gives time to fight fires, have friendships, and pay attention to horses

Who fears cancer, tourists, teachers

Resident of the Colestin, Colestin Road

– Pratt –

That says it all!
I love you,
Jennifer

The Butterfly Effect

A DOG STORY
by Janet Spencer

I had a dog named Fibber McGee that reminds me of Marley. Fibber got hit by a car—an accident which left her permanently paralyzed from the waist down. She was six years old at the time and spent the next nine years "confined" to a little doggie wheelchair. Although she was crippled for the rest of her life, I would hesitate to call her handicapped. She was pure hell on wheels. She actually had two wheelchairs, one with wheels and the other with skis so she could accompany me both hiking and skiing. She went with me all over Montana, canoeing, berry picking, swimming, and she trundled happily about in her little cart with never a complaint about her condition.

I spent much time wondering about the karmic and cosmic implications of her paralysis. What could be the good to come out of this situation? I admit that she attracted an enormous amount of attention—she was a real traffic-stopper. People may forget meeting me, but they NEVER forget meeting my dog in her wheelchair. Over the course of nine years, I explained thousands upon thousands of times what had happened and how well she was doing. Still, what was the purpose of this accident?

Then one day I found out. I was walking down the street on the way to the library with her tagging along as usual. A man in a wheelchair came down the street towards me and called out for me to stop. He told me that he'd been living on my street for many years and had watched me and my dog go by more times than he could count. Today he had to tell me his story. "I live on the bottom floor of this apartment building but I used to live upstairs. One day six years ago, I had too much to drink and I fell down the stairs. By the time I landed at the bottom, I was permanently paralyzed from the waist down and I've never walked since. I was real depressed when I came home from the hospital—but every day you and your dog would walk by right in front of my window. One day I said to myself, 'Dammit, if that DOG can do it, then I can do it too!' and I shook off my depression and got my life back together. So I just wanted to meet your dog and say thanks for helping me so much."

When Fibber died at the age of 15, I ran her obituary in the local paper because she had become quite a celebrity. We held a memorial service for her, and many people, including a lot of total strangers, showed up to pay their last respects and honor the spirit of this indomitable dog. I still dream about her occasionally. She doesn't use the wheelchair anymore.

"Never believe that a few caring 'people' can't change the world. For, indeed, that's all who ever have."

—Margaret Mead

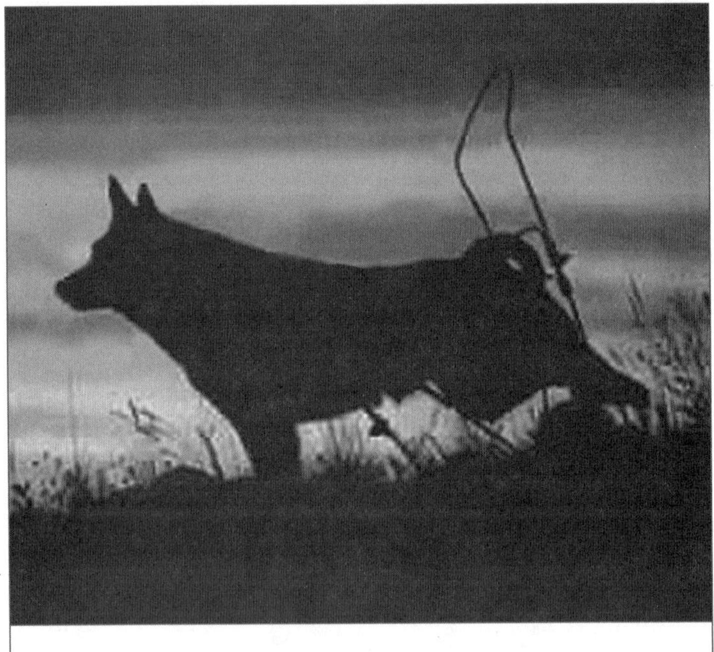

Fibber McGee Spencer

Photo: Janet Spencer

Sunday, August 18, 2002
Subject: "REUNIONS"

Dearest Marley fans,

It's a quiet Sunday afternoon. The kids went back to Drew and Cindy's last Friday for another two-week shift. I've come into town to help work on Marley's website, write to you, and to get a jump on this week's work load.

Catie, Marley, and I had a superior trip south to visit family (two back-to-back reunions). The first gathering was to celebrate my brother-in-law's 64th birthday. The Foster reunions are a summer tradition that include most of Steven's kin and non-kin family. The Foster clan comes from everywhere on the West coast to toast this long-toothed wise man for all the gifts he's given to so many. Steven has been suffering from a rare lung disorder for several years, and his health is rapidly deteriorating. This reunion may be his last hurrah, so we made sure it was a very special time.

The second reunion was to celebrate my sister's father's 90th birthday. Phil is frail, yet this old codger keeps on shuffling into the future. It is a rare occasion that all of my siblings gather together, for we are scattered across the globe. We had a grand time and took some great photos of the three generations. These are precious shots, because three of the clan (one from each generation) are not long for this life.

For years now, Steven, Phil, and Marley have been nudging each other in the ribs, taking side bets on which of the three is going to die first. (Black humor, at its finest.) It was sad yet heartwarming to watch the three of them live so fully and love their family true, savoring every exchange as if it might be their last.

During the return trip, Marley was riding shotgun in our beloved, deluxe Suburban, while Catie slept in the back. At one point, he turned down the music and matter-of-factly suggested we head to see his doctor Diane, ASAP. My heart sank, because I knew Marley knew something serious was up. He had just spent two weeks being incredibly social and active, rarely complaining. I pondered about why he had waited until the trip back to say something. Maybe being around Phil, shuffling slowly to-and-fro, and Steven, hauling his oxygen tank with him everywhere, made Marley feel like the healthy one! Maybe he just didn't want to ruin two great reunions.

As I tightly gripped the steering wheel, he described what he was feeling. The one tumor, on the lymph in his neck, hadn't changed much since the last MRI, but he complained his neck was feeling tight in certain positions. He pointed out a new, smaller one that's now visible, just below the existing one. He also said he was having fairly constant pain in both his right shoulder and hip. (As always, he complained about his knee, which always hurts, but we all know there's not much we can do about that.)

So…once we returned and saw the doctors, he started a new round of radiation. We're now halfway through the four weeks of zapping the two diseased lymph nodes. Surgery wasn't an option, because we needed to act fast and the risks were too high. A CAT scan of his shoulder and hip didn't show anything obvious, so an MRI was needed for a better look. I took Marley in on Friday, but the results aren't in yet.

His hip has had the "maximum radiation advisable," and replacement parts don't exist for that bone so, like his knee, it seems there's nothing we can do. We have to concentrate on alternative therapies for those areas. In the meantime, aside from the various cancer cure pills, vitamins, homeopathic remedies, etc., we have some other tricks our sleeves.

Alternative alternatives! Marley now has regularly scheduled massages with a big, beautiful, blind, black Brit. Marley loves this guy and apparently the feeling is mutual, because he has offered his services to Marley for free! If all goes well, Marley will also be meeting with a Karate teacher who is also a youth counselor. Hopefully he'll be working with Marley to find ways to deal with the ever growing frustrations of living.

Last week, Marley met the wonderful therapist I have gone to see several times when I needed to cry on someone's shoulder. Marley thought Dot was pretty neat…for a shrink. Dot is a 4'8" silver-haired woman with an ear-to-ear smile, deeply lined leathery skin, and twinkling eyes that look right into your soul. He fell in love with her a few days after their first meeting when he saw her speeding by the office on her bike, passing all the others on the trail. That impressed him so much, he now wants to meet with her regularly for counseling!

So now that we have his body and emotions tended to, we can concentrate on his mind. Marley is entering his junior year at high school. The spirits were smiling on our family when the Marley Man was accepted into The Wilderness Charter School. Of forty applicants, only twenty were chosen. This is an alternative school within a school at Ashland High. It's the answer to a decade of my dreams. This school rocks! Marley's in very good hands.

Know that we love you and I'm thankful you are all out there.

Check out Marley's new website. It's still under construction but it's fun to see the unfolding.

Oh my God, someone please tell me to shut up!!!

But…I forgot to tell you Marley has a very cool electric bike that was donated to him. I'll tell you the whole story later.

Good night!
Jennifer

"What is to give light must endure burning."

—Viktor Frankl

The Butterfly Effect

THE MARLEY FILTER
by Patty Foster

To think about Marley brings a smile to my face, yet to adequately express all the ways Marley affected me is difficult. It embarrasses me to think that I could possibly express the depth of feeling that goes with being lucky enough to have known him.

There are so many "Marleyisms" that have seeped into our family's daily life. Questions we often ask at difficult junctures are "What would Marley say?" or "How would Marley handle this?" We've learned that sometimes the absurd will make total sense if we put it through the Marley filter.

We have often used Marley's take on life to help guide our daughter Olivia through the hellish middle school years. We'd often look at each other and ask "What would Marley do?" Somehow the answer always became clear. That beautiful kid was the ultimate guide, especially effective since he did so without us knowing we were being guided. A teacher that teaches while making us think we are going solo.

We think of Marley every time we drive to Sebastopol, California, which is where we went shopping during the last Foster family reunion. Marley drove into town with us because he wanted to be where the action was. He was in a lot of pain, so he planted himself on a park bench and waited while everyone else ran around shopping.

In the park that day was the first time I spent time alone with Marley. I was taken back by the way he looked at life. He was so sure of himself and so calm. But mostly he was so honest and upfront about what he thought. He talked of what colored jelly bean he loved most and then, without warning, spoke of what he'll miss most and wished he could do. It wasn't what he said as much as *how* he said it—without caring what anybody else thought.

A POWERFUL GIFT

Energy in Motion

The one thing that Marley sorely missed was mobility. Getting around on his own steam was becoming a chore. Crutches helped with the leg, but hurt the shoulder, so he rarely used them. His manual wheelchair got him from point A to B, but was only viable if he was on relatively level ground. Working the wheels definitely buffed up his upper body but, again, it was really hard on his bad shoulder. When he was desperate he'd break out one of his six bikes and try to ride. Unfortunately, his knee didn't have quite enough strength or flexibility to pedal, and the muscles that were working over-time trying to keep his hip together would give him incredible amounts of grief. The iliam bone was getting so brittle, too much direct force could crack it.

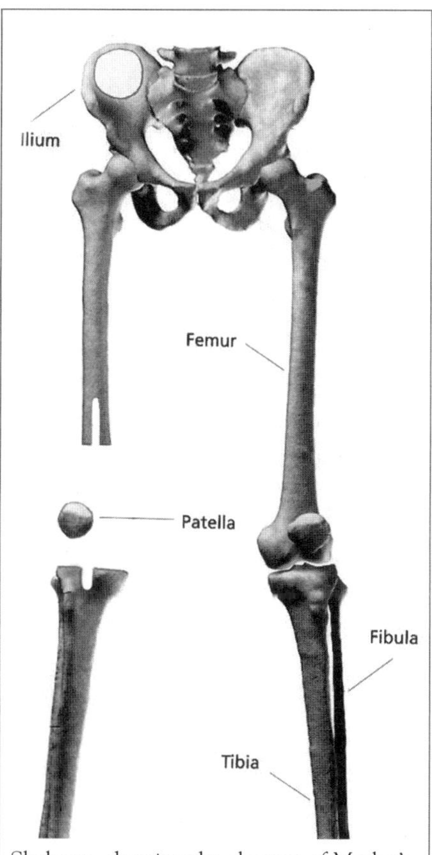

Skeleton, showing the absence of Marley's bone in both the hip and the knee where the prosthesis was placed.

Not being able to ride his bikes was the thing he missed most about the past. Lacking that feeling of freedom created a low level of depression that I worried about. Even though he couldn't ride them, he spent a lot of time fixing and reconstructing his bikes. He made some very funny contraptions, mixing and matching different parts. He made a bike with a large ten-speed wheel on the front and a small, BMX wheel on the rear, and added the handle bars from his old-fashioned cruiser, but positioned them tipped way down for a unique look. The finishing touch was to put stunt pegs on the back tire so Catie could stand behind him.

Through the window at the BRI office, I would watch one humorous test run after another. This particular contraption bombed badly when Catie mounted the pegs and her weight popped the bike into a permanent wheely. After lots of cursing and kicking the lawn furniture, he'd just start all over again. Tinkering with his bikes, trying to find the balance between functionality and originality, made him feel better about not being able to use them.

Positive Enforcement

Our little town is a progressive, inventive community that is not afraid to test local products. One of our businesses has invented and manufactured bikes with extended front forks. The comfortable chair-like seats are very low to the ground with the pedals positioned in front of the rider, like a paddleboat. Another local company manufactures a battery pack that can attach to any mountain bike. It's the same concept as a moped, but they have a governor that keeps speeds just below the requirements for needing a license.

Looking for new ways to satisfy his undying desire to move, Marley investigated both designs. He would study the low-riders every day as a crew of healthy seniors would cruise by on the trail in front of the office. At Evo's, one young guy would whiz into the parking lot with his electric bike to grab his cup of java, and then speed away at 18 miles per hour. Marley would drool. His final decision was made when his favorite cop, Terri, was seen doing her rounds downtown on one of these electric bikes. Marley knew he just had to have one. If the police department had adopted them, well, that was good enough for Mars.

Spoke-n-Truth

A few weeks later, I bumped into Brian, a friend I had known for many years. It was always a pleasure to chat with Brian, because our conversations were deep and honest. He had always offered to help Marley in any way possible, so his eyes lit up when he heard Marley was depressed about not riding bikes anymore. He was friends with the folks manufacturing the electric bikes and just happened to have a brochure in his truck. He said he could get us a discount. Being a skeptic, I thanked him and figured the rest was up to me. Just to play along, I showed him which one Marley wanted and took the brochure.

I didn't jump on the idea immediately. I figured I could buy some time handing Mars the fancy brochure. The delay technique worked for about an hour and then the pressure was on, double-time. Marley started nagging me. I'd stall and he'd whine, trying to convince me how important it was that I spend a lot of money to make him happy.

"Mom, ya know how much moor pleasant I am ta be awound when I'm ridin' and feewing fwee. Jus' do it and stop dwivin' yor litta sef cwazy!"

"Yeah, yeah, yeah. Whatever." Another nice stalling technique as I'd walk away. Luckily, Brian stopped by the office soon after and told me he had talked with the manufacturers and they agreed to donate a brand new bike, complete with the motor unit. Wow! I was blown away. This man actually followed through and created a reality that would change Marley's sometimes defeated outlook on life.

"He is rich who hath enough to be charitable."

—Sir Thomas Browne

Just in case something went wrong with the plans, I asked Brian if we could surprise Marley. I told Marley that Brian wanted to take him on a picnic the following day. With lunch in hand, Marley was ready for an adventure with a man he had met only once before. Mr. Social didn't care who Brian was, he was ready for any new experience. Little did he know what was in store for him!

Brian picked him up and took him to the storage unit which doubled as his shop. Mars thought it was a cool place to have a picnic, although a trifle unusual. Brian said it was really cute watching Marley's facial expressions as he tried to figure out what was going on as Brian rolled open the storage unit door. Brian had parked the bike front and center. Marley's eyes rolled wide when he saw it. He was twitching with excitement because he figured he might get a chance to try it out. Then Brian announced, "Marley, the folks who make these bikes thought you oughtta have one."

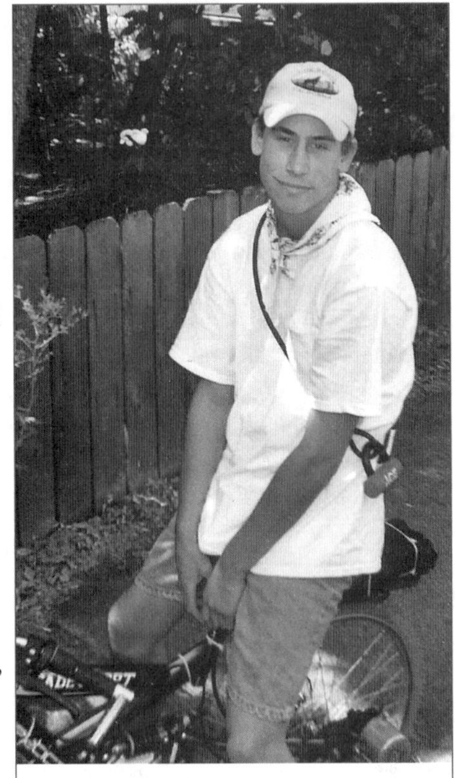

Marley on his new electric bike.

Apparently it took a minute before Marley picked his lower jaw off the pavement and said, "It's just like the one Offica Terwy has!" The best part was, there was some assembly to do, so Marley got to work together with Brian for the next few hours. I think Marley loved the one-on-one instruction just about as much as he loved getting the bike. I forever send my love and thanks to Brian for helping to make one of my boy's dreams come true.

Friday, October 11, 2002
Subject: "BREATHING EASY"

Hallo out there in Marley-land,

It's Friday night. Just passed the kids off to their dad, so I have time to write. We finished *Uncle John's Ahh-Inspiring Bathroom Reader* and it'll be in stores two weeks early! Yahoo...jump for joy! No more 20 hour days, six days a week. Now, we're back to the regular 10– to 12–hour days.

I *did* panic a couple of weeks ago, knowing there was no way I could be a mom and pull off the final week of deadline. So I pulled out my Marley Network e-mail list of local folk and posted a list of my needs. The response was phenomenal and everything worked perfectly. Catie was invited to live with our beloved friend Dee and her little son Kellar. She had a great time and even complained about coming back. Each day, someone different picked Marley up from school, took him to radiation, and delivered him to the office. I'd give him a kiss and someone else would pick him up to take him out to dinner. They'd drop him back at the office, he'd go into the back room, watch a movie, and go to sleep. I'd wake him up in the middle of night, drive him home, feed the goats, wake up at 7 A.M. and start all over. It worked out just fine!

Marley finished radiation a week ago. He had both tumors nuked, the new one on his neck and the old one, in his shoulder, that resurfaced. The doctor said that the shoulder tumor was like a smoldering volcano. It's the third time we've tried to zap the bugger. Fortunately, the area can be continuously radiated, because there are no "vital" organs in the line of fire. We only did five days of radiation in the hopes that we could reduce the pain and put out the fire again. The doctor also said that the scar tissue surrounding the place where the tumor has made the bone mush-like, may actually keep the tumor from spreading too much. (Sounds like wishful thinking to me.)

So this round has been completed, and all we've really had to watch out for was the skin on his neck. Last time, the skin blistered, oozed, and peeled off like it had been seared with a blow torch. This time I knew what to expect, so we began applying aloe and comfrey before the blisters could form. Although the radiation continues to cook the cells for two weeks after the procedure has ended, I'm pretty sure we've escaped the nasty this time!

Marley, Catie, and I checked out electric wheelchairs today. We found a really cool one called *The Blast*. Now I get to approach the insurance company and find out what the financial limit is. (It only costs $7,500.) Did I mention the ramp we have to buy to get the damned thing in the truck? (That's only $550.) I'm not too worried; our insurance company has been very cool since the beginning. I'll have to remind them about the first wheelchair that Marley thought was cool. It was called *Independence Day* and the base model cost a mere $23,000!

So I'm sure Marley's off with the Coyotes by now (his wild and crazy four-wheeling gang) and feeling good. How does Marley spell relief? C-o-y-o-t-e-s! I know they're T-r-o-u-b-l-e! But it doesn't matter…think about it…I'm one mother that can say I don't have to worry about my son running off and taking drugs…I feed them to him daily! (Sorry, I've been working too hard. Thank God it's Friday!)

I'm going to take the weekend off. I promise I will not set foot in the office until Monday. I'm going to build a rock wall and split more firewood. Gee, maybe I'll even do a month's worth of laundry to relax!

I love you all,
Jennifer

Ouch! The Day Had Come

by Catie Pratt, age 12

The day had come...
We did not know how or
where it had come from
but the pain said something!
Something we knew that had to go.

The night had come...
The pain struck hard and clear,
it was too much for the young man,
my brother, indeed.

Now today, as we sit and play
As we play, the cancer stares at us.
It comes to the touch
Hope it's not too much

We say to him, "It's all right."
But he tells us, "It's hard to fight."

Marley and his uncle Joseph wrestling

Friday, November 1, 2002
Subject: "CHANGING THE WORLD"

Dear friends and family,

At the end of this e-mail, I've included a letter from Marley's teachers. This will help you understand what Marley's education has been like this year. His teachers, Kate, Katie, and Jim, have developed an exceptional program that stands to impact us all. These students are bright, and they're going out into the world to use what they've learned.

Two weekends ago, I took a trip with Marley's class, the Wilderness Charter School (WCS). We drove to the San Francisco area for the 2002 Bioneers Conference, and learned about hundreds of actual ways people from all over the globe are healing various international social and environmental problems. It was truly inspirational. Since our return, it seems everything I do and say is filtered through an entirely new set of guidelines. I'm glad I went with these very smart and willing teenagers, because I know they aren't as likely to fall back asleep as most adults are. They came back ready to take action to change the world!

The special-ed programs Marley had been placed in for the past few years were discouraging. Marley was "mildly mentally retarded," but was put into the only special program the high school had available, one designed for developmentally disabled kids. As he couldn't read, write, or deal with the abstract nature of symbols, he certainly couldn't function in regular classes; but the special-ed classes frustrated the hell out of him and bored him to tears.

The Wilderness Charter School offers an entirely new set of options. These kids were from regular classes at the high school, but weren't thriving within the construct of normal educational techniques. The WCS is a haven for the artistic, poetic, hands-on learners that hated the box-like rules and regulations of the public high school system. They are creative.

As an example of one of the reasons I love this school: They started the school year with a two-week backpacking trip which included a solo. During this trip, these kids all bonded as a team in a very special way. Although Marley couldn't physically join them on the trip, as they were leaving, he gave the group a stuffed animal and asked them to take this symbol of him with them. They did, each of them taking turns carrying "Marley" on top of their backpacks. The result of the trip: These kids really love being with each other, and they love being a part of this program.

For the first time in years, Marley hasn't dragged his feet getting to school—even when he really hurts—and *that* says a lot. But recently, Marley's pain has been intense and he's only been to school one day this week. We went to the oncologist for the post-radiation checkup and everything looks good—except for the things we no longer have control over: his knee and his hip.

The following excerpt from a parent/teacher's e-mail illustrates one way the WCS has been dealing with watching Marley slip further away from them.

"Today we did a 'check-in' at the beginning of class and talked about how the students want to support Marley. Everyone agreed that if he's into it, we'd like to send him healing energy once a week (maybe we can get him in the middle of the circle and give him a big energetic POW!)."

It's one way to change the world!

I love you all,
Jennifer

GRASPING AT STRAWS

Scrambling for Solutions

Time seemed to be slipping through our fingers. Was there anything we could do to stop this pattern of new tumors developing? Drew, Cindy, and I started searching the Internet for any new therapies available. We no longer cared how outrageous they seemed. Since Marley had outlived his prognosis, he was a perfect candidate for *clinical trials* (using terminally ill patients as guinea pigs for new and untested drugs). Theoretically, folks like Marley have nothing to lose and if the treatment kills them, so what... they were going to die anyway!

We heard about a doctor in Argentina who was having remarkable results treating cancer patients. We investigated his program, but not only was the price astronomical, the travel commitment was intense. We would need to get from Oregon to Argentina four times in the first year. Drew, Cindy, and I concluded that just one leg of the journey would probably kill Marley, so we abandoned the idea altogether.

While hunting for other possibilities, we found a few new tidbits about this mystery we call cancer. I couldn't help myself from trying to understand how Marley's cancer was possible and what my role may have been. I know I'll never know, but the roller-coaster ride seemed to be occasionally necessary for me.

I started this investigation knowing that cancer is thought to be caused by DNA mutations. While reading, my stomach started tensing up as I learned some people inherit DNA mutations from their parents that greatly increase their risk for developing cancer. These defective genes either: 1) activate (turn on) *oncogenes*, the genes that promote cell division or 2) inactivate (turn off) the *tumor suppressor genes*. Then I read, "However, inherited oncogenes or tumor suppressor gene mutations are not believed to cause very many lung cancers. These gene mutations usually develop during life rather than before birth." Imagine the relief I felt, thinking to myself that I wasn't responsible.

But I wasn't off the hook; the roller-coaster took another

dive—"Although some people seem to inherit a reduced ability to break down cancer-causing chemicals, others may inherit an increased tendency to activate carcinogens, making them even more dangerous." That was the last straw. I gave up caring if I was responsible for Marley's cancer and focused on finding clues that might help Marley now.

We had learned earlier that the reason cancer cells can survive our immune system's defense is because these buggers are sneaky and can hide behind healthy cells until there are enough of them to form an army, becoming a tumor. Research is being done to alter lung cancers by injecting extra DNA so that cancer cells are better recognized and naturally attacked by the patient's immune system. Basically, this technique uses the same principle as homeopathy and immunization: Give a small dose of the invader so the body's immune system can recognize and attack the enemy. A sound theory, but I figured it was a little late to try this method on Marley; screwing around with his DNA seemed a little extreme.

The Marley Mystery

One little piece of information made me stop and read more slowly. I started to connect Marley's mental malfunctions and various physical oddities to his unusual cancer case. "Researchers have known for decades that squamous cell cancers of the larynx often have abnormally high levels of *growth factor receptors*, hormone-like substances that attach to receptors, signaling cells to grow and divide. Having too many receptors is one reason that laryngeal cancer cells grow abnormally." Bells started ringing in my head. Marley's neck was a hot spot for tumors; did this have anything to do with "growth factor receptors?" All I could do was once again try to review all of the clues.

• Didn't talk until he was 5 years old, • Had difficulty forming some sounds, • Had chronic stomach disorder when young, •Was always filled with gas, • Had extremely high tolerance to pain, • Cuts healed ultra-fast, • Rarely, if ever, bruised, • Hit puberty very young, • Was born with teeth, • Cut his wisdom teeth at 15 years old, and finally, • Had both exceptional hearing *and* problems with an abundance of earwax which blocked sounds.

Okay, so if Marley had high functioning "growth factor receptors," is that why he healed so fast? Is that why radiation wasn't terribly effective? Is that why the cancer was growing so fast? Like always, I asked more questions without finding any answers. An article on the American Cancer Society's website gave me even more info to chew on. It stated, "Several new drugs have been developed, intended to block growth factor receptors such as the *epidermal growth factor* (or EGF) receptor. By blocking the receptors, they slow down growth and division of the cancer cells. Some of these drugs may also make cancer cells more sensitive to chemotherapy and radiation."

High Hopes and Disappointments

Drew and Cindy learned that apparently several of these drugs were being introduced for clinical trials for people with non-small cell lung cancer, like Marley's. One of them was called Iressa. It had been recently approved by the Food and Drug Administration as a treatment for patients whose cancer has continued to progress in spite of chemotherapy treatment. There was a 10 percent chance of success, and *that* was looking pretty good.

We were very excited when we heard about Iressa and asked Diane, our beloved oncologist, to research the success rates. The reports were very disappointing, and the option was quickly discarded as the cons outweighed the possible pros. Once again, the only choice we seemed to have was to carry on and live life well.

"The goal is to live a full, productive life
even with all that ambiguity.
No matter what happens,
whether the cancer never flares up again
or whether you die,
the important thing is
that the days that you have had
you will have lived."

—Gilda Radner

Chapter Thirteen:
GRAVE HUMOR & TIDAL WAVES

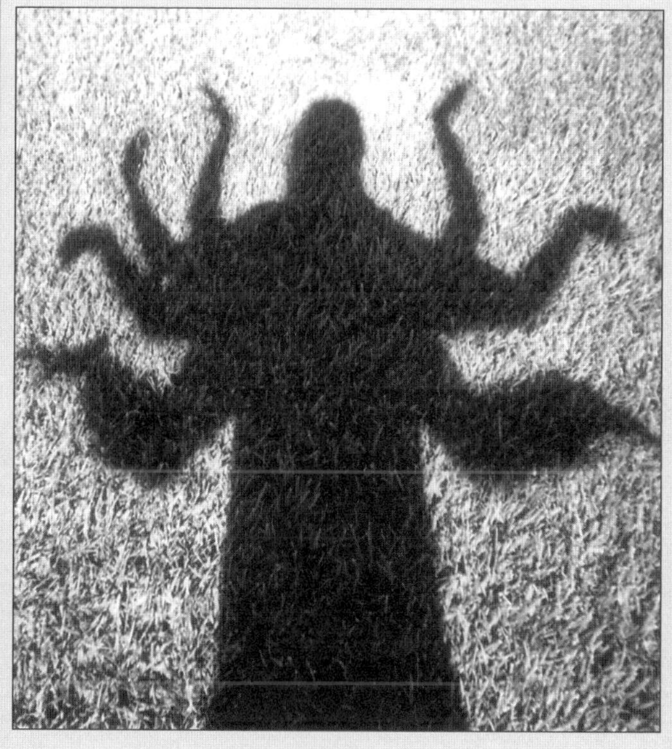

"Shadow Play"
Selene, Jennifer, Catie, and Laura
Photo: Jennifer

THE GUESTBOOK

Letters to Marley

Thanks to Debbie, no matter how hectic our lives were, Marley's revised website was always available whenever anyone needed a Marley fix. She made sure new photos were added, the Update Letters were posted for new readers and for those without e-mail, and that the "Guestbook" was ready for anyone to include notes. I would periodically print out the Guestbook and read these notes to Marley. As time went by, more and more people started to write letters to Marley. The entries became a way for all of us to log our feelings and thoughts, similar to a communal journal aimed in Marley's general direction.

I also noticed that people we didn't know were logging onto the website and reading everything. Maybe it was because Marley shared the same birth date as singer Bob Marley. If an Internet search was typed in as "Marley," our website would be listed. I guess that's one way strangers got hooked by mistake. They too would sign the Guestbook, honoring us all for our courage and ability to love and support each other. It was pretty cool when they said things like, "I feel like I know all of you, and I'm right there with you." I could feel the strength of our community grow even larger.

As Marley's life began to get more and more difficult, people wrote more and more in the Guestbook. Even I began to use it to write to Marley. It was like when I used to write him letters before he was born. It didn't matter if he ever read them or not—the expression is what mattered.

Often at the office, I would look across the room and see Jay or Thom reading the newest Guestbook entries instead of working on their stories for the upcoming *Bathroom Reader*. As their boss, what was I supposed to do? Tell them that writing about the history of the bra or compiling funny bumper sticker quotes was more important? I think not. I looked the other way. I figured helping my staff manage their feelings was an important part of my job description.

Monday, November 18, 2002
Guestbook entry from Uncle Joseph

Marley Man:

You have been in my heart and mind. You come to me like sunshine and shadow, so natural, so real, and therefore so alive in the moment. Your mother says that the recent tumors concern you. I know you have to wonder what might be lurking in your body. If you want to talk about it, we can…but I don't want to intrude. Sometimes there is no need to talk. I know this too. I know that for me, talk is good; it connects me and gives me reflection from someone outside myself.

When I was 22 years old, I met your grandfather Alden for the first time. He was the best friend I have ever had, and he died from lung cancer at the age of 55. I loved him a lot. I still do. Even though I have always been at peace with his death, in some very real way I miss him more and more. That's how it is in me towards you: I seem to love you more and more.

You bring a longing to my heart. Just thinking about you, my heart swells with pride and laughter, toughness and tenderness, and so much else. I am called back particularly to our time when you, Winston, and I took a walk together with you in your wheelchair—just being with you. There are so many reminders of how fragile life can be and yet how wonderful it is. You are filled with an energy and a desire that few people have ever known. You are so alive, Marley!! And so I say to you, from my heart to yours, whatever goes down, know that I am here and you are loved.

Joseph
Asheville, N.C.

GRAVE HUMOR

Comic Relief

You'd think our lives would have been sullen and depressing, witnessing the cancer feasting on Marley's body. Sometimes it's just plain embarrassing to reveal how much fun we had. I don't think I'm very witty or humorous, but I sure seem to think everything else is funny. Drew thought my sense of humor was totally inappropriate most of the time—at least that's what he expressed. He would shake his head and say, "Jesus, is everything funny to you? You laugh at the stupidest things." Inevitably I'd shrug my shoulders and laugh. I don't know about you, but when I smile and laugh, I find it much harder to let stress get the best of me.

Each new wave of Marley's disease was larger, and it seemed like there was much less time to recover before the next wave hit. His knee was always an issue, his shoulder always hurt, and his hip region was a constant pain in the ass…literally. The shadow of the wave was looming bigger than ever, and all I could do was lean on humor for relief.

"Laughter gives us distance. It allows us to step back from an event, deal with it, and then move on."

—Bob Newhart

When Marley's frustration got the best of him, I'd turn to him and say, "Well, I think amputation from the neck down is the only solution." Then I'd tell him about a movie I saw when I was a kid, called *The Brain That Wouldn't Die*. He'd grab his cane, expertly flip it upside down and use the hooked end to tip my chair over. I deserved it.

Choosing not to pussyfoot around his pain or our helplessness made everyone feel more comfortable. Like Drew, Catie didn't always appreciate my sense of humor, but Marley did. He shared my challenging nature, questioning everything thought to be sacred. Maybe it was a defensive fear of attachment, but it sure helped us not take life (or death) so seriously. Not walking on eggshells and getting a few good laughs in each day felt healthy.

KNEE-DEEP IN TROUBLE

Excessive Flexibility

It had been almost two years since Marley's right knee was replaced with a prosthesis. It hadn't healed right and always caused him grief, but Marley was convinced his femur was cracking. I took him in twice to get X-rays of his leg to prove he was right, only to have them say, "It looks all right to me." They looked at me like I was a hypochondriac on my son's behalf. We'd walk (or hobble) away feeling completely frustrated. We *knew* something was wrong. Why couldn't they see it? I completely trusted Marley's process of self-diagnosis. I wanted to jump up and down and yell at the doctor, "Your stupid machine just isn't good enough. We're wasting valuable time!"

Marley fell walking down the porch steps, once at Drew's and once at the office. Nothing happened, he caught himself both times, but after that he knew something was definitely wrong. He wasn't just imagining a problem. One cold, slippery wet day, he plopped down next me while I had my nose glued to my computer screen at work. He said, "Mom, my knee's not wurkin' right. It's like it's not holdin' me steady any moor. It goes one way when I'm goin' the otha way. I'm thinkin' it's not safe to walk on anymoor." *That* got my attention!

I swiveled around to face him, forgetting the BRI website completely. He nonchalantly said, "Check this out! I've gotta new twick." Without any delay he proceeded to painlessly lift his foot, that had been propped up on his other knee, toward the ceiling. With images of *The Excorsist* and Linda Blair's head spinning around, I completely lost my calm, cool, concerned mother routine. It didn't matter that I was in an office with three other people diligently working around me. I yelled, "Oh my fucking God! What the hell is happening?" Marley just cocked his head sideways and smiled.

Jay, Thom, and my new assistant Julia all turned around to see Marley's leg pointing straight up like it was broken at the knee—like a nasty compound fracture with no blood, no pain. Jay yelled at Marley, "Jesus Christ! Stop it! Put it down! That's disgusting." Julia was pale with her mouth hanging open. Thom's eyes were wider than saucers, staring at my boy who was beaming with delight. Jay yelled again, "Stop! Now! That's gross, Marley." Marley set his foot down on the floor and looked back at me. I was already on the phone calling the orthopedic surgeon for another appointment.

As it turned out, it wasn't his bone that was cracked, it was the cement that held the rod to his femur. The cement had let loose and was slowly grinding away, allowing the stainless steel fixture to rotate not only up and down but 180 degrees around too. Marley wanted a new knee—"One that wurks"— but by the time we identified the problem, getting another prosthesis was out of the question due to new tumors.

A Sure Bet

It didn't take long for Marley to figure out how cool it was to gross people out. Even I must admit I had fun nudging Marley a couple of mornings at the coffee house, saying, "Hey Marley, show 'em your new trick." All of my friendly neighborhood java junkies reacted just the way we had at the office. Debbie even screamed and covered her eyes like she was watching a scene in a horror flick. It was a sick trick unique to Marley. I seriously doubt this happens to a lot of people. If it does, I think the cement manufacturers better work on their product some more.

Marley loved the attention. He was proud to be able to disturb everyone, and no one was immune to the effects of this move. I've seen people who were double-jointed at the shoulder and could fold their arm behind their head and down their back—but that move, as weird as it looks, didn't hold a candle to Marley's malfunction. While at the doctor's office, Marley confided that he was making bank at school, betting unsuspecting kids and teachers $5 that he could touch his outstretched hand with his foot without moving his thigh. Suckers!

"If we couldn't laugh, we would all go insane."

—Jimmy Buffett

Friday, November 22, 2002
Subject: "KEEN NEW KNEE TRICK"

Hello My Friends,

Marley has a new trick that just can't be believed.... Follow these directions and you'll have a sense of what I'm talking about.

Sit down. Place your right ankle on your left knee. That's a normal position. Now grab your right ankle and lift it (just your ankle, keeping your knee in the same position). If you're limber, your foot will lift up about 12 inches. Marley can lift his so the bottom of his right foot faces the ceiling! It's like a weird circus act.

Watching the orthopedic surgeon's expression yesterday, while he watched Marley do his new knee trick, was too funny. After sliding limply into the nearest chair, he regained his composure and simply said, "That's just *not* right." Drew, Marley, and I howled with laughter. We like this guy 'cause he laughed with us. Hell, what else could he do?

This new abnormality is much more entertaining than when nurses have routinely tried to listen to Marley's left lung with a stethoscope. Drew and I find great pleasure sitting calmly, semi-sadistically watching as their faces slowly reveal their anxiety when they're unable to hear any breathing sounds. Finally, one of us takes pity on them and says, "His left lung has been removed."

My personal favorite was when one of his new oncologists, with an overly apparent superiority complex, tried to get a nerve reaction with that little rubber hammer. With straight faces, we watched as he kept tapping below and then above the right kneecap, getting no response. I almost applauded as Drew calmly said, "If you look in his chart, you'd find he has had a total knee replacement and you're hammering against stainless steel." Yo!

Life is so absurd!

Winter is definitely upon us. It's funny how sneaky this season can be, replacing fall's feeling of change and excitement with inward emotions and the need for solitude. It's so subtle yet so pervasive. I am in constant awe of how my stomach can clench with the fear of being unprepared to survive the winter months. While at the same time, I feel like Mother Nature has just wrapped me up in a cozy blanket and set me down to ponder the meaning of life.

Now I have some precious down time because it's switch day and the kids are with Drew for two weeks. I can't wait to spend the weekend knitting, sitting before the fire, and dipping candles—all great meditations. But alas, I must balance Being with Doing. I must play with the goats while I reroof their part of the barn that blew off last week in a windstorm. If I care enough to venture to town, I'll go get a massage and then I'll be able to split some more firewood too. Hmmm, does anybody think working really hard could be my coping mechanism?

I love you,
Jennifer

Tuesday, December 3, 2002
Guestbook entry from Reagan

I love Marley like the fog and the sun love to sit in the trees together outside my window.

Reagan
Ashland, OR

MOBILE MAN

An Uphill Battle

Helping Marley move about safely was our primary focus. Physical therapy wasn't an option, because Marley's hip was less functional than his broken, fake knee. His right leg was dangerously unstable. If his muscles and ligaments didn't exist, nothing would have stopped him from twisting his knee like a wet washcloth. The problem with muscles is, if you don't exercise them, they tend to atrophy and wither away. There wasn't a whole lot we could do about the fact that one leg was about as big around as my arm while its mate could be mistaken for a bike racer's. The doctor's only remedy was to hand Marley a deluxe leg brace with a heavy-duty hinge that only let his leg move forward and backward.

Even all this didn't stop Mr. Energizer Bunny from movin' top speed. He had been using his manual wheelchair at school, leaving it there at night. Whenever his shoulder tumor was acting up, he had to revert to mostly using one arm and his good leg to power the chair. The Wilderness Charter School was on a piece of property next to the high school. It was a swift downhill ride in the morning, but a painful uphill battle every afternoon. Before long, he had to rely on his classmates to push him up the hill in time for his other classes. It only took a few solo tries for him to beg me to get him an electric wheelchair.

Life's a Blast

It was December and I knew I had less than a month to get the insurance company to do the paperwork and agree to cover the costs of a high-powered chair. We had already met our deductible for 2002 and this new addition was going to be spendy...we're talking over $7,000. After a lot of research, paperwork, phone calls, and eye batting, the "Quantum Blast" was delivered to the office, accompanied by a team of two; one to custom-fit each part of the wheelchair for Marley's body, and another to teach Mars how to program the chair's computer to master all terrain.

Marley lovingly called his new chair "Masta Blasta" in honor of Mel Gibson's "Mad Max" movie, *Beyond the Thunderdome*. Masta Blasta was fast, clocking in at 8.6 miles per hour. Masta Blasta was beautiful: cherry red with rugged all-season tires, and a toggle stick to die for. The only problem was it was heavy—about 400 pounds heavy. It was a challenge to get in and out of my jacked-up Suburban (even with a ramp) and impossible to move if the batteries went dead.

Marley mastered the use of this machine lickety-split. He made it look so easy to manipulate, I thought I'd give it a try one day at the office. I nearly killed myself even though I was outside. That thing went so fast that whiplash was a consideration. As I was just about to crash into the fence at 8 mph, I pulled the toggle switch back with force and slid right off the seat. I learned why it came with a seat belt.

It didn't take long to learn that Masta Blasta was not only smarter and more responsive than I was, it was much stronger. I plowed into a fold-up chair and couldn't stop myself before I rammed the chair into a stone wall, crushing it. Masta Blasta didn't care, it was just following my orders. I was completely out of control, having the time of my life, laughing so hard my tears were blinding me. Marley was lying on the grass, clutching his gut, laughing so hard he couldn't breathe. I had a newfound respect for Marley and his ability to manipulate this incredibly responsive robot.

> ***"A youth is to be regarded with respect. How do you know that his future will not be equal to our present?"***
>
> **—Confucious**

Ho! Ho! Ho!

Even with Masta Blasta, Marley's mobility continued to be a serious issue. To keep the wheelchair charged, Marley either left it at school or at the BRI office overnight. While he was in town, he got around on his electric bike and his wheelchair. At his dad's he had his Kawasaki Mule. But up at my place, he had only his cane and the riding lawn mower. The mower wasn't bad, but it sure didn't go anywhere fast. His trips to visit the neighbors became downright embarrassing for him. He said, "Ridin' that thing makes me feel like an owd man."

He was right. I knew he was right. There was only one thing left that he REALLY wanted…an ATV. Now he *needed* it too. I knew his desire to live was threadbare; the walls of death were closing in on him rapidly. So, the week before Christmas, I grabbed Selene and said, "Come on. I've got to go do it!"

"Do what?" she whined.

"The only thing left to buy for Marley!" She looked at me and her eyes lit up on that cold, dark, winter afternoon.

She squealed with delight, "You're going to actually get him an ATV?" And off we went to Dreadford.

I ended up getting a deluxe model—an Arctic Cat 400. It was big and beautiful with plenty of room for two. Selene and I were naughty; hoping to get a good deal, we told the young salesman we were shopping for "a young thrill-seeker who was dying and running out of road." Our sad story worked—not only for a lower price tag—he also said he would personally deliver it on Christmas morning!

Everyone in the clan knew about the surprise and they all wanted to be there, so it was a full house on Christmas morning. I was cooking up a storm, and there were so many gifts that even the kids needed to take a break midway. When the last gift was opened, it was hard to keep straight faces. I knew Marley well enough to know he was secretly disappointed his dream hadn't come true, but he didn't show it. He was content sitting in his recliner surrounded by wonderful friends on a beautiful morning. Outside, the ground was covered with a thin layer of snow, and the sun made it look like billions of tiny crystals had been scattered around our cabin. Delicious smells filled the house along with music, laughter, and loads of love. It couldn't have been more perfect—until a big truck drove down our road.

From the kitchen I exclaimed, "Damn, who's that?" I yelled towards the living room, "Hey Marley! Catie! Do you know anyone who drives a brand spankin' new white truck? Go out and tell them to go away, will you?"

That meant excitement to Marley. He grabbed his cane, threw on his cowboy hat and was hop-skipping out the door, right behind Catie. We were all jumping up and down in the kitchen with tears running down our cheeks as Marley and Catie were gawking at the ATV in the back of the pick-up. The driver got out, and before either of the kids could say anything intelligent, he opened the tailgate and started to pull out the ramps. At this point, Marley and Catie both completely lost it! The rest of us joined them in the snowy driveway, yipping and hollering. Everyone was in a frenzy, boinking up and down, hugging each other, and feeling very proud of ourselves. Once again, I felt successful...I made Marley cry with joy on Christmas!

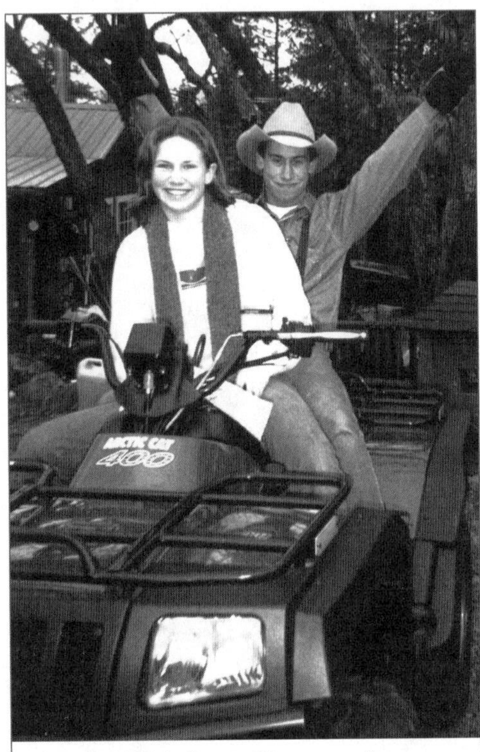

Catie and Marley on Christmas afternoon

Before he even took it for a test drive, Marley "ran" into the house, plopped on the couch, and grabbed the phone. He could barely contain himself as he called his fellow Coyote, Lucas.

As soon as Lucas answered, Marley bellowed with sheer glee, "I got an Autic Cat Fowhundwed sittin' in my dwiveway and I'm gonna wip dis vawee up!"

Friday, January 10, 2003
Subject: "CONVERSATIONS WITH MARLEY"

• From: Llyn

Dear Marley Network,

I'm writing a letter on behalf of Jennifer because, what with holidays and her work schedule, there hasn't been an update since November. I've been friends with the family for about 20 years, and I just happen to be passing through Ashland this week. I thought another perspective might be refreshing.

Marley just went for his regular checkup with his primary care physician three days ago. He seems to be in solid good health. No new tumors have surfaced since the ones in his neck last summer. Marley's hip and knee still give him a lot of ongoing pain. There's still a tumor in his hip, but it doesn't seem to be growing, which is good because it's already been radiated about as much as his hip can withstand. He walks with a knee brace and doesn't need crutches. When he's at school he uses his electric wheelchair.

Marley is in good spirits. He got a new "Arctic Cat" four-wheeler for Christmas that he's keeping at Jennifer's house. He took me for a ride on it last night when I arrived and it was great fun! We drove on a logging road down to the creek below their house, through the woods, and looped back on the main dirt road. This was similar to the route he led me on when he was three years old. I was amazed then at his ease in the woods—the familiarity he had with the wild surroundings of his home—and that ease has continued to this day. Marley says, "My Cat can go up to 60 miles per hour but I've only taken it to 45!" It was a strange and wonderful sensation to be hanging onto the back of this man-child who, it seems, was a babe in my arms not so long ago.

This morning Marley and I took his motorized wheelchair out

for a walk along the bike trail that cuts through Ashland. Here are some of the things we talked about:

...Graduating from high school: This is scheduled to happen in spring of 2004—if all goes according to plan. Marley's excited about it. He loves his Wilderness Charter School classes and the reading he's doing—the story of a shepherd who goes hunting for treasure. He also loves the two elective classes he takes at the mainstream high school; wood shop and photography.

...Search and Rescue classes: Marley's looking forward to going with his sister Catie as they begin Emergency Medical Training in a few weeks.

...Demolition Derby: Marley would like to enter into competition and smash up other peoples' cars for the fun of it!

...College? "I doubt it," says Marley. (I think he'd rather be a cowboy, fireman, or a Search and Rescue guy.)

...Girlfriends? "Not really. Though there's a girl who's my friend who lives on a ranch behind Emigrant Lake."

...The Coyotes: Marley, Luke, and Lucas are four-wheelin' ATV buddies. Marley says, "We like to get into just about as much trouble as you can imagine!"

So, as you can see, in spite of the life-altering, life-threatening ordeal that Marley and his community have been dealing with for three years, Marley continues to stay in close touch with the things that bring him joy and make his life meaningful. It's been a joy to spend time with him as well as with Jennifer and Catie. I am reminded of the preciousness and tenuousness of this gift we call Life.

Love,
Llyn

JUST SAY YES!

The Drugs of Choice

It's a good thing painkillers affect us differently when we're in pain than when taken as recreation. The amount of drugs Marley had been ingesting was increasing slowly but surely. If taken without need, he would have been a basket case. He could have been downing twice the amount around the clock but, for better or for worse, we all somehow agreed to use the minimal amounts until he really needed them. When *that* was going to be, none of us knew.

At one point, his radiation oncologist said we should be more generous with the meds, hinting that no one should be dealing with the amount of pain Marley must have been in all the time. He looked at Drew and me like we were abusing Marley, deliberately withholding the drugs. Maybe he figured that we were worried about Marley becoming addicted, because he kept reassuring us that the dependence issue wasn't a part of this picture. We reassured the doctor that Marley was in control of what he took and when. We explained that it seemed to be more important to him to be clearheaded, so when using his electric wheelchair, he could avoid slamming into people and things. Maintaining clarity to operate his beloved Kawasaki Mule at his dad's, or the Arctic Cat at mine, was key in his survival plan. Marley knew well enough that he couldn't carry passengers or trek to the mountain ridges if he couldn't see straight.

Celebrex, Vicodin, Percocet, and Oxycontin were all available to him depending on his needs. Celebrex was used daily to help with the severe stiffness of his fingers, elbows, shoulders, hips, knees, and ankles. Every joint always hurt. The kid was riddled with cancer, and what the cancer hadn't attacked, the radiation had. He would choose between Percocets or Vicodin for spiking pain and he knew when the time came to begin taking the Oxycontin—a slow acting, time-released dose of morphine that lasted 12 hours. For me, he didn't need to use words to describe his pain level. I knew just how he felt by the drugs he asked for and how often he'd moan for them. Another symptom of increased pain was when he'd go spin donuts in the mud on the ATV—he'd go 'round and 'round endlessly until I swear he was in a trance.

On his ATV he kept his cane securely tucked under a special seat—a padded camouflage seat complete with storage compartments for gloves, a first-aid kit, duct tape, and extra clothing. When he was too tired to continue, or it had gotten too dark to see, he'd rely heavily on his cane and limp into the house. He'd flip off his mud-caked shoes or whimper until I'd help unlace his boots, and then he'd flop onto his chair at the counter and ask something benign like, "What's for dinner, Ma?" or "Catie, wanna wrestle?" Watching him deal with his pain made my heart crack open. Aside from giving him painkillers, there wasn't a damned thing I could do to make life easier for my child except remain calm and behave as though everything were as it should be.

"Live as if you were to die tomorrow,
learn as if you were to live forever."

—Gandhi

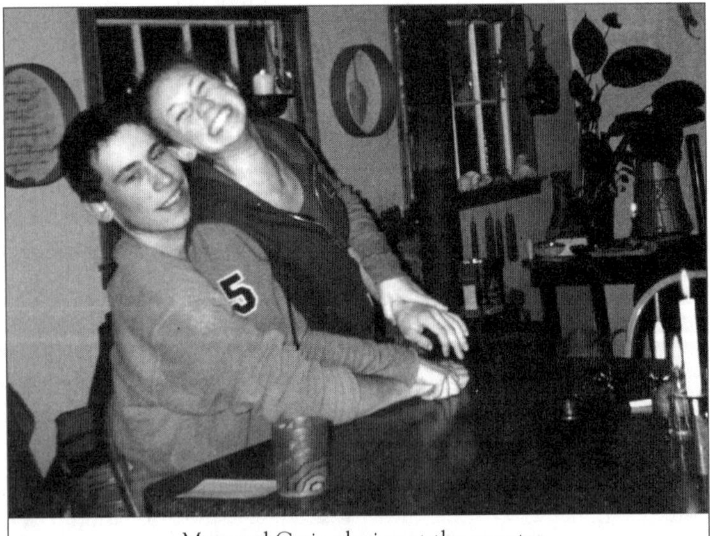

Mars and Catie playing at the counter

Monday, January 20, 2003
Subject: "A STATE OF GRACE"

Dear Network,

Once again, a new year has been awarded to our little family. I thank "All That Is" daily for the time—precious time—to be with Marley as he so gracefully lives his life. Once again, I thank you for your involvement in this story. Just knowing you are out there helps me find the strength required to keep smiling and working hard.

Marley's Network consists of family, friends, those who know *of* Marley via a third party, and those who have stumbled across this story by accident. Regardless of how you were drawn to our family's adventure, you now act as our witness. Just *that* has been a tremendous act of support. I'm beginning to understand why the marriage ceremony includes witnesses. It is harder to shirk the responsibility of commitment when others are watching. When things go awry, these witnesses also act as support to help the couple remember their vows. I think the same kind of "ceremony" spontaneously happened when I wrote the first letter to Marley's Network. I cannot thank you enough for sharing this journey with us.

UPDATE

Marley continues to amaze all around him. He says he's "falling apart" and indeed he literally is, yet he keeps going. It is extremely hard for him to walk, but he does. He hurts all the time, but he still laughs and always wants to do fun things.

Just like last year, on New Year's Eve, we rented a room at a hotel in town. A constant stream of people came to socialize with Marley. Laura joined us for the night, and the three kids played endlessly in the pool and the Jacuzzi. We ate pizza and watched TV until just before midnight.

Our pyrotechnician friend had planned a firework extravaganza at a lake, a ten-minute drive from town. Laura and Catie stayed in our room while Marley, our faithful dog Zipper, and I jumped in the Suburban to join Eric, Rhys, and many others for the light display. Eric had put a couch in his van for Marley's viewing comfort and the rest of us stood close by, waiting for the countdown.

When the first firework went off, poor Zipper flipped out. I put her in the Suburban, but I didn't know the passenger window was open. We were clapping and cheering as the fireworks went off, one after another, not knowing that Zipper was running as fast as she could back to town. Afterwards, Marley and I spent hours searching for her but…she was gone.

The following day we searched again and found her by the side of the road, half a mile from the lake—victim of a hit and run. We picked her body up and took her home. On the first day of the year, there was work to be done. Fortunately the ground was not frozen, and digging a hole for our shepherd mix was possible. Catie, Marley, and I each laid our hands upon her familiar soft fur to say good-bye. The tears started pouring forth as we realized this was the last time we would ever touch her.

Saying farewell to Zipper hit Marley's core. It wasn't just about the dog—it was personal. He was saying good-bye on multiple levels and he started questioning what happens after a body dies. It was the perfect opportunity to talk about how each of us want our bodies treated after we die and what we want our funerals to include. Marley said he wants people to gather around him like we were gathered for Zipper. He also said he wants to be cremated. As a mother, I cried, not for my dog but for my boy's realization that this same process would take place in his honor. I cried watching Catie weep as she felt her brother's fear of the unknown be unearthed for the first time. I cried for me, not knowing if I could survive Marley's death, knowing I would never be able to touch or see him again.

GOOD GRIEF!

A few days later, Marley and Catie decided the cure for our grief was to find a replacement for Zipper. I wasn't thrilled about the concept but knew I didn't stand a chance against both of them. Lo and behold, at Evo's Coffee House the following week, four puppies needed a home. By the end of the day, only three puppies needed a home! Gracie became the newest member of our family. Marley's in seventh heaven because he has a source of constant entertainment and unbridled love.

Drew and Cindy have just gotten a new puppy too. Although Dinah is an Australian shepherd, she has been honored as a family member, not just another working cowdog like the others. When Dinah and Gracie met, it was love at first sight. It wasn't planned, but it has been a saving grace for Marley and Catie to have puppy energy at both houses—a symbol of new life.

I hope this new year brings to each of you symbols of playful life and that you too can live in a state of grace.

With much love,
Jennifer

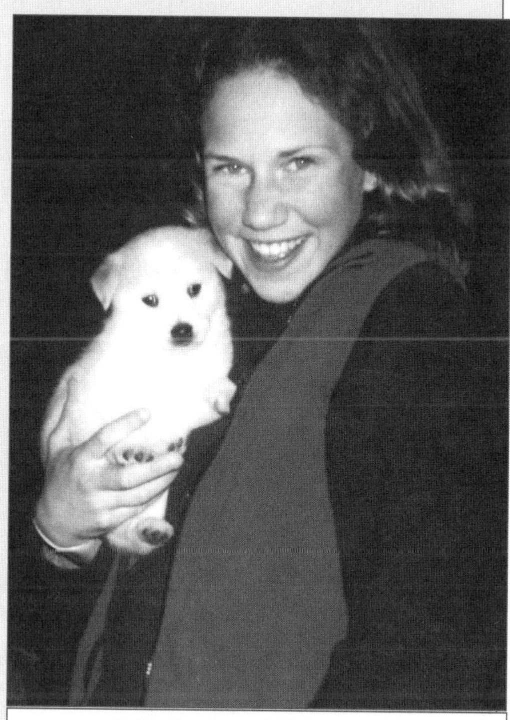

Baby Gracie and Catie, age 13

WILDERNESS REPORT

Put to the Test

Since Marley was very young, no one seemed to be able to peg what was different about him. There were no existing labels to slap on him and no aid that educators could use to help him learn. It was also flat-out impossible to *make* Marley do anything he didn't want to do. The end result was that this young man had managed to slip through the fingers of the traditional educational system's requirements. I mean, this kid was a junior and had only done two reports in his life! (I wish I had been so lucky.)

The first report was done in the 10th grade—the oral speech and video presentation on the surprising history of the Colestin Valley. The only other sample of Marley's compliance with regulation education was a midyear report done at the Wilderness Charter School. They had spent the first part of the year studying and practicing sustainable living techniques within a community setting. Even though he dictated all of his answers and all the spelling was accurate, I had to laugh at the way Marley made sense of the world.

Marley Pratt's First Semester Final Report
Wilderness Charter School

1) What were your goals? Method of achievement? Obstacles?

• *Goal #1:* To attend as many classes as possible. *Method:* Doing it! *Obstacle:* Cancer.

• *Goal #2:* To be more tolerant of others. *Method:* To listen. *Obstacle:* Me.

• *Goal #3:* When physically able, to work on the [school] property, support others, and supervise. *Method:* Being put in charge and explaining about safe tool use. *Obstacle:* Radiation.

• *Goal #4:* Contributing to discussions on fire practice and forestry. *Method:* Presenting ranching perspective. *Obstacle:* Being reckless (as a habit or hobby).

2) Which speaker influenced you most at the Bioneers Conference three months ago? What did you learn?
Julia Butterfly Hill, who sat in a tree for two years to protest clear-cut logging. She stopped the logging and had the courage to stay up in the tree. I see that her courage gave her the strength to stick it out.

3) Name three critters in your garden and how you would solve the problem.
Critters: Bunnies, gophers, and bugs.
Solution: Dogs, cats, cayenne, and my .22.

4) If we cannot maintain or improve a given system, what should we do?
Rip down the system and rebuild it. You usually do better once you take things apart.

5) What have you learned about yourself so far this year?
• I can't push myself up the hill without hurting myself.
• Vegans are more fun to pick on than vegetarians.
• The biggest thing for me this year has been cancer. I can't ride horses or BMX anymore, and I'd like to. I would like to ride down the new stairs at the college because you're not supposed to. If you tell me I *can* jump off the Mark Antony [Ashland's only high-rise], I won't do it. But if you tell me I *can't*, I will.
• The cancer has kept me alive. It's kept me from trashing myself bike riding down places like Pinball [a very steep trail]. But I'm still going to jump the quarry this summer on my bike.
• I want there to be no more cancer for the rest of my life.

6) How have you contributed to the Wilderness Charter School?
It's really fun when we're doing check-in and someone's whining about their life and then it comes around to me. Then everyone realizes someone has bigger problems than they do—someone who has *real* problems with their life.

7) How does it feel to be a part of this community?
Being the biggest meat eater feels a little weird.

EIGHTEEN AND I LIKE IT!

Becoming an Adult

Marley's 18th birthday was special. I never thought this day would actually arrive. I felt like I could exhale for the first time since Marley was born. I realized I had been holding Marley's 18th birthday as a milestone marking his ability to survive humanhood and my ability to survive parenthood. It was as if on this special day, *I* had succeeded. My boy had made it to an invisible threshold. But he hadn't crossed it—not yet—we still had twelve hours to go…and what a twelve hours it turned out to be.

Due to new pains, on his birthday, we had to go to the hospital to get X-rays of Marley's foot and pelvis. After finishing up in radiology by mid-afternoon, Catie, Marley, and I went back to the BRI office. The energy of that place was filled with an air of expectation and nervous excitement. No one could concentrate on work. The only thing I managed to do was to write an extremely short, uncharacteristic Update Letter informing everyone that it was Marley's birthday. I couldn't even bring myself to let the network know we were in a state of limbo and the twentieth shoe was about to drop.

Thursday, February 6, 2003
Subject: "BIRTHDAY WISHES"

Yahoo!

Marley turns 18 years old today!!! Amazing.

Let's all light a candle at 6:00 P.M. tonight to honor his will to stay alive! Wish or pray for six things for Marley to receive during the next six months. May we all have the will to live and die with grace and courage.

I love you all,
Jennifer

If No News Is Good News…What's News?

It was always hell waiting for the test results to come in. We all knew that whenever Marley had X-rays done, nine times out of ten, a new tumor or two would be found. Right after I sent the e-mail, the radiation oncologist called. The doc was apologetic that he was calling to give us the official bad news on Marley's birthday. Everyone in the office stopped talking when they realized who I was on the phone with. I sat down at my desk and braced myself as I listened to what the doctor had to say. It was a brief call, and I thanked him for relaying the results so quickly, hung up, and immediately called Drew and Cindy. All ears were flapping, waiting to hear the other side of the conversation.

Two tumors were chewing away at Marley's right ankle (the same leg as both the hip and knee problems). One tumor was on each side of the *talus*, a part of that complicated little bone structure that holds the bulk of our bodies upright. Another tumor was attacking the bottom of his heel bone (*calcaneus*) on the same foot. But the really bad news was the iliac wing in his pelvis was on fire again and there wasn't much left of that bone to begin with. These four tumors were growing so fast we had an appointment at the hospital the next morning to start the all too familiar process of radiation prep. Uggh. Happy birthday Marley.

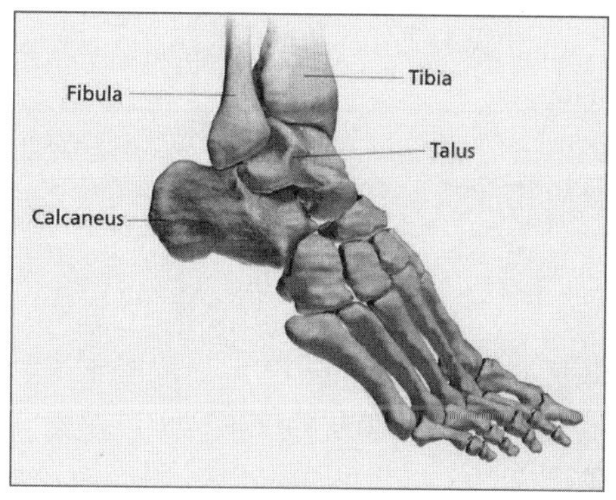

Everybody's whirlwind energy ceased as if caught in the eye of a great storm. Just then, Marley's best friends Luke and Lucas blew through the office door bringing with them the winds of youth and celebration. They entered with no regard that the office was a place of business. One announced his arrival with a loud whistle while the other yelled, "Hey Mars!" Marley heard their grand entrance and came hop-skipping out of his back bedroom, crashing into everything in his path. Whooping and hollering, they clumsily hugged each other and slapped each other's backs. It was like having three Great Danes greeting each other in a very small hall that amplified the decibel level. Marley was big and loud, but Luke was bigger and louder! Everyone else had to work hard to be heard over the three boys as they lumbered to the back of the office. Their excitement was contagious, and quickly we were all giddy with life once again.

Under Pressure

Luke and Lucas had been dropped off after school in order to join us for Marley's party that evening. The event just wouldn't be complete without them. I had agreed to drive them back to Lucas' house in the Colestin Valley after the party. The arrangements had been made long before I knew the impact this day would have. With the new news, I had a sneaking suspicion that this was going to be a very long night.

Jennifer S., who had worked at the BRI years before, was now writing feature articles about unusual women for a local magazine. She was focusing on my story—a mother's coping techniques under pressure—and she wanted to use Marley's birthday party as a photo-op. The article was to be used as a follow-up article for a piece the newspaper had printed about Marley's Monster Bash, two years earlier. I was supposed to meet the photographer in just an hour—there was still much to do—but first things first....

Little Thom, Gordon, Julia, Jeff and Jay—the office eavesdroppers—all wanted a detailed explanation of what the recent test results meant. Time was running short before we had to go to the restaurant, so I rounded everybody up to let them all know what was going on. My five co-workers, Catie, the Coyotes, and I all squeezed in the cozy 12' x 12' room used as BRI library. I relayed the results and explained that these new tumors could put a significant hamper on Marley's mobility.

The Coyotes groaned in displeasure because it meant the fun times, "rippin' the valley up" might be limited. However, it didn't take long for them to start elbowing each other, challenging that maybe four tumors wasn't such a big deal. Lucas said, "Nothin' like this has slowed Marley down in the past. Why should these new tumors have any effect on him? We're talkin' about Marley here...It can't be *that* bad!"

Let the Party Begin!

The Coyote's whirlwind energy started to swirl again, so the discussion was kept short and direct; the boys had better things to do than to listen to me babble. Besides, it was time to go downtown to have fun and celebrate Marley's birth. This event was well planned—with a few surprises—and chosen to be a simple rite of passage into the adult world.

Meredith and Steven had driven up from their home in the California desert just in time to attend the party. Some of Marley's most special people had come to this dinner, and he was glowing in the limelight.

The Kat Wok was a classy Asian restaurant by evening and a balls-to-the-wall dance hall by night—generally a place that kids didn't frequent. It had a cool layout with two levels. The upstairs dining area was an open loft, overlooking the dance floor and the first floor dining area. I had rented the entire balcony area and had pre-planned a three-course meal for forty people to be served buffet style. The space was stylish, but tight, which meant everyone had to hug and touch a lot in order to move around.

Marley was looking a little more ashen-faced than normal. I could tell he was drained and feeling pain, even though he was milling lovingly amongst those who came to honor him. I didn't want to interrupt his gracious socializing, so I caught his eye, nodded to my cupped hand, and just walked by him offering the opportunity to take some painkillers...just in case. Without missing a beat in the conversation he was having with his Aunt Meredith, he grabbed the drugs from my open palm and slugged them down with a Mountain Dew chaser. He gave me a secret smile that wordlessly said, "Thanks Ma, you want one too?" Instead, I raised my glass to toast him and sipped my shot of tequila—a feeble attempt to act as graceful as he was being.

The magazine photographer was busy, taking pictures of a small sample of Marley's Network. We had a great time; everyone was in a good mood. That morning, I had been given a "birth giving" gift called Angel Snot. It was like Silly Putty, but was translucent, of a lighter consistency, and would stretch realistically with its own weight. I had been practicing all day, putting bits of the goo at the corner of my mouth, perfecting various expressions to give the impression that I was drooling. My climactic performance was applying a string under my nose, sneezing, and looking up at unsuspecting souls just to wipe the fake snot off on my sleeve. It was fun watching everyone, all dressed up, belly laugh and play with it like sixth-graders.

"He who laughs, lasts!"

—Mary Pettibone Poole

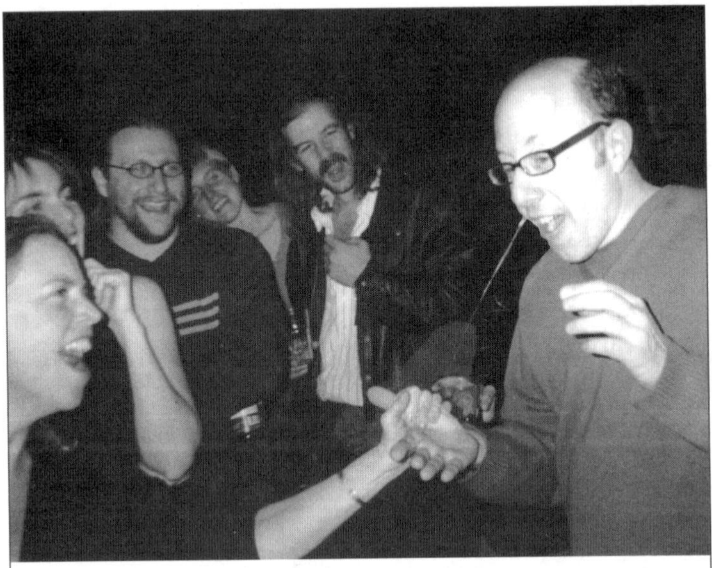

Jennifer, Annie, Jeff, Selene, and Rhys watching Gordon play with Angel Snot during Marley's party.

Photo: Debbie Thornton

As the dining and drinking subsided, we gathered in a large circle to hold hands and focus our energy. Four pillar candles were held in the four directions and lit as I invoked the benevolent spirits of all those who had gone before us. I asked them to join this celebration in order to help Marley during the coming year. I reminded this circle that Marley's Network extended much wider than this group and to take a minute to include all those who could not attend. The power was palpable as I asked everyone to silently focus on six wishes for Marley. The silence ceremoniously concluded with coyote howls and hugs.

Conversing With Coyotes

When all was said and done, Rhys took Catie and Marley home while I drove Luke and Lucas over the mountain. It was the first time I had ever been alone with these two extraordinary young men. They had served as the best and most powerful medicine Marley could have hoped for during the past three years. I thanked them sincerely for being there for Marley and for sticking by his side through thick and thin. They both started talking about how important being with Marley had been for them, how much he had taught them, how much fun they had while together, and how worried they were.

Lucas was riding shotgun while Luke was leaning forward between the captain's chairs, with his face illuminated by the dashboard lights. Luke, the older of the two, showed me his serious side. He used the time we had together in the Suburban asking very technical questions about Marley's cancer and the "cures" used to date. He was a sponge and wanted as much hard-core information as he could absorb during the 25-minute drive as we wound through the gravel back roads of Mt. Ashland.

These boys were hungry for the truth—they were starving from lack of details. It was the opposite of what they displayed in the tiny library earlier. I held no punches and spoke to them like I would to any of my kin. I figured they needed to know exactly what Marley was up against; a very limited chance of survival, a whole lot of pain, and probably little time to play in Life's light.

It was a difficult conversation to have, but I was deeply grateful for their willingness to listen. Marley's three sisters had the benefit of this information being distributed gently, over a three-year period of time, along with the rest of Marley's Network. I hadn't realized that these boys weren't on the e-mail list. They knew only what Marley told them and possibly whatever information their parents may have heard from gossip floating around the Colestin. From the nature of their questions, I gathered the info they had was extremely limited.

Marley probably shared the bare minimum: facts about new tumors and procedures that happened while at my house. He would have certainly shown his small tribe the countless war wounds he had acquired, but he apparently didn't want to focus on details, feelings, or projections. He was too busy having fun with them. But Luke and Lucas had eyes—they could see how his body had been changing. They were closer to him than most. They knew what was happening wasn't good, but I don't think anyone was telling them that their best friend was dying.

"Tis strange—but true; for truth is always strange; Stranger than fiction."

—Lord Byron

They both thanked me for being open and honest with them. I asked them both to watch Marley's back when they were off four-wheeling in the woods and when they did the grueling all-day instruction while training to be firefighters. After that conversation, I knew that they would take care of Mars. These boys were being asked to grow up fast as they faced the reality of mortality in a very adult way.

I also knew that they should be put on Marley's Network e-mail list so they could get any new information firsthand. I laughed when I learned that Lucas' e-mail address was "SpeedFreak" and Luke's was "LucifersChild." There was something intensely special about this small pack of rabble rousers. I drove away feeling honored. I had been fully embraced by each of the three famed Colestin Coyotes.

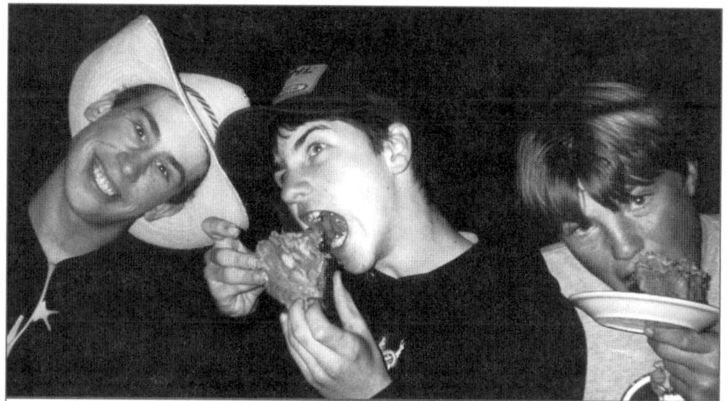

Marley, Lucas, and Luke – having their cake and eating it too!
Photo: Elizabeth Morgan

COYOTE LORE

"A long time ago when the animals could still talk to each other…four of the mightiest animals had a disagreement…While most of the animals felt that the bear deserved to remain the chief, others sided with one or another of the animals challenging him.

One of the challengers was the buffalo…Another challenger was the eagle…The other one to challenge Bear's right to be the chief of the council was the coyote. Coyote said, 'I am the trickiest of all of the animals. I can survive anywhere. I have the ability to teach things to all of you whether or not you want to learn. Because of the growth I bring about, I deserve to be your chief.'"

In the end, the Great Spirit settled the conflict by assigning each animal to be chief of one of the four directions. Bear in the west for strength and the ability to think before speaking; Buffalo in the north for renewal and purity—its paradoxical power of providing new life cloaked in death; Eagle in the east for clear vision, wisdom, and illumination, bringing the awakening; and Coyote in the south with its ability to teach and survive, helping to bring growth and trust into being. Unified they would create Life's powerful Medicine Wheel.

—This story excerpted and summarized from *The Medicine Wheel*, by Sun Bear and Wabun

LIFE IN THE FAST LANE

Misery Needs Company

Marley was officially an adult, and I had theoretically done my job as a parent. Experts say that by the time a person has reached 18 years of age, their cellular patterns have been established and they have formulated their basic belief structure; that's not to say things can't change—simply that they have everything they need for survival. But I guess if someone has cancer and is "mildly mentally retarded from 9 A.M. to 3 P.M." a parent's job is never done (at least during daylight hours). Mine sure wasn't.

My best friend Andrea had flown in for Marley's birthday and was soaking up Marley's demonstrative way of loving. The day after Marley's birthday, she, Marley, and I had arranged to meet Steven, Meredith, and Selene in order to spend as much precious time together as possible.

Steven and Meredith were on a journey north to visit all of Steven's relatives. Steven's health had become extremely questionable during the previous months. Because he was having difficulty breathing, they were moving from the high desert to the low elevations, just north of San Francisco. He figured this was possibly the last chance for traveling. Steven was determined to say good-bye to all those he loved…just in case.

As sisters, Meredith and I had bonded in a new way over the past few years due to the fact we were both caring for our closest men, both of whom were unique, powerful, and independent. They were both fighting their final battle. We would talk for hours on the phone about the endless demands we were experiencing, both physically and emotionally. We could be fiercely honest with each other about feeling like we were being pushed into a dark tunnel that kept getting smaller with each new day. We would ponder how caring for the terminally ill felt like caring for the very young except without the benefit of a light at the end of the journey. We shared how even though we loved these men more than any other, we hated them at times too for making us feel their pain. We couldn't judge each other harshly, because we were in the same boat. We felt free to share feelings other people just wouldn't understand.

During this brief visit, Steven and Marley bonded in a way that quietly broke my heart. The kids and I hadn't seen Steven since the reunions the summer before. His health had taken a serious dive—so had Marley's. They both swapped stories, laced with wry humor, about what it was like to have their once robust bodies slowly malfunction, limiting life's pleasurable activities such as hiking, driving, going to movies, etc. I'm sure it was a relief for them to be able to freely gripe about the new pains associated with life's activities that, up until recently, had been taken for granted; simple things like breathing and moving. They both complained about feeling useless, and dealing with other people's pity and desire to fix the unfixable.

A Picture's Worth a Million Words

The day after Marley's birthday, we had to go to the cancer center in Dreadford to get scans of the two areas (foot and hip) the radiologists planned to aim four beams of radiation at. They used 3-D digital images to measure and test the best angle of attack to avoid unnecessary damage to neighboring cells, organs, and joints. This appointment was a long one, because there were four tumors to focus on. The tumor on his heel bone was pretty simple, but the two tumors on either side of the ankle were problematic due to limited room for error. The ankle is an important, weight bearing joint with a relatively small diameter. They also used this time to "block" the area, creating molded casts for his foot that would hold it in the exact position—a different mold for each angle of radiation used.

This process was actually fascinating. We had found the more we learned about it by watching and asking questions, the easier it was for the technicians and doctors to communicate with us. It was also easier to understand and visualize what was happening inside Marley's body. Marley was training to be an EMT, so he loved this stuff—it was better than watching a program on the Discovery channel. For me, it was like having the opportunity to go to medical school without the tests, grades, and expense.

Andrea, Selene, Steven, and Meredith had never witnessed this, so we met at the cancer center and asked the technicians if we could all watch. I think they actually liked it when they could show off what they knew and when patients took an interest in their art. With their permission, we all slid sardine style into the tiny darkened room aglow with the image of Marley's pelvis. The technician helped us to recognize the skeletal structure, scar tissue from previous nuked tumors, and the current army of invading cancer cells.

By that time, I had much practice asking "intelligent" questions, like: "Are we looking at his head or his butt?" "Is this view from the top or from the side?" Or, "Is that what the bone is supposed to look like?" Generally speaking, the professionals were patient and never turned to me in disgust or cruelty, snidely saying, "You can't be serious!" Looking dumb was a small price to pay for the pearls of knowledge I acquired.

"Let us be thankful for the fools.
But for them the rest of us could not succeed."

—Mark Twain

So I asked, "Aren't we supposed to see more beige colors where the iliac bone is supposed to be?" I'll never forget the way the tech's body tensed up as he tapped his pointer on the monitor and responded, "There's no bone actually left except the outer rim and a few fragments that the cancer missed. All that orange you see isn't supposed to be there."

Selene, not so calmly, said, "Jesus Christ!"

It was a perfect opportunity to ask my next really dumb question. "So what exactly is keeping his leg attached to his torso?"

As he swiveled in his chair to face me, he rubbed the back of his neck, raised his eyebrows, and stammered, "Well...um...it's hard to know for sure, but Marley's mobility seems to rely solely on his strong muscles and ligaments."

Meredith whispered under her breath, "Damn!"

Molehill? Or...Mountain?

All of a sudden, the little room was overwhelmingly stuffy, so we peeled ourselves off each other and spilled into the hall, shaking our heads in amazement. Boy Wonder announced he was starving, which we all welcomed as something new to focus on. The goal was food, and the closest food was located at a restaurant in the hospital. The cancer center was a separate building from the general hospital, sharing the same grounds—an easy and short walk for the healthy, but an uphill challenge for our two survivors of terminal lung disease.

Just a few years ago, with their long strides and enormous lung capacity, these two men could have circled the hospital twice by the time the rest of us could reach the restaurant. Now it was a whole different story. Marley had a brand new, shiny black cane for support while Steven had the rolling support of the dolly that held his slender oxygen tank. The journey was slow and laborious yet rather humorous. It took them about 20 minutes to travel 50 yards! Every five steps, toward the final incline, Marley would lean against the outer wall of the hospital and Steven would slump against the nearest parked car. There was a slightly competitive edge to both of these guys and the last one to temporarily collapse was grateful the other gave out first. Even they would have laughed at the sad state of affairs if they'd had the lung capacity to do so.

"That was the day Steven told Marley that they were in a race to death. Steven was determined to win so that he could be there to catch Mars."

—Meredith Little Foster

After a wonderful and well-deserved lunch, we sat out on the grass. We only had a few minutes to be together before Steven and Meredith left to continue their journey. As a seasoned wilderness rites-of-passage guide, Steven had a remarkable ability to probe into the heart of hearts of any soul brave enough to be close to him.

As Steven slowly settled on the ground, he asked, "So, Marley, what happens if they have to amputate your leg?"

With a sideways glance at the puffy clouds set in the pale blue sky, Marley matter-of-factly stated, "Ahh, I dunno, I guess my leg will hurt less. But they'd have to go pwetty high, wouldn' they? Couldn' be wurse than what I'm deawing wif now."

Marley had just talked to a friend who knew someone who had a similar operation, and described the amputation included the whole buttock area on one side.

He pulled up a handful of grass, tried to stuff it down the back of my shirt, and after my giggling and swatting his arm away, he continued seriously. "You know, alls we'd have ta do is weld some stwaps on my Atick Cat so I could attach my body to it—then I won't fawl off goin' 'round fas cornas. Thad work!"

Steven nodded, staring at the freshly cut green expanse, with a blade of grass wedged between his lips. "Yup, it sounds like you've been thinking about it and have a pretty good plan."

There was no place even Steven could dig to get more honesty out of Marley. This young man wasn't in denial and he wasn't side-stepping reality. Marley did, however, redirect the conversation to how he was looking forward to "slammin' thwew the biggest mud bog in the Colestin." Life, according to Marley, just keeps on going until it doesn't. In the meantime, there's always ropes and pulleys to help get through the tough times.

"A wounded deer—leaps highest."

—Emily Dickinson

It was a great visit, even though we only had a few hours together. Selene returned with us as Steven and Meredith left with kisses of hope and mutual admiration and heartfelt hugs that lasted an eternity. From that perfectly manicured lawn, next to the parking lot of the hospital, we waved good-bye. Andrea, Selene, Marley, and I just stood there with arms woven around each other, watching their car disappear in the afternoon traffic. For all of us, save his daughter Selene, that was the last time we ever saw Steven alive.

Chapter Fourteen:
IT'S THE LITTLE THINGS

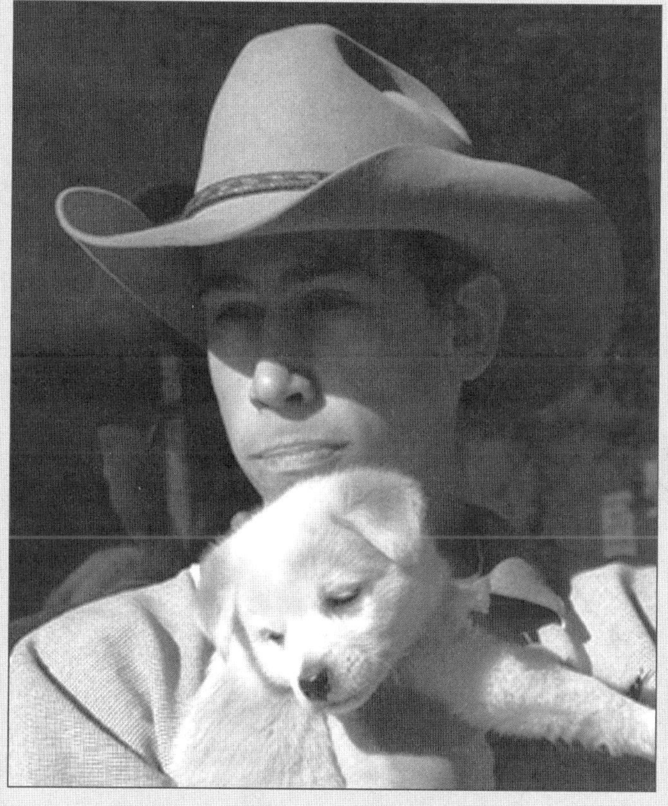

"A Boy and His Dog" - Marley and Gracie

Photo: Debbie Thornton

Tuesday, February 26, 2003
Subject: "TUMORS–R–US"

Dear friends,

I've been negligent in keeping you all up to date. Please forgive me, I'm swimming as fast as I can. Now it's catch-up time. In a nutshell: I'm always busy doing something, Catie's depressed that the ski season is prematurely over, and Marley says, "My tank's been running on reserve for a year, and now I'm running on empty."

Marley is in his third week of a new round of radiation. Yup! More tumors. The diagnosis was confirmed on his birthday, but I just couldn't bear to focus on it as I was writing the quick update sent that day. It was a whirlwind day filled with doctor visits, X-rays, and CAT scans. An hour before his birthday party was to commence, as people were gathering to celebrate, I received the dreaded phone call—the test results were not good. None of us were prepared to deal with this. We just had to grin and bear it—celebrating his birth was far more important than moaning over new tumors.

This type of lung cancer really seems to like the squishy, soft middle parts of Marley's bones. (I'm learning more about the skeletal structure than I ever wanted to know.) This time, there are two new tumors in his right ankle, one in his heel bone, and the tumor in his pelvis has flared up again for the third time. Damn! There's nothing to do but keep nuking his poor hip and the three new tumors, which are also inoperable. Double damn. Other than radiation, we have no options that produce an immediate effect. The radiation does not cure the cancer, or replace the bone that has been eaten away, but it reduces the pain by stopping it in its tracks, at least for a while.

We have been warned of the risks of continued radiation: a secondary cancer, extremely brittle bones, arthritis, poor circulation, and malfunctions of organs that have been partially nuked in order to zap whatever tumor they're aiming at. Marley continues to push the bounds of what "they" think the limits are and has miraculously avoided most of these risks. We keep exploring alternative options, but the pickin's are slim.

Alternatives

Saturday is Marley's third year anniversary of dealing with this disease. So, like duh, we're gonna have a party! The theme is "Stayin' Alive!" This one is an informal outdoor party at our place, around the fire pit. Hopefully it will be a healing, relaxing, and fun time. Life's pretty stressful right now. (That's the understatement of the year!)

Marley's Uncle Joseph (my brother-in-law) is flying in from North Carolina next week to help out. Marley is receiving some high levels of radiation to three different areas over a three-week period (five days a week). The effects are cumulative, and no one knows what to expect anymore. Small raft, big ocean. It will be nice to have backup help. Joseph will help cook, clean, cart kids around, and chop wood. It's like importing a temporary combination of a husband, a wife, a nanny, and a laborer. Thanks, Julia, for loaning me your husband!

Brittle Bones

Today we spent lots of quality time in the emergency room. Not! We were trying to figure out why, after Marley lay down last night and heard a small pop in his hip, excruciating pain commenced. The only logical conclusion was that he had cracked his pelvis (*iliac crest*). I was worried because Marley was worried. I've seen Marley *really* scared only one other time during this whole process, and that was three years ago when he couldn't breathe due to pneumonia.

He was spending the night with his buddy Luke when this new horror happened. Luke lives in a trailer in the woods a short but steep hike from his parents' house. Marley simply shifted his position, heard the pop, and then couldn't move without feeling intense shooting pain. Luke had to carry Marley to the main house so Luke's mom could drive him to where I could meet them halfway. Last night, when I asked him to describe his pain level on a scale of 1 to 10, he replied, "50!" But all he wanted to do was go home. What can I say. I gave him a Percocet and took him to the ER early this morning.

A special thanks to Sunny for driving all the way up to my house at 8:00 A.M. He felt his job was to make Marley laugh, to relieve the tension from fear and searing pain. As far as I was concerned, his purpose was to help me carry Marley to the car and, as gently as possible, hoist him into the Suburban without killing him. Once we got to the hospital, two large male nurses "helped" get Mars out of the car with the finesse of gorillas.

I want to praise sister Catie for rising to the occasion, doing all that she could, and being incredibly patient. It was a tough day, and she was a tremendous help. We spent four hours in the "emergency" wing just to get CAT scans and watch the doctors scratch their heads. All I know is as soon as we walked in the hospital and sat down in the waiting room, Marley began to throw up. When he started retching, I grabbed a nearby industrial-sized trash container and dragged it over to his wheelchair. Catie curled up in a ball and covered her ears as Mars yorked in the trash. As it turned out, puking in the waiting room was a highly effective method of being quickly escorted to a private room. There are pros and cons to everything!

Once again, I was shocked at how slow "emergency" care is. I did a good job of politely demanding attention, but it didn't seem to matter much. We waited for two hours in our sterile 10' X 8' cubby before his blood pressure was even taken. The room was so small that when the on-call doctor tried to open the door, I had to move my chair out of the way first. Catie was sound asleep, lying face down, stretched between two grey plastic chairs like a lion draped across tree branches. Marley was lying down and remained calm as I informed the poor doctor what was going on and suggested the only logical thing to do was to get pictures taken…NOW! It took a while but that's what happened.

Basically, the scans showed that there's no solid bone left to break, so their best guess was that two pieces of the remaining iliac crest rubbed together, causing the pain until they repositioned spontaneously. Marley walked out feeling better and the only procedure done was the CAT scan. What a waste of time.

We didn't bother reading the official report, but I suspect it would have read as follows: "Something happened that caused a dramatic increase in pain at approximately 10:00 P.M. which, for some reason, decreased in severity by 2:00 P.M. the following day. The patient was released."

Marley thought he should get an award for escaping without getting any shots. I thought he should get an award for once again confusing the hell out of the health professionals.

I got a very real taste of what my future could look like. I began to seriously doubt my ability to independently care for this 6'2", 162-pound baby boy. Like: how would I get him out of the bathtub if he could no longer propel the lower part of his body? Marley got a taste of a possible future too. Last night he whimpered in the wee hours, "I just can't stand not being in control of my body." There was very little for me to do except say, "I love you" and give him a reassuring and very gentle hug.

I guess we'll all be out of control someday. In the meantime, I hope you all celebrate STAYIN' ALIVE!

Love,
Jennifer

COMMUNICATION

Comfort Levels

As much as I hate computers, I loved the ease of communicating with Marley's doctor, Diane. She had signed herself up on Marley's ListServe, and received all the Updates so, even without visits, she knew what was going on. Whenever we had questions, we communicated directly via e-mail.

Wednesday, February 26, 2003
Subject: "EMERGENCIES"

• From: Diane – Marley's oncologist

Jennifer,

How is Marley??? I did receive a phone call from the ER saying that the hip wasn't fractured. Do we need more pain meds? If his pain issues get too bad, we may need help from home health nurses and/or the Hospice people, since they are some of the best pain specialists available.

Diane

That benign little e-mail took days to fully comprehend. It was the first time Hospice had been suggested. Was this her gentle way of saying we were heading into some rough water? Did that mean she thought we were close to the end? Did we need more help? Marley didn't think so and continued to plow ahead. My job was to sit tight and hope for the best.

"The human body experiences a powerful gravitational pull in the direction of hope. That is why the patient's hopes are the physician's secret weapon. They are the hidden ingredients in any prescription."

—Norman Cousins

MEDICAL INVENTIONS

Morale Booster

A few days later, I looked at the Guestbook on Marley's website and read an entry that warmed my heart and gave me hope. Once again, I was reminded that our little circle was much wider than it appeared.

Friday, February 28, 2003

• From: Carolyn

Dear Friends,

I'm a nurse and a friend of your sister, Constant. She's been forwarding your Update Letters to me since the beginning of Marley's illness. After reading the last Marley Update, I wanted to let you know about the Hoyer Lift.

This device is a pneumatic sling that has a base on wheels that go under a bed or wheelchair. The patient is placed in the sling and the attendant turns a crank and lifts them, then wheels them to the bathroom or chair and lets them down without the attendant doing any lifting. This nifty invention is commonly available from medical equipment suppliers.

I also wanted to tell you about pain patches. You may have already used them, but if not, they are placed on the skin and the medication is slowly absorbed—lasting for up to 72 hours. This gives steady pain relief. Then liquid or oral meds can be used for "breakthrough" pain, for quick relief.

Hope this is helpful. It sounds like you are doing a wonderful job in a very difficult situation.

Love,
Carolyn

Inventions

I did some research and found that the Hoyer lift was similar to what auto mechanics use to lift an engine block from a car. The sling can be positioned on the person without having to move them much (even in a wheelchair) and then it's attached to a sturdy tripod on wheels.

I replied to Carolyn immediately via e-mail.

Friday, February 28, 2003
Subject: "RE: HOYER LIFT"

Very cool, Carolyn,

Thank you so much! I had no idea either of these inventions existed. I hope I never have to use the sling, yet it's a great comfort to know I don't have to hire a man with big muscles to live with us should Marley become immobile. Thanks for the mental relief.

Pain patches? You've got to be kidding me. What will they come up with next? I will do more research on this one!

I was just interviewed for an article based on community support and the healing process. One of the comments I made was that Marley's Network was like having an invisible army of loving support standing shoulder to shoulder. Receiving your Guestbook entry was one of those great reminders.

Thank you very much,
Jennifer

"Success is not measured by the position one has reached in life, rather by the obstacles overcome while trying to succeed."

—Booker T. Washington

Friday, February 28, 2003
Subject: "AN INVITATION TO STAY ALIVE"

Dear Marley Fans,

CELEBRATE STAYIN' ALIVE!

It's not every day we have the opportunity to rejoice about a young man's third-year anniversary of staying alive as he continues a warrior's dance with lung cancer. It's not every day we have the opportunity to rejoice about our own efforts to stay alive as we face our world at war. Now is the time to come alive and party!

WHEN? Saturday, March 1st

- 2 to 5 P.M: We'll gather wood, hike, ride, prepare, and Be.
- 5 to 9 P.M: We'll eat the food we bring, gaze at stars, gather 'round the fire pit, and tell stories.

A RITE TO LIVE

- Prepare to share what "staying alive" means to you.
- Bring an object to burn, symbolizing what you're ready to let go of. (Please, no old recliners or hazardous materials!)

COME PREPARED

- This is an outdoor event. Bring warm clothing.
- Bring gloves for gathering firewood.
- Bring food, drink, blankets, and/or chairs. You are responsible for your own comfort.
- Silence, song, music, performances, costumes, and truth are welcome. (Electricity not available.)
- Prepare to share on video how Marley has affected your life and how you think he is unique. This is optional. Reagan is producing a video and has invited your participation.

What you bring represents who you are in our society.

BE ALIVE!

STILL ALIVE!

A Time to Party

We had a great time at the "Stayin' Alive" celebration. It was a gathering designed to lift wilting spirits. With only a few days of planning, a grand event was executed. It started raining the day the invitation was sent out and didn't stop until several hours before the party started. Rhys and I had been working hard, thinning the undergrowth of the woods on my land, and had collected an enormous pile of slash to burn at the party. We had filled the 30 tiki torches on the property, and the house was clean and stocked with provisions. All Rhys and I could do that day was to sit on the couch on the front porch and pray the rain would stop. Just before the party, it did. It was perfect weather for a great big bonfire.

One of the first things we did was to fuel the fire with things that people had brought to symbolize what they wanted to be rid of in their lives. Drew and Cindy had arrived with the X-rays from the first year. They ceremoniously handed them to Marley and asked if he would like to torch them. He gleefully agreed.

Reagan used this event to video tape interviews with the people in Marley's life. She set up her makeshift studio in our guest house. One by one a trail of people were snagged away from the fire to answer the question, "What makes Marley so unique?" Meanwhile, back on the porch, one of my dearest friends, the pyrotechnician, taught Marley how to make BIG fireworks. As soon as it was dark, Marley told Reagan he had something special to include in her movie. As we all stood facing the pasture, they set off their professional grade four-inch fireworks. The display was incredibly dramatic, and could be seen from miles away.

Marley had turned the pasture into a mud bog for his ATV and, after the fireworks display, he challenged Rhys to a daring game of tug-of-war. Rhys just couldn't say no! Marley hooked a heavy 8-foot chain to the front ends of his Arctic Cat quad and Rhys' Toyota 4-Runner. We all stood around the firepit, and watched the two sets of headlights illuminating the mud spewing in all directions. The two machines did their best to maintain. Both engines were being pushed to their limit, with the pedals to the metal. After about ten exciting minutes listening to the whine of stressed engines, they called it a Mexican stand-off. Neither rig had managed to move the other more than a few inches sideways. It was rewarding to watch the people who love Marley experience firsthand what makes Marley tick. This was one of those stories Marley would tell and no one would have believed, but this time, most everyone Marley knew was there and Reagan got it on film!

During the pulling event, Rhys was in his truck so, other than his head, which he had to stick out his window, he was fairly clean. Marley, on the other hand, had no windshield to protect him from the mud Rhys' truck was spraying in his direction. Mud was everywhere! As Rhys and Marley walked to the house, Marley draped his arm around Rhys and said, "Mud…it's good medicine."

Just before midnight, it started to snow. Those of us around the fire marveled at how the fire not only melted the snow but turned it to steam before it could touch us. It was a great night that left us energized and very happy we were all still alive.

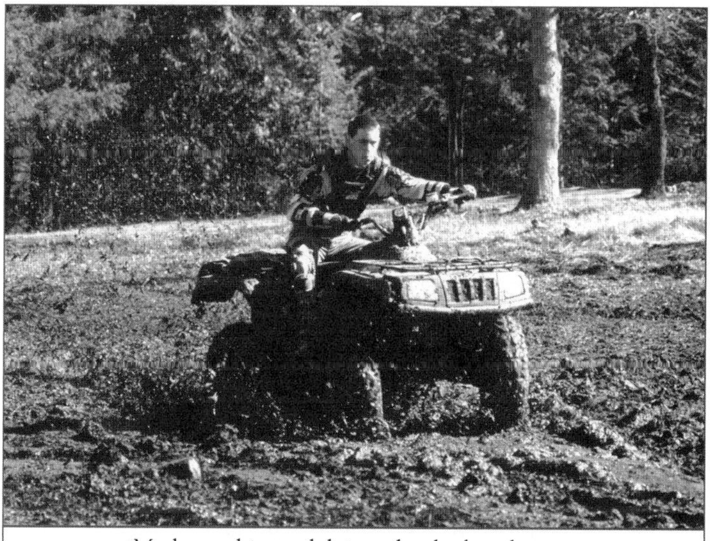

Marley on his quad doing what he loved most.

Thursday, March 21, 2003
Subject: "IN THE NEWS"

Happy Spring Everyone,

Marley and Catie just returned to me for another two weeks! Catie's grown yet again. I swear my neck gets tired from looking up at both of my children's faces as they tower above me.

Below is the article Jennifer S. wrote for a news magazine, called "W-3." It came out on Wednesday and includes a sidebar description of the video that one of Marley's special ed teachers is putting together (titled: "Healing Through Video").

Enjoy!
Jennifer

Printed in *W3 Magazine* (*Words, Wit, & Wisdom*),
March 2003 – Theme "Hope"

The Mother of
ONE AWESOME TEENAGER
is learning lessons about life through dealing with death.
She's Learning…
MARLEY'S WAY
by Jennifer Strange

When hope is based too much on a future that may not materialize for a child, what does a mother do? An Ashland publisher whose son was diagnosed with terminal cancer three years ago, has learned to live in the present and to value each day spent with a growing circle of supporters.

Jennifer's 18-year-old son, Marley, has defied all common knowledge when it comes to cancer. Although he was given six short months to live upon his diagnosis in 2000, Marley—minus one lung, half a rib, and many lymph nodes, and supplemented by a prosthetic knee and a few two-foot scars—continues to laugh, walk, and ride his ATV all over the Mount Ashland area.

Jennifer attributes Marley's unexpected quality of life to his lack of fear of death, his sense of humor, and his strong will. It's also due, no doubt, to her bottomless well of advocacy and love. "It's kind of the cowboy mentality of 'okay, you just got kicked off the horse, time to get back on,'" says Jennifer. "There's no room to fall apart here. We all have careers. We're all running farms. Kids still need to be fed, and kids still need to go to school."

Keeping Marley in school despite his medical trials is important to create a sense of normalcy and to provide stress release for child and parents alike, says Jennifer. And constant communication with loved ones is also critical to her and her family's emotional well-being.

Finding the best way to spread news to her circle of support was at first a dark cloud that later showed a silver lining. Until Jennifer's niece, Selene, landed in Ashland to help the family out, information was disseminated in a haphazard fashion, resulting in more misunderstandings than solutions. Selene helped develop a ListServe that started with 50 people and soon grew to 150. The list just kept getting longer and reaching farther.

"This revolutionized our lives," Jennifer says. "I post a letter that says we have to get to Boston in two weeks and have no idea how to do it. Within three hours, I've got 40 letters from people donating frequent flyer points and volunteering to organize the flights."

Soon, the ListServe became known as "Marley's Network," and a website was created, with regular updates and photos. At the same time as Marley and Jennifer's world started to seem smaller, it was actually growing. People all over the world were responding to calls for prayer, to calls for hope, to calls for ceremony, and to calls for good old-fashioned help. The magic just kept on happening....

"When Marley required a knee replacement, he needed a

wheelchair," Jennifer remembers. "Three days later I got a call from the bus terminal in Ashland saying there was a wheelchair waiting for me. Somebody in Marley's Network who had a wheelchair and didn't use it sent it via Greyhound to Ashland. It was instant."

Jennifer refers to this amazing system of support as an example of the "build it and they will come" theory. And it has taught her the simple beauty of making simple requests. "Results don't happen unless you ask," Jennifer says. "And I don't know how many ears and concerned hearts are around us, but it feels like an invisible army."

Two months before Marley's 16th birthday—which coincided with the one-year anniversary of his cancer diagnosis—this invisible army took up formation to create Marley's Monster Bash. A core of ten volunteers met every Sunday to plan what was to become a huge party for 400 people. They gathered every item as a donation, from banners to food to five live bands to the Ashland Armory as a venue.

Marley's "pebble pool" was unveiled at this event. "It was the technique that my family used as a way to build ceremony when my father got cancer," Jennifer explains. "We did a meditation every evening, and each pebble received in the mail that day was placed in the pool. It worked then and it's still working now." Jennifer calls it a tangible form of prayer. "The fountain serves like an altar, where every day I look at the fountain, Marley looks at the fountain, and we remember we're not alone."

Marley's Network also netted hundreds of alternative healing ideas, which turned into a blessing and a curse. Whereas Jennifer wanted to try everything that sounded good, she had to learn to listen to her son. And what a lesson this was for a mother. "When it's your own child, you want a little more control," says Jennifer. "But when he's saying, 'No, it's my life; it's my death,' well, it was a fast lesson, realizing that he is truly his own individual. We cannot make him accept any cure."

That's not the only thing Jennifer has learned from her odds-defying son. "Marley is so unusual that I had to pay attention to many of his lessons," says Jennifer. "At the beginning I thought, if my 15-year-old can cope with this so well, what does he know that I don't? So I started asking him questions. I'd ask, 'Are you afraid?' and he'd respond in complete innocence, 'What of?' I'd ask, 'Dying?' He'd say, 'What's so bad about dying?'"

This bold and simple philosophy has changed Jennifer's life, allowing her to "live in the now"—both for her son's sake and for her own. She says she has learned not to worry about the things she has no control over and to focus, instead, on what's right in front of her. More often these days, she finds herself sitting against a tree, writing down her thoughts, or watching the birds and clouds.

"I like myself now a whole lot more than I did three years ago, because I'm a whole lot more present in all my dealings," Jennifer says. "And, as I learned Marley's way, I had to re-evaluate what I was wishing for. Now the consistent line is to pray for what's right for Marley. I don't know whether that's for a graceful dying or a healthy living—and I don't know if he knows, either."

So—for now—Jennifer and Marley and their huge fan club are letting the present guide their days. And what does today say to this miracle-maker of a mom? "Be available. Breathe. Laugh. Be ready…ready for whatever happens," Jennifer says with a smile that's just a little sad. "If I'm going to be like Marley, he's going to play, he's ready for action, and so must I be."

Healing Through Video

When Reagan Burrell met Marley Pratt 10 years ago, she never imagined her life would become consumed by his story. Sure, he was an unusual kid who challenged every standard, but, as a special education assistant, Reagan met a lot of unique kids. Now, a decade later, Reagan had reacquainted herself with Marley and his family and is making a video of his life, inspired primarily by his current battle with terminal cancer.

Reagan's video project began as an offshoot of a music video she did for a class at Southern Oregon University, where she is an art major. The movie has become her main focus in study and in life, inspired, she says, by Marley's mom, Jennifer.

"What made the movie happen in my head was Jennifer," says Reagan. "I just thought of how Jennifer's energy changed Marley's opportunities and life—she never allowed him to be mislabeled and always gave him a safety net to be himself."

The film will feature interviews with Marley's teachers, peers, family, friends, and doctors, all of whom have been asked the same question: What makes Marley different? "The more I ask the question, the more profound and intense it becomes," says Reagan. "No one can deny they've been touched by Marley."

Reagan's goal is to introduce the film to the medical field, which she hopes will use it as a tool for people living with cancer. "I'm trying to show that this thing is bigger than just the world of cancer," she says. "There's something really particular about the fear that comes with a diagnosis of cancer. Others see only the disease and not the human who has it."

To bring the person into the picture is her directive. "I want to show that Marley has figured out how to manage his pain and how he has gained this freedom from fear," says Reagan. "I would want others to know that we can all try for that. I want others to see life through Marley's eyes."

The video is called "On My Horse," the title to a poem Reagan found while poring through a stack of Marley's grade school papers. The short verse written by Marley reads:

i am on my horse
i ride all night and day
i ride against the wind

"Challenges are what make life interesting; overcoming them is what makes life meaningful."

—-Joshua J. Marine

BRIAN'S MOM

Dis-Ease

Our family didn't have a corner on the market of pain and suffering. Marley was not the only sick child in town. We had plenty of company—too much company, as far as I was concerned. One of the kids in trouble became a close friend of Marley's. While I was watching my 18-year-old hyper-age, becoming an old man before my very eyes, Brian's mother Martha endured something very different—and yet, it was strangely similar.

Just before Brian's 18th birthday, he had a heart attack and fell from a tree, and was in a coma for almost two weeks. When he decided to re-join the world of the living, he had to face re-learning everything: how to speak, how to remember, how to move…everything. It was like he was born again as a toddler.

> Friday, April 4, 2003
> Subject: "MOTHER TO MOTHER"
>
> • From: Martha – Brian's mother
>
> Hi Jennifer,
>
> I just read the piece about you and Marley in "W3." It reminded me of all the times I have wanted to stop by and wish you well, give you a hug, and ask "HOW DO YOU DO IT???" In the year and a half since Brian went down, in the daily struggle to help him cope with all his losses, I often think of you and Marley. I am learning more about patience than I thought was possible, more about faith and hope. And more about how TIRED a person can get when it seems that the whole world is nothing but stress and pain. When I look at Brian, I know I cannot give up. I know I will never give up. I don't know how you do it each day—and yet, I do. What else is there, but the beauty of each morning and the spirits of our sons?
>
> Thank you,
> Martha

The Butterfly Effect

THE MARLEY EFFECT
by Martha Hammon

I first met Marley at Ashland Middle School in the spring of 1998. I was a volunteer math teacher working with the special education department. Although I knew Jennifer, I didn't know she was Marley's mom. All I knew was there was this lanky kid who did NOT want to do math and was planning to charm and grin his way out of it. He disarmed me completely, and he is the only kid from that class that I remember. At some point, I put Marley together with his little sister Catie, who had been a student in the last class where I had done student teaching. Again, Catie was about the only child in the class who had made an impression. Then I put Jennifer in the picture, because she used to pick Catie up from school. Suddenly, I had this great family.

My next encounters with Marley, other than seeing him around and having him say a friendly "hi" while riding past on his bike, occurred after his cancer arrived and my own son, Brian, had nearly died from a cardiac arrest. Brian and Marley connected in a way only young men who have been at the threshold can interact. They had a special bond. There were also the inevitable "family" connections that happen in a town like Ashland: I know Jennifer from music and dancing around town; Marley's stepmom Cindy was one of the first people I had met in Ashland, 25 years ago; and my dear friend and "little brother," Thom, worked with Jennifer. It felt as though we were a big family, pulled together by our love for this remarkable young man.

Marley's strength has helped me in subtle yet enduring ways. Brian also looked up to Marley, as a hero and an inspiration. Now, Brian realizes that he carries Marley with him as a part of his own strong soul. I will always remember seeing Marley at the high school, wearing his cowboy hat and long Outback raincoat, laughing and zooming around in his wheelchair. It is Marley's joy I want to hold within me, the grin I saw that first time in a math class, that grin that said, "I'm gonna do exactly as I please."

THE FLIP-SIDE OF HOPE

Chaotic Harmony

I've looked in life's mirror trying to figure out why Marley's illness never swept me off my feet or made me lose my mind. I battled feelings of guilt when other mothers held me and said, "I don't know where you get your strength from. I'd be a basket case." Was I crazy? Was I in such a state of highly developed denial that I was bullshitting even me? Why did Marley's story make such sense to me?

Why wasn't I in a state of rage that my boy contracted such a bizarre disease for a 15-year-old? Why didn't I react like my brother, outraged that it seemed like Marley was just giving up and letting the cancer kill him? But Marley was still alive and kicking hard in his own way. I had to just keep asking myself, "What is it that determines which side of the razor's edge life falls on?"

In a journal entry, just months before my father died, he reflected on living through the mirror of dying:

> "I believe this morning that the major contributing factor to my illness is my continuing loss of enthusiasm, for with enthusiasm has always come an abiding and sustaining sense of determination and confidence."

Definition:

Enthusiasm

"...comes from the Greek entheos, meaning literally 'in God,' and is defined as 'the power actuating one who is inspired by a divine or superhuman power.'"

—Virginia H. Hine, *Last Letter to the Pebble People*

Inherited Gifts

I realized that, for better or for worse, this trait of requiring enthusiasm in order to endure living was mine as well. It was Marley's trademark from day one. He lived BIG!

It is a core belief of mine that it doesn't matter *what* we do but *how* we do it. I feel like I came to this planet with a sense that the world is in total chaos. This makes me very uncomfortable, because I simply don't understand why this insanity is necessary—yet, simultaneously, I accept this as perfection and, in a weird way, harmony.

"…born with the gift of laughter
and a sense that the world is mad."

—Rafael Sabatini

Once it became apparent that my father wasn't going to survive his cancer, he wrote;

> "Without enthusiasm, at least in sustaining amounts, so many things can erode the ego and damage what confidence is left. Enthusiasm and confidence are a strong combination; for with them, the petty arguments, disagreements, and misunderstandings are either impossible or irrelevant."

I believe defeat and hopelessness occur when a lack of enthusiasm toward living overwhelms. I think this is what ultimately kills most of us. Developing a powerful will to constantly create that which enthuses has been my personal method of embracing all the crap this planet has to offer. I think hope and attachment to an outcome, like staying alive—which is, in itself, an illusion—is what makes most of us fear death.

Facing Death as an Ally

One conversation with Marley I'll never forget. We sat alone, under the stars, after watching the movie *I Am Sam*, starring Sean Penn. Sam was a single father who had to fight Child Services to retain custody of his young daughter. It didn't matter that he was incredibly loving, he had some mental abnormalities—a round hole in a square world.

I don't know what got into me, but the movie affected me so deeply that I shared with Marley, with a gut-wrenching honesty, my fears about his ability to live as an adult in our society, if he should survive the cancer. He didn't hear the point of my concern; all he heard was "if he survived" like he hadn't even considered what might happen if.... I was shocked. Death was a baseline reality that we had talked about intellectually, but it seemed like all new information to him on a soul level.

Our commitment to openly communicate with Marley was a requirement from the beginning. When doctors tried to tell us what we were up against by escorting us politely into the hall or another private room, we firmly declined and let them know that Marley needed to hear anything they had to say because it was, after all, his life. We felt it was important that Marley be able to hear information firsthand so he could pick up all clues, including body language and subtle verbal cues.

We went through the tedious process of researching and understanding doctor's jargon with all the children. Granted, each child's grasp of this information was absorbed to their capacity to understand our interpretation. In the beginning, for instance, we would explain what "stage 4 terminal cancer" meant by saying, "'terminal' means you can die from it, and 'stage 4' is like how they rate white water rapids in levels of danger (except the highest level of danger in cancer was a 4, not a 6)." Because it was put in terms they were familiar with, all the kids would nod in understanding.

Marley had a really unusual way of dealing with having terminal lung cancer. I could never tell what he was thinking or even if he thought about dying much. It wasn't part of his script to battle cancer cells; his role was to carry on with normal teenage activities. All I could do was try to follow his lead.

Just when I thought he had a wicked case of denial, he would surprise me. Every once in a while, in an offhanded, matter-of-fact way, he would say something like, "I hope I die from somethen excitin' like a wattlesnake bite, wipin' out on my bike, fawin' off a cliff, or even gettin' munched by a couga. Anything but cansa." He trained me well to be prepared for him to die at any time, by any means, regardless of the cancer. I knew if a cougar did kill him, he'd be happy, so I never spent much time worrying about his safety or keeping him from doing what he loved. Why protect him by thwarting his desire to live fully—in order to keep him alive long enough to die?

> ***"When a man knows how to live dangerously, he is not afraid to die. When he is not afraid to die, he is, strangely, free to live."***
>
> **—William O. Douglas**

Marley knew better than any of us that his body was riddled with cancer which was eating away his bones, organs, and lymphatic system. He had admitted he didn't want to die, twice before, yet he never bemoaned the fact for more than a few minutes. I was always honest that his body probably was not going to be able to stand much more of the effects of cancer. He understood, and yet there was some invisible line his mind refused to cross when it came to facing the fact that he was, indeed, dying. I began to notice that he wasn't alone.

The Ostrich Theory

I didn't know if Marley was going to survive the nine months in the womb or if he was going to wake up on any given morning. From the minute he was conceived, Marley trained me to love and "be here now" because life might be short. It took me a long time to figure out how many people saw Marley's cancer as an enemy to fight because it might kill him.

> ***Definition***
>
> **Hope**
>
> "A feeling that what is wanted will happen; desire accompanied by anticipation or expectation."

As each tumor came, they were seen as obstacles to overcome so Marley could live. Each success increased the level of hope, and the goal of Life became increasingly important. Marley, on the other hand, only seemed to see what was right in front of him. One of Marley's doctors reported a statistic that those with mental abnormalities survive terminal disease longer than the average human with normal mental faculties. Maybe it stems from their way of living in the present rather than focusing on the possibilities of the future.

With a need to invest in unrealistic outcomes, such as living life while refusing to accept death as a part of it, comes hope. Somewhere deep within me, I knew hope was one way to combat the fear that death would occur. I think I was more scared of disappointment than death. Although I felt too realistic to hope for my son's continued life, I could, however, hope that Marley would die with honor, dignity, and grace.

In her book, *Last Letter to the Pebble People*, my mother wrote:

> "I believe now that a recurrent problem for any family facing death, oddly enough, is the issue of hope. Hope is the bright bird we must always keep in sight, shining through the darkness of the jungle. To follow it, we must learn that its plumage changes. What we hope for must evolve."

It seemed to me that, as people focused on the hope that Marley would survive the cancer, we lost sight of fully experiencing Marley in a perfect state of having cancer. He was going to die even if he survived the cancer. It seemed to me that if we hoped for anything other than his dying well, we were setting ourselves up for failure.

An excerpt from John Cagle's essay, *It Ain't a River In Egypt*, describes an alternative way to see our inevitable death.

> "Sometimes, it is helpful to shake off denial and face death head-on. As a Hospice social worker, I am probably more aware of my own mortality than most people. But, when I reflect on my ultimate fate, it enhances my experience of the present. Knowing I will witness a finite number of sunsets makes the colors of dusk more brilliant. It makes the words 'I love you' take on a new and sharper meaning. New York cheesecake begins to taste creamier. Tears are saltier. And springtime thundershowers are more spiritual."

INVISIBLE ARMS

Glen, On Dying

One of the most remarkable things about my job was the dedicated readers who joined the Bathroom Readers' Institute. I corresponded with the same customers year after year. Many of us will continue to communicate long after "Uncle John's" products cease to exist. Glen was one of those customers. During our business calls, we would check in on the personal level. Both of us were caring for loved ones with a terminal illness. After his beloved wife let go of her tenuous hold on life, he sent the following e-mail.

Wednesday, April 30, 2003
Subject: "TRUST AND LOVE"

• From: Glen

My dear friend Jennifer,

Janese's decline was rapid but followed a very predictable pattern. Hospice gave me a booklet, called "Gone From My Sight," which was wonderful in helping me to know what to expect during my wife's last couple of months—and I'd be happy to send it to you.

As Janese's condition worsened and she weakened, she grew immeasurably stronger in spirit. She had dozens of visitors, and the support around both of us was truly wonderful. During the last week of her life, her pain increased to the point where she was up to 1000 mg of morphine per hour. On Saturday the 26th, at 5 P.M., she was beyond the point where I could help, and so I decided to have her taken to the hospital. Her body did relax a bit as she was carried out.

At the hospital, I conferred with the doctor, and I decided to have them administer "terminal sedation," which basically meant they were going to treat her as though her pain level was at a 10 on a continual basis—and administer medication accordingly. She received over 25,000 mg of morphine from 5 P.M. until her death at 10:08. Still, the nursing staff was shocked that she went so quickly—apparently from a blood clot in her brain due to the cancer.

How did I prepare? Well, I allowed God to guide me and friends to support and love me. At the encouragement of the minister who married us, I gave Janese permission to die when she had about two weeks left. I reaffirmed that permission with love and encouragement many times after that. We'd go on spiritual meditation "test flights" together, where I'd speak to her of flying all over the planet in her beautiful new body. I told her of things I would hope to do when she was gone—basically a continuance of the spiritual path we'd shared up to that point. And—I thanked her—and I apologized to her—and I loved her with all of my heart. And I cried and cried and cried.

So I was as prepared as can be—but when she finally died I wasn't prepared at all for a few seconds. She had gone through a sort of slow motion seizure and was struggling for her final breath. I called the nurse and she came in and said "What happened?"—as if I'd know. And then Janese simply relaxed (for the first time in many weeks), and stopped breathing. I asked the nurse if she was gone, and she checked her and told me she was.

I think I'd still be standing there in shock—but the nurse, after a minute, said, "Thank God!" I realized then that I had not taken Janese to the hospital to get a cast put on, I'd taken her there to die—and the fact that she passed away after only five hours was truly a miracle.

Jennifer, the miracles keep happening! And yes—I cry a lot.

Love,
Glen

Grace

I cried, sitting in front of my computer at work, as I read Glen's words. Even though I felt his heart breaking, I could also feel the lightness of release surrounding him. As everyone in the office gathered around me, reading the letter over my shoulder, I explained my tears were flowing because I knew just how he felt. After each of my parents had died, I felt a magical and overwhelming joy at the same time as an unfathomable pain.

Deep inside, I knew I was also crying because it couldn't be long until I would be writing words like his. Yet, at that time, all I could feel was pain. Maybe I was a bit jealous of his freedom, too. One thing is for sure; I knew that I was scared. After I dried my tears, a wash of peacefulness swept through my being. Glen's recount reminded me how beautiful and loving the death experience can be. It was like I was invited to remember what a state of grace felt like. I replied immediately, knowing a true friend that I had never met was waving at me from across the finish line, saying, "It's all right, Jennifer. It's really all right!"

Dearest Glen,

Thank you so much for your courage! Your heart is true and open, and it's a pleasure to share the planet with you. I know I'm prepared for what lies ahead. That little, continual voice is always with me, assuring me everything is as it should be. Although I've felt heavy for the past two days, I trust.

I have a major deadline to contend with for the next month, a new school year beginning, and a very strong boy facing more pain. I question what the hell I'm doing. It's a very bad time to take a sabbatical, yet I don't want to miss out on making Marley's life really enjoyable. Tough choices I make. I guess it will become clearer over the next few weeks what the right action is.

I'll keep asking and I'll keep listening.
Jennifer

WHEN IT RAINS, IT POURS

A Call from Selene

Selene had moved to Oakland, California, to go to art college. She was also closer to her parents, Steven and Meredith, who were now living just across the bay. She was totally stressed out. This particular spring was challenging the very fiber of her being; she was finishing her first year, felt too far from Marley, and was watching her dad's health disappear. I adored Selene, and during our many phone conversations it was hard to feel her pain.

One day she called me at the office, and I was surprised to hear a new tone in her voice. Although she was obviously scared, she sounded strong as she told me Steven was dying. My heart sank as she told me that he could no longer take in enough air. The next day, he died at home. I prepared to travel south to say good-bye to his body and to help with the cremation ceremony.

I had never had an easier trip to San Francisco; the time flew by as I thought about Steven. I arrived in record time and met Meredith, her brother Jay, and his fiancée Laurie at a blues bar. Meredith looked like she had just returned from a vision quest—her eyes were clear and she felt solid. She told me how amazing it was to be by her husband's side as he took his last breath. She told me how hard it was watching his pain, and what a relief it was when it was all over.

The following day, about ten of us gathered at the crematorium to send Steven's body off. He was in an open, waxed cardboard coffin. Each of us brought something to be burned with him. Standing in a circle around him, we held hands. I stomped my left foot three times and then asked the others to join me. I told the spirits to watch out because Steven was coming their way! I gave him a pack of Spirit cigarettes because I knew how he had missed smoking the last few years, and maybe he could use them if he needed to do any trading with the gods and goddesses. Then I said good-bye to his body, holding his face in my hands and kissing his cold forehead one last time. One by one the others said their good-byes too. After the oven doors were closed, we went outside to watch the heatwaves rise from the chimney as we bid farewell to Steven's body.

A Call For Thom

After I returned to Ashland, we had to work hard at not letting the intensity of Marley's situation depress us, especially after Glen's letter and Steven's death. But sometimes, when it rains, it pours, and there's nothing you can do about it. I'll never forget watching Little Thom pace around the yard just outside the window by my desk talking on the phone. Something was wrong. When he walked in, we all turned to face him, silently questioning what was up. He said his oldest sister had a cancerous brain tumor and he wanted to go be with her. After a few minutes of shock, we all independently thought, "So who's next?"

Marley responded by hugging Thom a lot and tickling him more than usual. Thom said he started to understand how Catie felt losing a sibling. There was a real sweet connection that was made between Thom and Catie as he prepared to go be with his sister Nancy. It was then that I realized, as much as I had been around death, I had never had a sibling die. I had no idea what Catie was going through. I'm glad Thom and Catie had each other.

It was hard watching Thom leave town. We all felt safer when we were together. All Thom could do was to stay close, while he had the chance. He kept telling Marley how much he loved him. No one knew how long Thom would be gone. One day, just before his departure, Thom and I were redesigning his schedule so he could continue to work from Colorado. It was then that it dawned on us—he might never see Marley again.

"When change is accepted—no, more than that, embraced— it catalyzes our lives, expands our understanding, and shifts our perspective from one of fear to one that affirms life. For life is change."

—Gloria Karpinski

Chapter Fifteen:
THE HOME STRETCH

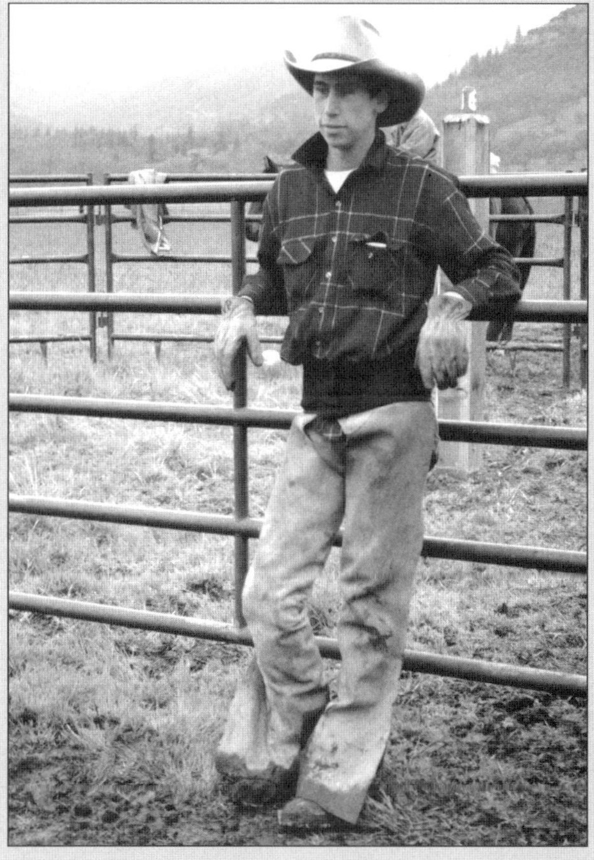

Marley at the Colestin cattle round-up, May 2003
Photo: Cindy Norton

RITES OF PASSAGE

A Guiding Light

Marley had become an untrained, non-traditional rites-of-passage guide of the highest calibre. He somehow inherently knew how to lead his local network through self-generated ceremonies. It began after his first hospital adventure, when he wanted to have a hospital gown burning ritual. After which, we had various theme parties: celebrating the end of a course of radiation, the beginning of chemo, Marley's birthdays, general survival, etc. At first, I thought he just wanted to be social, but now I'm convinced it was more than that—he was purposely creating these ceremonies so his changes could be recognized and felt by his community.

Traditions

In this country, some traditions are recognized: house warming parties, stag parties, weddings, anniversaries, birthdays, baby showers, and funerals. (The Jewish tradition also includes coming-of-age ceremonies.) But there are other life-altering transitions that our culture generally fails to acknowledge, let alone celebrate.

Modern Life Transitions

Life passages to celebrate (** indicates rites currently honored by many.)

Being born
Becoming a Mother**
Becoming a Father**
Becoming a Sibling
Becoming a Grandparent
Getting a Drivers License
Menstruation
Adulthood
Changing Residence**
Employment change
Registering to Vote
Loss of Virginity
Planting / Harvest
Cohabitation
Preparing to Marry**
Marriage**
Pregnancy
Miscarriage
Abortion
Divorce
The Four Seasons
Birthday Anniversaries**
Wedding Anniversaries**
Deathday Anniversaries
Retirement**
Old age
Dying
Death**

Aging and dying are two life passages Americans like to ignore. They're most often viewed as dishonorable or private. Some changes happen gradually and therefore are hard to define. At various times throughout Marley's illness, my sisters asked me, "Is it time? Should I get on a plane to be by your side? Do you think he's in the final stages?" I never knew how to answer them. I had never watched Marley die before. How was I supposed to know when he was officially dying?

Shift Happens

Not all of our life passages are dramatic, but they do make a difference by changing us. The seasons affect us all, yet most of us don't recognize this. The majority of our lives no longer revolve around them. Regardless of whether we stop to recognize that fall has ended and winter has begun, a shift *has* occurred. Maybe if we honored our fragile mortality, we'd be more likely to stop to acknowledge life's subtle changes.

> ***"As nightfall does not come at once, neither does oppression. In both instances, there is a twilight when everything remains seemingly unchanged. And it is in such twilight that we must be most aware of change in the air—however slight—lest we become unwitting victims of the darkness."***
>
> **—William O. Douglas**

Relatively speaking, our lives are easy, automated, and consistent. Every Monday seems the same, every year seems the same…and then you die. So what? Our modern culture operates at a mind-boggling pace 24/7. The work week is no longer Monday through Friday from 9 to 5. For many people, Fridays no longer represent a reason to celebrate the weekend, and Sundays are no longer considered a day of rest and relaxation. These kinds of rituals used to (and still can) give us something to look forward to. That's why Marley's Network found excuses to have parties. Our rituals made our lives special. They memorialized the precious passage of time and created sweet memories we will all take with us to our deathbeds.

Ritual

It's pretty simple. Every ritual is a ceremony consisting of three components: severance, transition, and reincorporation. Closing your eyes, sleeping, and waking up could be a ritual if its significance is acknowledged consciously. Everything we do, including breathing, can be acknowledged as a rite of passage. But let's face it, if I made a big deal out of every time my heart did its thing, I'd be completely dysfunctional, wouldn't have any friends left, and would probably die from a heart attack!

Andrea, our network's unofficial "goddess of ceremony," always sent *me* a card on both Catie and Marley's birthdays to celebrate my "birth-giving day." She has reminded me how easy it is to forget how important those two days were for me—not just for my kids. Ceremony doesn't have to be elaborate to make something special. Ceremony can be as simple as a hug or saying, "Thank you" as long as it's mindful and sincere and is powered by intention and purpose.

Severance

One of the most dramatic and meaningful severance ceremonies I've ever been a part of was performed for logical, functional reasons instead of for ceremonial reasons. It didn't seem to matter—the impact was incredibly significant. I had been determined to hire Rhys to remodel Marley's room and add on a new room for Catie. The prospect of this project was daunting and had been postponed for several years for many reasons. I knew Marley might be confined to a wheelchair soon, and I had better get my act together before that happened. I decided the only smart thing to do was to prepare.

Catie could remain in the loft while a new room was built for her, but Marley had to vacate his room for the remodel. Thus the project had to be completed during the two weeks that the kids lived at Drew's. It was a small window of opportunity that had to align with Marley's health, the weather, and Rhys' availability.

First things first: clean and pack up anything Marley didn't use on a daily basis. Marley's belongings were stored in twenty plastic containers neatly stacked in the barn.

Meanwhile, back on the ranch…Drew and Cindy had determined that it was time for Marley's room to be moved to the first floor of their house. He was having trouble managing the stairs, so they figured they'd swap bedrooms. It was not planned this way, but they too were packing all of Marley's belongings in boxes. The process in both houses was the same; Marley had to review every object he had, keeping only what was critically important to him. Throwing things away was incredibly therapeutic—it was a superior method of preparing all of us to let go. This process turned out to be a physical reminder that big changes were approaching and that life would never be the same. Packing Marley's stuff and cleaning his room was our spontaneous severance ceremony—a death of the old Marley.

Ways of Marking Severance:
(leaving something or someone behind)

Burning
Breaking
Smashing
Tearing
Crying
Closing
Cutting
Untying
Packing
Burying
Throwing
Blowing
Extinguishing Light
Cleansing
Yelling
Undressing / Taking off

(Anything that reminds us that letting go is the intent.)

"To those who fear change, evolution is the enemy. But to those who respond consciously to the steady beat of evolution, it is the essence of life summoning us to become all that we can be."

—Gloria Karpinski

Transition

In terms of recognizing the three stages of ceremony, *severance* would be the "preparation" stage while *transition* would be the "doing" phase. The process of moving his furniture downstairs or moving the boxes to the barn was our way of symbolizing the transition from the old to the new.

On some of my crazier days, I couldn't believe I was actually going to work and not staying home to focus on and cuddle my kids. I'd chant to myself something like, "I'm going to work in order to make money so I can stay home when they *really* need me." It made me want to work harder because I had a goal. Doing this kind of conscious act helped me retain my sanity and kept me off of the shrink's couch.

Ways of Marking Transition:

(going from one form, stage, place, etc. to another)

Speaking vows
Solitude
Dancing/Chanting
Silence
Changing style
Lifting up
Enacting desired change
Fasting
Nakedness
Traveling
Changing name

(Anything that symbolizes the intended change.)

"Power resides in the moment of transition from a past to a new state."

—Ralph Waldo Emerson

Reincorporation

When we were done with Marley's room, his way of completing our unceremonious ceremony was to flop on his newly made bed and howl. Quick and simple, yet effective—the deed was done and everyone within earshot knew it! Marley never had a problem letting the world know when he had completed something. He marked his transitions loud and clear. For instance, he always announced when he was leaving a hospital with, "I'm outta here!" and when he was outside, he'd yell, "I'm free!"

Reincorporation can be the most difficult of the three stages of ceremony, because even though it feels like a change has been made, it may not look like it from anyone else's perspective—you may still look and act the same. The task is to incorporate our new Self into our daily lives before it becomes real. As Black Elk, a Lakota medicine man spoke, "A man who has a vision is not able to use the power of it unless he has performed the vision on Earth for the people to see."

Just a century ago, outward symbols of change were commonplace. When someone died, mourners would wear black, or when a boy become a man, he would wear pants instead of knickers. These days the symbols acknowledging a rite of passage are harder to identify. One obvious tradition that still exists is wearing an engagement or wedding ring.

Ways of Marking Reincorporation:

(to combine the new with something already formed)

Crossing over a rope, threshold, line, etc.
Stepping on
Unveiling
Fusing or Joining
Tying or Knotting
Exchanging gifts
Building up
Embracing
Forming a circle
Filling up
Drinking in
Feasting / Ingesting
Lighting candles or lights
Unpacking
Dressing / Putting on

(Anything that symbolizes adding on or completion.)

"Change is the constant, the signal for rebirth, the egg of the phoenix."

—Christina Baldwin

Decision Road

The choice to live without purpose is somewhat new. Many of us are not driven by a collective desire—the "American Dream" is an elusive myth unraveling at the seams. Living to make money, forsaking our heart's desire, just doesn't make sense to many of us anymore. However, we're so well-trained that even when we hear the internal call to live differently, few will find the courage to listen. It's much easier to ignore desires that require a commitment to living a life of meaning.

Steven Foster and Meredith Little describe this process as "decision road" in their book, *Roaring of the Sacred River: The Wilderness Quest for Vision and Self-Healing.*

> "Every person who elects to participate consciously places his feet on decision road, the way that leads ultimately to the purpose circle of death.... Most people would simply prefer not to think about decision road, or their inevitable deaths. Better to hide the absolute certainty of it with illusions of present safety, comfort, and convenience. Better to put the feet anywhere but on decision road. Hence, they are captured unaware by all the symbolic deaths the living of their life brings. At every transition they must sacrifice something of themselves. Giving up a part of themselves while at all costs avoiding decision road invariably turns them into victims, problems, liabilities, imbalances in the social order."

I had grown up as an anthropologist's daughter, sometimes having the concept of "rite of passage" shoved down my throat. Even so, I chose to become a wilderness quest guide, helping people enact self-generated rite of passage ceremonies. (So much for rebellion!) I decided the last thing *I* was going to do was to shove the fine art of ceremony down my children's throats. Nevertheless, Marley became the prince of ceremony as he traveled down decision road, picking up hitchhikers along the way.

"Hitch your wagon to a star."

—Ralph Waldo Emerson

THE PARTY'S OVER

Fateful words

Rhys and I went to an annual party designed to celebrate the host's birthday. The kids were with Drew, so letting go and partying up in the mountains seemed like a great plan. I needed to have some fun, and missing one of Joska's birthday parties was sacrilege.

As soon as we arrived, we located Joska's booming voice coming from the four-foot long grill. I bounded up to him to give him a big hug, and when he saw me his party mood softened immediately. He laid down his spatula, turned squarely toward me and said, "I am so sorry to hear about your son." I was confused. Joska knew Marley had cancer…what was he saying? I said, "What? Marley's still alive…." He sighed in relief and said he had heard Marley had recently died. I said "Not yet, dude, all is well!"

Little did I know that at that very minute, back on the ranch, Marley had "broken" his hip a second time. Rhys and I got back to my house very late, and it wasn't until the next morning that I picked up multiple messages on both my home phone and my cell phone. At that point, I realized I needed to stay available and within phone range at all times.

As it was, there was nothing I could have done anyway. I called Drew and told him I was on my way. When I got to their ranch, I went upstairs and found Marley lying in bed. With him was Laura, Vanessa, Catie, Luke, and Lucas. The lava lamps were glowing and the music was blaring. I held my head and asked if someone could turn down the decibels—I had a hum-dinger of a hangover. Lucas explained what had happened.

> "Marley was helping me paint my dirt bike. He spent the night at my house, and at 10 in the morning we took the muffler off the Mule and we drove up the road, we were only going about 15, but it sounded like a Harley…it was badass! Anyway, he was coming home from my house, driving the Mule and he just bent over to spit. He said a huge shock went through his body, and it was the most pain he had ever felt."

I went downstairs and talked with Drew and Cindy about whether to take him to the emergency room. I said his symptoms were exactly like the first time his hip "popped," causing excruciating pain. We decided not to cause him more pain by moving him and to wait it out, hoping that it would pop back on its own like it did the last time. It was two days until he could get up out of bed. That was the last time he attempted to walk without his crutches or a wheelchair, even in the house.

That Saturday was a turning point for Marley. New pain relating to the lymph zone in his groin worried him. He said it was like a band of pain around where his leg attached to his body. He complained that his hip kept "popping" at times unannounced (not caused by any specific action). His intake of pain meds doubled from the last time he was with me, and his need for them continued to increase. By the time he and Catie came back to my house, he was asking for painkillers every four hours, like clockwork. He said they weren't working. His oncologist prescribed Neurontin, which helped.

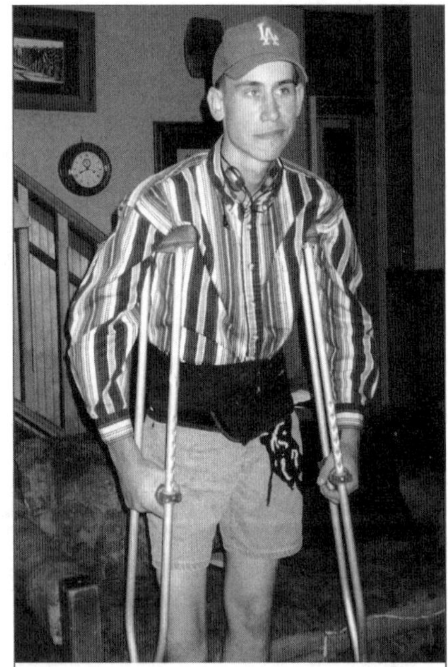

Marley at Drew and Cindy's (June 16th)
Photo: Cindy Warzyn

It was all happening so fast. Joska's words rang repeatedly in my head. I didn't tell anyone but Rhys what Joska had said. I was afraid to admit that my little world was now out of control. There was an invisible knot growing in my solar plexus as I realized that Joska's premature condolence was practice for what people would soon be saying to me.

Thursday, June 19, 2003
Subject: "ROLLER COASTER RACING"

Howdy Gang, (Hold on to your hats!)

Let it be known that I write letters to you every few weeks but no longer seem to have what it takes to get them in digital form. Until now, I've compared my life to a merry-go-round that is spinning way too fast, but now it feels like I've graduated to a roller-coaster! Big life changes have occurred since the last round of radiation in March. Marley was incredibly active in April and May, living life to the fullest and full of outrageous stories. After one has reached for the stars and touched them there seems to be nowhere to go but down.

The Ups…
For some reason, Marley seems to be taking some unusually high risks. Three weeks ago, he rolled his ATV down a steep hill and miraculously survived without a scratch. Unfortunately, the ATV didn't fare as well, and much to Marley's dismay, it is now in the shop for repairs. He gets it back tomorrow—which should help to get Marley back on the trails of life again. (He lovingly calls his quad his "little painkilla.")

Just after that event, Marley got kicked in the head by a calf during a cattle roundup in the Colestin. Other than a sore jaw, Marley reported that he's been thinking more clearly and can now remember people's names better. Strange kid. Maybe "calf kicking" is a new remedy for neurological malfunctions—let's all try it! I'm sure the way my brain feels, I could use a good swift calf kick to the head.

Catie ends the school year with a 4.0 GPA—that makes two years running on the honor roll! (I'm not proud.) She's also been spending her time loving soccer and track. I never thought the day would come when I would be called a "soccer mom" and have it mean something positive. Catie's totally cool and she's so much fun to be with. I drag poor Marley to all of Catie's soccer matches, propping him comfortably in reclining lawn chairs. Although it's often a painful process, he likes watching his little sister kick ass.

...And the Downs

Last week while at Drew's, dear Marley "broke" his hip again. He was laid up for a few days, unable to move without experiencing intense pain. We knew from the last time there wasn't anything to do but control the pain and wait for the bones to separate. BUT, just after the hip righted itself, he started to throw up violently for no apparent reason, causing excruciating pain. The pain meds wouldn't stay down long enough to be effective, and he ended up getting dangerously dehydrated. This landed him in the hospital, as an outpatient, for an infusion of liquids and some tests.

The test results were not good. Marley has been diagnosed with *hypercalcemia* (too much calcium in his blood). Too much calcium is toxic and can be fatal. Apparently this condition is due to two things: As his bones disintegrate, the waste matter is filtered through his blood stream, overloading his system with too much calcium. At the same time, his body has been trying to regenerate the bones the cancer has destroyed, thus his body is producing extra amounts of calcium.

The hypercalcemia now requires constant monitoring and probably regular infusions to flush his system. Throwing up is the symptom we need to watch for. Our world was rocked as we read the statistics of increased mortality rates when malignant tumors and hypercalcemia join forces. The stakes are definitely much higher now.

He's now taking Neurontin and Oxycontin on a regular basis. Oxycontin is a time-released morphine to help combat the constant pain level while using Vicodin and Percocets for extra relief. He's questioning what his life is going to look like without ever riding ATVs or walking again. He confided, "the box just got a little too small, Ma."

How Low Can You Go?
Marley and Catie's Uncle Steven died last month. Looks like Steven won the race on "decision road." We just made the journey to the desert (Owens Valley, California) for the weekend memorial celebration in honor of Steven's life. It was a long, hard trip but it was full of heart.

We're all still swirling in an altered state, having to adapt to the new rules. We have to live without having Steven in the flesh, and we have to live with Marley facing a fierce reality shift. How much can one family withstand? We're meeting with Hospice case workers this afternoon—maybe they can help us transition to accepting death as a possibility.

Marley is off with his beloved Brianna today. Brianna is four years older than Mars and has been a cross between neighbor, sister, and best friend to Marley since he was less than a year old. With the new diagnosis, Bree has dropped her regularly scheduled life to move to the Colestin Valley to add "nanny" to her list of roles. Marley's as happy as a clam deep under the sea because he adores being with "his Bree."

I'm having a terrible time concentrating on work, so I thought I'd take a few minutes during lunch to fill you in. Thanks so much for being out there in cyberville—just knowing you're there to write to, gives me strength. You have become my lifeline. I need to get back to work. Know that we love you and will keep you posted.

I love you,
Jennifer

"The doctors gave me six months to live and I gave 'em three and a half years of living!"

—Marley Jacob Pratt, age 18

Thursday, June 19, 2003
Guestbook entry from Thom

Yo Marley, Little Thom here.

I'm in Denver!! And I'm writing in your Guestbook for the first time. Just went through your website (again) and I've got the sniffles and everything. Dang it! I miss you buddy. Sorry you got laid up and think that your "box just got smaller." It doesn't look or feel smaller to me, my friend. It seems bigger and bigger all the time and still is not big enough to hold all the love and care that I feel for you and from you and from all these good people. Knowing you, I won't be surprised if you have some more rolls on that four-wheeler coming in the future.

I'm hanging out here with my sister Nancy. As you know, she also has cancer, and is doing the routine; get up, drive forty miles to radiation, drive home, take a nap, take the chemo pills, sleep, and get up—just to do it all again the next day.

You know, I can't help thinking about you an awful lot while I'm here. You've been a big help to me as far as being with my sister. Marley, you've helped me know what to say, know what to ask, and know—to a degree—what to expect. Thanks for that, and for smiling smiling smiling through this like you do. You have a very special place in my mind. (That all goes for you too, Jennifer darling.) I'll be home soon, I hope you can meet my sister someday. I'll try and get her to Oregon.

See you in July, love love love and what the heck, some more love to you.

Your friend,
Thom

The Butterfly Effect

THE LAST WILD RIDE

by Lucas Morgan

The day that Marley came to my house on his Arctic Cat wasn't too good of a day for it. The first thing we did was to ride up on my property. Marley tried to do a pretty challenging hill climb and rolled over backwards. He stopped when the front wheels came off the ground. All I heard was, "Fuck!" I turned to see the ATV crash down on top of Marley. It was lucky for him that he didn't die and only slightly bent the handlebars. Later, we decided to do the 40-mile run through the woods to the Hilt store. We came upon a new trail and wanted to go on it. I followed Marley up the trail, leaving the road far down below. There was a sweeping part of the trail—a steep hill with rolling bumps.

Marley stopped and I said, "Go ahead, Marley, you can go across it."

He said, "I dunno Lucas, that's a pwetty steep hiw." He had Luke's little brother Sean riding with him…an inexperienced counterweight on the back of his ATV.

My quad was small and low to the ground while his was tall and top-heavy. "Ah bullshit, you can make it!" I said.

So he continued forward. He hit the first bump and then the second. That's when the tires came off the ground on the uphill side. I heard him scream, "Jump, Sean!" Marley stayed on until Sean had jumped clear but by then it was too late for Marley to bail. And once again, the quad rolled on top of Marley. Except this time, it rolled down the hill about three times and the bars smacked the ditch! I jump off my quad thinking, "This is bad…." Just then Marley leapt to his feet to make sure Sean was okay. I was amazed no one had died! The cushion of the seat protected Marley until the last roll when the frame hit his leg, leaving only a bruise. The ATV wasn't so lucky. The steering stem was bent so bad that Marley couldn't steer it any more. So I went for help. Six miles down the road, I found the first sign of civilization. A truck passed and I asked for help. We loaded up the quad and went back to my house. That was our last wild ride.

WAKE UP CALL

"Life should not be a journey to the grave with the intention of arriving safely in an attractive and well preserved body, but rather to skid in sideways, champagne in one hand, strawberries in the other, body thoroughly used up, totally worn out and screaming, "WOO HOO—What a Ride!"

—Author Unknown

Milk...Does a Body Good?

When communicating with Marley's Network, I shared only a brief, unemotional synopsis of the report: "Hypercalcemia can be fatal." The details were learned while Drew, Cindy, and I sat by Marley's side during the infusion. We were reading a five-page printout about hypercalcemia by Dr. Robin Hemphill. I was slowly plowing through it when Cindy came over and silently pointed to one paragraph, and then looked me in the eye. I'll never forget that look. She was scared. Before I even read the information, I knew we were in trouble. It read:

> "Mortality: Prognosis of hypercalcemia associated with malignancy is poor; the one-year survival rate is 10–30%. In one study, 50% of patients died within one month of beginning treatment; 75% died within three months."

Excuse me? After reading this, Drew sat with his head bowed in the darkened room. I couldn't see his face, but his body looked as if someone had drained his life source. It was the only time during this whole affair that words weren't needed. And it was the only time, since the very beginning, that we didn't share the details we had read with Marley or anyone else. Was Marley going to be one of those statistics? If so, which one? How long did the boy have before he joined his Uncle Steven?

Fostering Love

The annual Foster clan gathering was right on time, except it was missing the reason for these summer reunions...Steven. For his memorial, people came from all over the globe to honor the gifts Steven had given to so many throughout his life. Marley was not in the best shape to be traveling, but we just *had* to help send Steven off. Marley, Catie, and I drove down in the Suburban while Drew and Cindy drove down separately.

My sister Julia, her husband Joseph, and their oldest son Winston flew in from North Carolina for Steven's final ceremony. Winston was three years older than Marley, and it was wonderful witnessing the bond between them. One afternoon, Winston, Meredith, Marley, and I talked about what we wanted our memorials to look like. Winston described that he wanted to be buried in a stone tomb decorated on the inside with graffiti. Marley thought that was very cool, but he wanted to be cremated. When Meredith asked him, "What do you want done with your ashes?" I was shocked when, without hesitation, he answered, "I want 'em put in a giant firawurk and shot high, high up in the sky. I have a fwend who'll do it too!" We all nodded in agreement, thinking, "Wow! That's a really cool idea!"

"Genius is an African who dreams up snow."

—Vladimir Nabokov

On the final evening, dancing and feasting was planned in honor of Steven's playful side. Several bands entertained us, torches were lit, and everyone looked beautiful. It felt so good to dance and laugh after a sobering trip down memory lane. We all cut loose. Marley was having fun on the dance floor in his wheelchair as the rest of us danced around him. During a slow dance, Drew picked Mars up and held him like he was holding his little boy. Marley wrapped his long legs around Drew's waist and leaned his head against Drew's. It was such a heartfelt moment that Cindy and I stopped dancing, burst out in tears, and held each other. Constant and Julia had the same reaction.

The following day, Meredith gave Steven's belongings to family and friends; she gave Marley the portable recliner that Steven had used the last year while escorting groups into the desert wilderness. Marley was honored to inherit Steven's "field throne."

PREPARING FOR THE END

Hospice Meets Marley

During Steven's memorial weekend, when Steven's Hospice doctor found out Marley had developed hypercalcemia, we had to promise him we would call Hospice as soon as we returned home. Making sure Marley's final days were *not* spent in a hospital was a no-brainer. Nevertheless, contacting Hospice was an incredibly hard decision for Drew, Cindy, and me. Just the process of calling them felt like an admission that our efforts to help Marley survive the odds had failed. This was unfortunately the reality. Ugggh.

Hospice serves adults and children during the end of their lives, when a cure is no longer possible. In other words, when the focus is no longer on prolonging the patient's life, but instead on the quality of life, Hospice will supply their expert "pre-fatal" care. Hospice provides superior medical, nursing, emotional, and spiritual care right in your own home. The coordinated team of professionals includes several nurses, a home health aid, a bereavement counselor, a spiritual counselor, and a social worker.

It was Thursday, June 19th—a bright, perfect day at the very beginning of summer vacation. People were roller-blading by as we sat on the fresh cut, lush grass in the park located across the street from the BRI office. Cindy, Laura, and Vanessa had joined Marley, Catie, and me to await the arrival of Dahna, the Hospice coordinator.

While we waited, to break the nervous tension, we played. Laura was practicing driving Marley's super-duper, high-powered electric wheelchair, with Catie on her lap. They spun around in circles and tried to follow the lines on the basketball court at top speed. Marley and I stopped wrestling to enjoy their show. Because they were laughing so hard and Catie was blocking her view, Laura was driving like a crazed woman.

As we rolled around, clutching our sides, laughing at their negotiation skills, a woman was parking her car in front of the office. She looked somewhat official as she got out of the car with her clipboard. Cindy assumed it was Dahna and called the girls over. Laura aimed directly for us. Cindy waved Dahna over as Vanessa brushed grass off our backs. Marley and I kept a close eye on the girls' too-fast approach, and were just about to roll to safety as Laura skidded to a stop, dumping Catie on the grass.

Surely this wasn't the scene Dahna was expecting. It looked so healthy, probably not like other appointments with cancer patients on the brink of meeting Death. She plopped down on the grass next to us, obviously approving of the attitude and the chance to sit on thick spongy grass, surrounded by laughter and sunshine. It turned out that she lived in the mountains, "just around the corner" from my property and had seen Marley whizzing by on the ATV as he headed into the woods. She was tan, healthy, ready for action, and down to earth. We all liked her immediately.

"When love and skill work together, expect a masterpiece."

—John Ruskin

After listening to why we had decided to call for Hospice's help, Dahna spoke with both knowledge and heart about what we were facing. She was in charge of coordinating whatever Hospice had to offer Marley. She told us a nurse would be arriving shortly to do an in-depth evaluation of Marley's current health status. Dahna explained that, after this initial evaluation, Marley would be assigned a team of three nurses who worked our backwoods territory.

Then she handed us an Advance Directive booklet and a DNR (Do Not Resuscitate) form. While Cindy and I glanced at the questions Marley was to answer, we must have groaned, because Dahna launched into imaginary scenarios of what could happen if these directives were not filled out.

Because she had seen Marley riding his ATV, she accurately painted a grim picture of what could happen if Marley wiped out and badly gashed his arm. If an ambulance were called to transport him to a hospital and critical complications arose due to, let's say, massive blood loss or his remaining lung deflating, the rescue team would do *everything* within their power to resuscitate him. She asked, "Do you want that?" We all numbly stared at her with our mouths hanging open.

She painted another picture of Marley being at home, close to death, and having a well-meaning but panicky relative call an ambulance to "do" something. Without this form, signed by Marley, they would do *everything* within their power, including taking him to the hospital, even if he were fully conscious and said, "No." We slowly understood that situations beyond our control could happen that might land Marley in exactly the wrong place, at the wrong time. Emergency doctors could cause more damage by not knowing the situation.

Marley didn't read, so I spent the next few days reading the questions and explaining them. The first question was, by far, the hardest, "Who do you appoint as your health care representative?" You cannot appoint your doctor or any of your doctor's employees. They suggest that you avoid people so close they may not be able to honor your directives due to their own emotions. Marley didn't view this as a difficult decision. He chose me as his representative and Cindy as backup, in case anything happened to me. He felt like a traitor for not choosing Drew but justified it by saying, "He's just too emotional sometimes."

Eat Your Heart Out

We were sitting in a Mexican restaurant, waiting for Marley's favorite beef sandwich, as I made my grand speech interpreting the two biggest questions he had to initial.

"As your representative, you're saying that I can decide whether 'life support' and 'tube feeding' should be given. Life support means using all the ways doctors have of keeping you alive, including surgery, machines, and medication. If you say you don't want life support, that means they won't try to save you, but they will keep you 'clean and comfortable,' including giving you any pain meds you need. The other kind of life support you need to decide about is if food and water should be 'supplied artificially.' If you can't eat on your own, they want to know if you want to be fed through a tube to stay alive. This tube is either inserted in your arm through an IV, down your throat, or into a hole in your belly that goes directly to your stomach."

Marley's face screwed up as if the room was instantly filled with rotten eggs. "Simple," he said, "No way! Not if I'm gonna die anyway. Besides, that's what *you* get to decide!" I knew I was losing his attention, but with determined perseverance I plowed through a few more of the questions so I could get a sense of what he really thought. "I mean, like duh, as your representative, I'm supposed to know what you want, right?" He moaned and laid his head on the table in frustrated surrender.

Basically, the remaining part of the form asked the same questions for four different scenarios. The three possible answers were: A) Yes, I want tube feeding / other life support…, B) No, I don't want…, or C) Only if my doctor recommends it….

1) If you are *Close to Death* and life support would only postpone the moment of your death,

2) If you are *Permanently Unconscious* and it is very unlikely that you will ever be conscious again,

3) If you have an *Advanced Progressive Illness* that will be fatal and is in an advanced stage, and you are unable to communicate, swallow food and water safely, and care for yourself, or…

4) *Extraordinary Suffering*. If life support would not help your medical condition and would make you suffer permanent and severe pain.

These are heavy questions for any of us to answer, but Marley, dear Marley, said, "Geez, Ma, didn' I jus' say you could make all the decisions fo me? Aren't all these questions jus' askin' the same thing? I'm jus' gonna say, 'No, I don' want 'em to keep me alive if I'm supposed to die.' If I do that, can we be done with this? When's my food gonna come?" I swallowed hard and put an "X" by all of the "No life support" answers. He initialed them, rubbed his hands together, closed the booklet, and slid it to the side. End of discussion. His beef-stuffed Mexican sandwich was delivered, and all was right with the world.

THE BEGINNING OF THE END

Break Through to the Other Side

The day after Hospice did their initial evaluation, Marley started feeling new pains in his chest. He kept saying, "Feels like someone's sittin on me." This was a little awkward, because no one knew if Marley was under the care of Hospice or the old system. Our oncologist said she didn't care who called the shots as long as Marley was cared for, so she ordered a blood test to make sure the calcium levels were still under "control." They were not high enough to warrant another infusion, so we went home to wait.

By the next morning, Hospice announced we were now officially under their care and gave us a list of contact numbers. Marley's pain level was increasing rapidly. By Sunday night, I had to try out the new system. It was about 10:30 at night and Catie was asleep. Marley was in too much pain to relax and had come to rest in my bed. The Oxycontin was taking the edge off the constant pain, but the Vicodin and the Percocet just weren't doing the trick for numbing the pain fast enough. Waiting twenty minutes for the Percocet to kick in just wasn't cutting it.

I called Hospice and was instantly connected to one of the three nurses on our team. She was already familiar with Marley's case. She was absolutely wonderful and behaved as if she really loved her work. She asked lots of questions and listened carefully to my answers. She asked about everyone's emotional status and what Marley's pain level was. She said it sounded like we needed to get some liquid morphine to take orally for faster "breakthrough" pain.

She said she would normally drive to the hospital to pick up the order and would deliver it directly to us, but I had called on the one night that the other two nurses were doing house calls, and she had to stay available by phone. There was no cell phone reception where I live so she couldn't deliver the drug; but she could go to the hospital to pick up the morphine if someone could meet her once she returned to Ashland. I couldn't leave the kids, but many in Marley's Network had continually offered their service, and now was the time to call on them. I scored on the first call—Rhys was more than willing to do the deal.

I felt very alone. It was one of those times the silence of the night was deafening. The Percocet had carried Marley off in a fitful slumber. Finally Rhys pulled down the driveway around midnight. I realized, with a sigh of relief, I had barely been breathing since the phone call. I can't tell you how nice it was to have another body close by. Rhys slept on the couch that night just in case Marley woke up and we needed more help. I slid snake-like under the covers next to Marley and listened to him breathe, knowing I was armed with a liquid fix if breakthrough relief was needed to get him to the other side of pain.

Stormy Monday

The morning came and Marley was not a happy camper. It was getting hard for him to breathe. I took him in for an X-ray. He had three views taken at the hospital in Ashland before they diagnosed the problem. The good news was that it wasn't pneumonia, but the bad news was fluids were collecting in the mediastinum, filling the cavity around his lung and heart.

We'd been here before, way back in the very beginning. I had images of foot-long syringes darting through my brain. I wanted to run away and hide, but there wasn't enough time. We were meeting Drew and Cindy for an appointment in Dreadford later that day to get two more X-rays before the *thoracentesis* (the method of extracting fluids from the thoracic region around the lungs).

The kids were with me at the office. Catie had been talking to Laura and Vanessa on the phone. They said they wanted to come to the hospital with us. Cindy's brother Steve was visiting from Wisconsin, and he and his best buddy Chet were also meeting us at the hospital. It had become a full-blown family production, and Marley loved it.

As we all piled in the Suburban that afternoon, Jay, Jeff, Julia, and Gordon all came out of the office to wave good-bye and wish us well. I had no clue what was going to happen or if I'd be back—and they knew it.

WATER WORLD

Feeling Drained

We all met in radiology for a few more X-rays, and then we were directed downstairs for the thoracentesis. We were in the bowels of the hospital, on the basement floor. We had gotten to know that hospital pretty well over the past three and a half years, but this territory was new for us. It was creepy walking down halls that all looked alike (I seriously feared getting lost). They were painted with a high-gloss grey coating that reflected the stark florescent lights that occasionally flickered. Because we were in the basement, there were no windows anywhere. There was no sense of time, and it was cold in more ways than one. It felt like we were probably next door to where they kept the recently dead in giant refrigerators.

The girls didn't want to watch the doctors stick a long needle in Marley's back that would poke all the way into the thoracic cavity. So the three of them went to see if they could find their way back upstairs for some ice cream, while we watched a doctor and his assistant draw out the thick liquid causing the pressure in his chest. I sat in front of Marley so he would have something comforting to focus on while they filled up three quart jars with what looked like frothy beer. At that point, some very funny jokes were told which considerably lightened our moods during that awful procedure.

After an hour of being in the cold dungeon, we had forgotten that it was a beautiful, hot summer day outside in the "real" world. We were all relieved that the puppies hadn't died from the heat as we gathered around the cars in the hospital parking lot to figure out what the next step would be. I had to return Laura and Vanessa to their dad's and go back to the office, because Marley said he wanted his electric wheelchair to be moved to my house. After that, we decided to meet up at my place to have some real beer and some good food.

This day was reminiscent of the first hours of the first day on Leap Day 2000. It felt too close to full circle for comfort. Marley was worn down; we were all tired from the various tests and the procedure. No one said anything about how defeating this felt. We had done what was possible, relieved the pressure in Marley's chest, but we all had a sense it was a temporary fix. No one yet had the guts to say that out loud.

Homeward Bound

Once we arrived at the BRI office, there was a sickly sweet taste in my mouth, but I didn't have time to think about it. Marley was tired and I had to get him home, but first we had the task of loading the wheelchair into our trailer. Doing manly-man kinds of things always perked Marley up. The gang came out of the office to find out how it went. I think they could tangibly feel our drained energy field. Just the fact that Marley had decided to transport the wheelchair to my house told them he might not be coming into town anymore.

Jay helped Marley and me load the wheelchair. We laughed, but nothing felt funny. CJ, one of Cindy's best friends, drove by and asked how things went. We said that everything came out okay and that we were going to gather at my house. She said she'd bring a salad (which was great, because preparing food was my last priority). Then Sherry, another of Cindy's great friends, stopped by on her way from the hardware store; same conversation. She said she would pick up some food, then swing by and pick up Bridget, the wonderful woman who taught the girls how to ride horses. Jay and Jeff said they wanted to come up too. Marley started to slowly melt like a beautiful candle left in direct sunlight. It was time to get him home.

Once home, Marley had a few minutes to rest before everyone started to arrive. Marley loved parties, and his energy level rose as he drove around on his Arctic Cat telling people where to park and giving them rides down to the house. He was amazing. His leg felt like it was falling off, his chest was drained just hours before, and yet he was out there welcoming people on his beloved quad. It was always difficult for all of us to realize the gravity of the situation when Marley would insist upon rising above the pain. I mean, we were all gathering around a young man that was seriously ill, yet he was gleefully transporting containers of lasagna.

A Swiftly Tilting Planet

He soon notified us that he couldn't sit atop his ATV anymore and needed a hand. Steve and Chet supported him as he hopped to our summer living room—a grassy area next to my house under the drooping oaks. There we had a carpet laid down in front of a futon, lots of giant cushions, several folding camp chairs, and Marley's place of honor—the portable green recliner he had inherited from his Uncle Steven.

The lasagna was put in the oven; CJ's big salad arrived. Drew brought a case of beer, Rhys brought the ice chest, and Jeff brought his guitar. I brought out the photo albums and everyone gathered around the couch to look at pictures of Marley's life. It was an informal gathering of heartfelt proportions.

It was an amazing, spontaneous mix of people that gravitated toward Marley that night. It had been over six years since I'd had the chance to hang out with Cindy's family and friends. It felt strangely like I was home with my family again. Two worlds were coming together around Marley. This is just what he always wanted to happen, and he felt very proud of himself. He was the reason for all of us to remember how much we loved each other.

> ***"Family isn't about whose blood you have. It's about who you care about."***
>
> **—Trey Parker and Matt Stone, *South Park***

Sweet Sirens

As happy as he was, twilight had fallen and Marley began to drift away. It was time to get him to bed and get everyone fed. We set him up in my bed all tucked in with his painkillers. We all joined him in the bedroom. People filled their plates of food and sat on and around the bed in chairs and on the floor, telling stories of various Marley adventures. The star of the show went into an otherworldly state, and Jeff started playing his classical guitar as a background to continued conversation.

Marley's eyes were closed, but every once in a while, he'd smile at a story or lift one of his long fingers to let us know he was listening. Yet it seemed he was not altogether with us anymore. The way his face looked a trifle hollow and the way his arms were folded across his chest felt different. Marley was ascending. Marley was dying and we all knew it. He had just crossed that invisible threshold.

My way of not falling completely apart was to play hostess, making sure everyone had what they needed before they needed it. I was in a super state of hyper-awareness. It felt like I needed to do earthly things in order to not be swept away with my son. For most of the evening, Drew sat in the chair positioned by Marley's head like a papa dog guarding his sick pup. As the night was coming to an close, Drew made way to let others sit close and gently lay their hands on Marley's quiet form before they left.

Slowly, most everyone started to depart, quietly kissing the sleeping boy. Catie, who had been curled up next to Marley, said she needed to go to sleep, so I took her upstairs to her loft. One side of her loft overlooked my bedroom and the other overlooked the living room. Divided by only one rail on both sides, the loft was illuminated by scores of candles burning steadily below us.

As I put Catie's hair into braids, we could hear Annie start to sing "Swing Low, Sweet Chariot," accompanied by Jeff's guitar and several other voices. As my fingers slid through Catie's silky hair, my feelings started bubbling to the surface. Annie's voice was clear and strong as she sang "Amazing Grace." I cried silently as I finished braiding my little girl's hair. I knew Annie would soon be singing that for us at Marley's memorial.

"Who has seen the wind? Neither you nor I;
But when the trees bow down their heads,
The wind is passing by."

—Christina Rossetti

WORDS UNSAID

A Mom's Farewell

Marley was leaving me, and I wouldn't be able to follow him for very much longer. He was approaching the final threshold. After everyone but Jay left, it dawned on me that it was a good time to consciously honor Marley's journey Home. I knew there was nothing to fear—I just had to find ways of letting my son go.

I prepared to write a severance letter to Marley, as he slept peacefully in my big bed. But first, I sat quietly next to him, watching him slowly breathe, looking at every line in his face. The candles flickered and I remembered everything—the way he so fully expressed himself before he was able to talk, teaching me communication skills far beyond words. I could almost feel the way he hugged me, sometimes pulling me forcibly into a pocket of his soul when I thought I had better things to do. Sometimes gently inviting me to be hugged. With his long arms outstretched, puppy-dog eyes, and big pouty lips he'd say, "Mama, commere—ya need a hug."

I sat on the bed, filling myself to the brim with all the memories of our past as tears made tracks down my cheeks. He loved me like no other and I was losing him. Yet, I was thankful, really thankful he was thoughtful enough to give me just a little more time. Time to sit next to him and breathe him in. I wondered if he really knew how much I loved him. Had I really been the best mom I could be? Did he really know that I loved him beyond measure and that I felt as though we had spent lifetimes together? Could he see beyond my tough loving mother act? Was he aware that every time I pushed him to go further than he wanted, I really wanted to say, "Oh my darling little one, forget growing up, just come sit in my lap and let me smother your sweet face with kisses as I rock you back and forth." I never admitted how much I wanted to keep him from being touched by the world, how many times I bit my lip with mind-bending restraint as I sent him off to school.

I knew he knew everything there was to know about me. He

knew me better than I knew myself. As I watched his ancient face, I knew he was being swept away, beyond my ability to comprehend, and yet I still had to pretend he was my son. But sitting next to him, late that night, no one could hear my thoughts or feel the immensity of my feelings for this being from another world. No one except for maybe Marley.

"Toto, I've a feeling we're not in Kansas anymore."

—Dorothy (Judy Garland),
The Wizard of Oz (1939)

He was leaving me. I had been left before. My dad left me when I was sixteen, after giving me a speech about using my best judgement at all times. My mom left me when I was twenty-two after giving me a copy of *The Secret Teachings of All Ages*. My nephew Sean left me without warning. I had been left by my dog Sage, my best friend, who was simply old. Now Marley was leaving me with no words—he didn't have to say anything. I knew.

So I looked at his hands and remembered the story behind every scar—the times he fell off his bikes, the circular saw accident, the porch nail when his sister pushed him off the deck, the barbed wire, the rocks, the knives, and the scores of other scars that just were. The wrinkles that he inherited from me, signs of an age beyond years, the mark that he was mine. With an artist's eye, I studied every line and hair follicle like I used to when he was a newborn. I was in awe that he existed. I thanked my lucky stars and slid out of bed.

The Last Letter

I had spent the last three years writing to Marley's Network, but I hadn't written anything directly to him for a very long time. It was time to add to the book of letters I had started just before he was born. It dawned on me: He would never receive this book as his 21st birthday present as I had planned 18 years ago. For this I cried. He already had one foot in the other world, and I knew he wasn't coming back. I knew I needed to say good-bye and do my best to clear the canvas for whatever lay ahead. There was no use giving him the book now—it was too late—he no longer cared about such things. I knew he knew and loved me all the same. It was the last letter that I wrote to him. It was the last piece of paper I would ever place in the three-ring binder. When I was done, I cried again as I snapped the metal rings shut. I placed the book back on the shelf, dried my eyes, and slid into bed next to my pain-filled boy like a timid cat not wanting my master to stir.

Monday, June 23, 2003

IN THE END

Is there anything left unsaid?
Have I relayed how proud of you I am?
Have I honored enough, your courage or your persistence?
Have I told you how handsome and strong you are?

Is there anything I've left unsaid?
Have I told you how grateful I am that you chose me?
Or how I love when you fling
your enormously long arms around me?
Have I mentioned how safe you make me feel?
Or how thankful I am that you challenge me—
the one that challenges all else? Bravo!

Is there anything I've left undone?
Yup. Plenty. Oh well.

Have I ever thanked you for being so forgiving of who I am?
Have I ever apologized for all I am not?
I know you love me still and
this is what I am most thankful for.

—Mom

Chapter Sixteen:
No Place Like Home

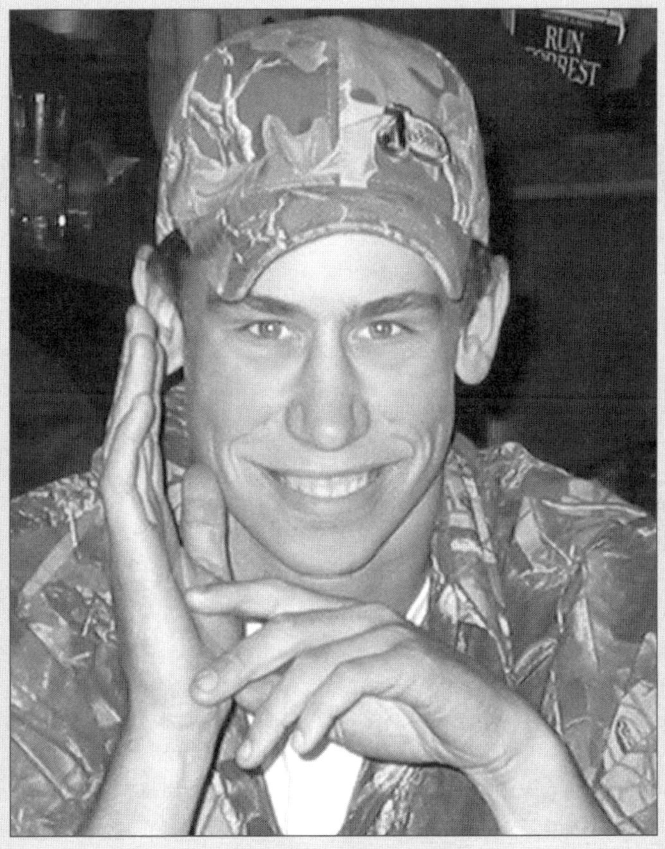

The Marley Man

Photo: Mandy Little

THE FINAL SWITCH

Shifting Sands

Switch days were generally always on Fridays, but we decided to move Marley over to Drew and Cindy's ranch four days ahead of schedule—we were going to need electricity. When Jay heard that we had changed the plans for switch day, he announced that he was going to spend the night. Marley and Jay had always acted like brothers—Marley lived to bug the crap out of Jay, and Jay loved dishing it right back. But that evening, my heart melted as I witnessed how tender Jay was being with Mars. The instant that Drew left Marley's side, Jay slid right into the chair to hold Marley's hand until everyone else left.

I don't remember falling asleep, but the pillow was still damp when the daylight nudged me to awareness. Marley was an early riser and was already awake beside me. He nuzzled his big face into my hair and said in the sweetest voice, "Good morning, Ma Ma." Neither one of us wanted to start this day, so we stayed as quiet as possible.

We heard Catie climbing down the ladder from the loft, and I started to scoot over. She slid into bed next to me without saying a word. Our peace was shattered when all three of us thought our bladders were going to burst—the day was official. Jay groaned from his bed on the couch.

I made tea and breakfast so Marley could take some Vicodin in preparation for the car ride to the Colestin. Marley had positioned himself close to Jay on the reclining couch. Each time I walked into the living room, their heads were touching as they quietly talked about the future. I think it was the first time I had seen them sit together without poking each other or joking and laughing. It was really sweet. Something had definitely changed.

Cindy arrived and we stood in the driveway and talked for a few minutes. She and Drew suggested I should spend the night at their place. I jumped at the offer. I was really happy to feel Cindy's warmth, not just as a friend, but as a co-mother.

"God could not be everywhere and therefore he made mothers."

—Jewish Proverb

This transition was much easier knowing I could stay close to Marley and Catie. And I was surprised at how comforting it was to know Marley was going to have three parents to look after his needs.

It took the four of us to get Marley safely inside Cindy's truck. My heart melted as Marley gave us a feeble smile and a sad little wave. Jay promised to visit him the next day. I kissed him and assured him that Catie and I would be by his side again in just a few hours. As the truck drove away, the three of us stood in the driveway feeling empty and alone.

The Payoff

After packing the car with items I thought would make Marley more comfortable, and throwing some clothes into a bag, Catie, Jay, and I drove into town. I dropped Jay off at the office and told everybody I didn't know what my future looked like or when I would be back. I was thankful I had spent months preparing my assistant, Julia, to fly solo—even though it might have been a surprise, it wasn't a shock. I knew this day would come, and I was glad I had worked so hard accumulating sick days and vacation time. All of my attention was now aimed directly at Marley's comfort and my entire family's well-being.

Catie and I picked up Laura and Vanessa at their dad's and did some last-minute shopping for their yearly vacation at Cindy's parents' home in Wisconsin. None of us knew what to make of the new circumstances and how it was going to affect their travel plans, but we figured they should be prepared anyway. Then we headed for the Colestin—we were in the home stretch.

"When crossing over fences, carry water with you and tend the grass wherever you may be."

—Robert Fulghum

THE GIRLS GROW UP

Assuming the Position

The first day we had moved to Drew and Cindy's, Marley made himself comfortable in his new room (the master bedroom on the first floor). My cot had been set up against the wall near the foot of his bed, and a TV had been brought in. His lava lamps and CD player were under the two full-length windows to the left of the double bed, and a few folding chairs had been brought in for visitors to sit on. They were already occupied by some of the Colestin volunteer firefighters.

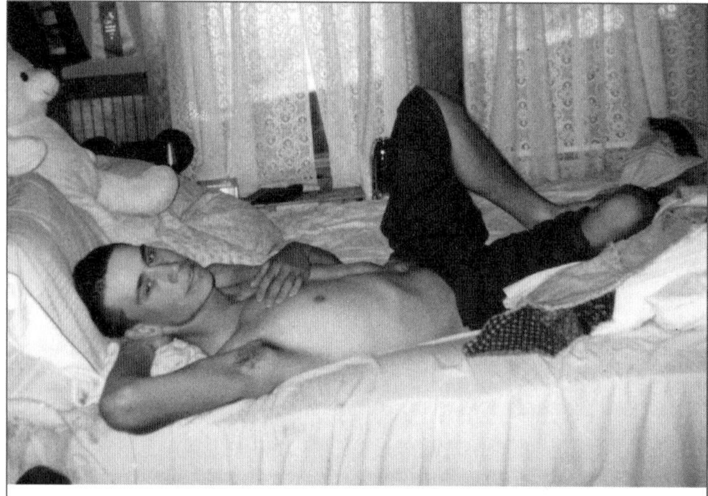

Marley taking it easy between visitors

Marley hadn't eaten in two days and had absolutely no desire to expend his limited energy even thinking about food. As twilight approached, his breathing became more labored and shallow. A combination of fatigue and pain made Cindy and me consult with Hospice by phone. They carefully listened to all of our clues and had us do an inventory of all medications, since the stashes from both houses had been combined. They said that the following morning a nurse and a spiritual advisor were going to come out to tend to our needs. They would also bring with them more morphine and an oxygen tank. They planned to talk to us about what we could expect as Marley entered "the final stages."

Cindy and I knew we had to get organized. We agreed to act as a nursing team, keeping not only a detailed log of times, drugs, and amounts given, but to tell each other what we did and when. We made a schedule of when different drugs would be given, a way of measuring how much he was drinking, and brought out the urinal that had been used after his surgeries.

Our brains had become mushy from the shock of how fast things were happening, and we instinctively knew we had to rely on each other to avoid critical errors. Drew and Steve took up a post at the long table between the kitchen and living room. Many neighbors had delivered food, but none of us had much of an appetite. Cindy knew enough about shock that she demanded we all eat protein-rich foods, whether we wanted to or not.

Decisions, Decisions

After dinner, some tough decisions had to be made. The girls were scheduled to leave for Wisconsin in a few days. All three of them were upstairs in Laura and Catie's bedroom, weighing the pros and cons of staying home. When Cindy and I walked in to help them, the tension was visible. Catie was on her neatly-made bed, while Laura was sitting on the floor amongst piles of her clothing, CDs, shoes, and books. Vanessa was sitting in neutral territory next to the closet with her arms folded across her chest.

Cindy sat on the floor near the door, and I sat on the edge of Catie's bed. Catie started to cry as she explained her feelings about traveling to Wisconsin. She was too scared to leave. For her there was no choice; she did not want to leave Marley. Laura, it seemed, was working her way into a major case of denial, not wanting to focus on the fact that Marley might not live until they were scheduled to return four weeks later. She wanted to continue on with the trip as planned. Vanessa was undecided.

Cindy and I shared everything that we knew. We told them that given the new circumstances, it did not look like Marley would be able to survive until their return. We gave them the option of going to Wisconsin for a week instead of a month, and explained if they chose not to go at all, their tickets could still be used at a later time. We also explained if they did go for a week, there still was no guarantee that Marley would live until their return, because it seemed that the fluid around his lungs was already starting to form again.

Cindy's friend CJ walked into the room. She could feel the gravity of the situation; she quietly slid into position on the floor next to Vanessa. CJ was a good friend to all—one of the family. She had an easy-going air. Maybe it was having her sit so close to Vanessa that allowed the oldest of the three girls, a beautiful seventeen-year-old, to vulnerably break down. As she spoke through her tears, she decided she didn't want to leave. That left only Laura to make her choice.

It was so hard watching Laura stay in control, keeping her emotions completely in check. As she verbalized her thoughts, I remember CJ, Cindy, and me catching each other's glance, acknowledging that we might have a serious problem. If Laura continued to deny her feelings about Marley's impending death, we were liable to have an emotional implosion on our hands. This could be a disaster.

As Catie witnessed her sister's reaction, I could see even she was looking worried. But then Catie lost her cool and spat, "Laura, don't you have any feelings? Don't you get what's happening here? What's more important?" We knew we were in for trouble—the room fell beyond silent. Laura was picking mindlessly at a spot on the carpet. Then she quietly started to cry. We all sighed.

CJ innocently asked, "Have you all talked to Marley about this?" Cindy and I looked at each other, silently saying, "What a novel concept. Why didn't we think of that?" Everyone blew their noses and agreed to ask Marley what he had to say about the girls leaving. We all went downstairs to Marley's room. He was quietly lying with his arms folded across his chest with his favorite stuffed animal tucked under one arm. He woke up and listened to the overview of the debate and suggested he and the girls go out on the front porch.

It was a moonless summer night, and the country stars seemed to be closer than normal. Cindy and I helped him into one of the overstuffed chairs by the front door as the girls gathered near. CJ, Cindy, and I walked into the darkness just beyond the circle of light cast by the glow of the house. We wanted to be close, yet afford them their privacy.

Marley was sitting up straight, listening to each of them in turn. Cindy and I knew what strength that must have taken. At one point, Laura doubled over in tears and we watched Marley tenderly lay his hand on the back of her head. Ten minutes later, we saw him motion for them all to stand and come close in a circle. He held out his hands to the girls on either side of him and they all held hands. He spoke to each of them as a priest would to his flock. They had a four-way hug and headed back into the house.

Staying Home

Whatever he said, it defused the tension. Laura said he told her that he would still be there until she returned if she really wanted to go. She decided to stay. Cindy's mother, Pauline, was called. She in turn called the airlines and postponed the girls' tickets for thirty days and made reservations for herself and her husband Dick to fly to Oregon the next day. Everyone was satisfied, though emotionally drained.

The girls crawled onto Marley's bed with him. With only the hall light and the lava lamps illuminating his room, they quietly shared their world. CJ, Cindy, Drew, Steve, and I broke out the giant bottle of tequila that the folks at the Hilt store had brought down as a gift. We toasted the wisdom and the love of our four children.

"Life's a voyage that's homeward bound."

—Herman Melville

UNCLE JAY'S ALERT

A New Dialog

The following morning, I knew it was time to rally the troops for the final battle. Although Drew and Cindy had a computer, I just didn't have the time or the energy to draft an e-mail Update to Marley's Network. So I called Marley's Uncle Jay and asked him to send out an e-mail via the ListServe, letting people know it was time to say good-bye to the Marley Man.

Most of the future communication was done through Marley's website with messages being posted on the Guestbook. The dynamics of our network's communication were changing. I was no longer feeding the network information; instead, members of the network began to inform and feed each other.

Wednesday, June 25, 2003
Subject: "TIME FOR GOOD-BYES"

• From: Uncle Jay

Hello to all in Marley's Network,

This is Jay, Marley's uncle, writing to you on Wednesday night. I just talked with Jennifer, and it seems like forces are really stacking up against Marley in an even more pronounced way. She said, "It is the time to connect with Marley."

Jennifer suggests the best way to do this would be to visit his website's on-line Guestbook and write to him. Write your fondest Marley story, a creative reminiscence, or a simple greeting in any form. We will all be able to read your stories there.

We all know that our bright star Marley makes his own rules and follows a unique path. No predictions, just love.

Lots of Love,
Jay

DECISION ROAD

Quantity VS Quality...One Last Time

By midmorning, the tension was increasing rapidly. Everyone was on edge as we waited for the Hospice visitors. Drew was not okay. He was quiet and withdrawn as he went out to "feed the animals." They had already been fed—it was his way of escaping. Cindy and I walked toward the barn. The three of us *had* to talk. I can only imagine what it felt like for Drew to see his current wife and the mother of his children walk toward him side by side. It must have been scary as hell, especially when he knew what the conversation would be.

As we approached, Drew bowed his head and, with his hands in his pockets, started kicking at a clump of grass. We stood facing each other in a triangle.

Drew asked, "So what do we do now? Do we take him to the hospital to get the fluid taken out again?"

I figured Cindy would have a better time responding than I. It was going to be harder for him to attack her out of frustration. She simply said, "Drew, I don't think that's such a good idea."

He argued, "Then what exactly *are* we supposed to do…just let him drown?" It was a hopeless question.

I said, "My main concern is if we take him in to get another thorocentesis—which will probably buy him another couple of days—something will go wrong and they won't let us leave. My fear is he'll end up dying in the hospital."

Cindy chimed in, "I'm worried that just the car ride may kill him. Is it worth putting him through the torture of the drive and the procedure for the temporary benefits?"

Drew bit back, "I'm his dad, I'm supposed to *do* anything and everything I can to keep him alive as long as possible."

My heart melted into a pool of internal tears as I calmly said, "Drew, we can't take the risk of hurting him more just so we can say we *did* everything that we could. It's just not fair to him to keep him alive longer for our sake."

He looked to the ground. Cindy and I shut up to let him

process that one. It was a delicate balance between husband and wife and mother and father. He knew the battle was over. The tears stung his eyes. He pressed his thumb and his middle finger to both eyes to staunch the flow. Then he gave up and he let the tears roll.

Through a gulp of air he helplessly admitted, "I don't want my son to die." Both Cindy and I burst into tears and nodded. There was absolutely nothing we could do to stop Marley from leaving us and we knew it.

The Right to Life

A calm washed over me as I knew I would not ever be faced with having to make the decision to "pull the plug" on my son. I could keep Marley safe at home and make sure no one interfered with his right to live his final days, without anyone sticking needles in him or inserting feeding tubes in his belly. I knew the three girls could be with him until the very end in the privacy and comfort of our own strengths and weaknesses.

Marley deserved not to live longer, but to live well and with dignity. He deserved to die on his own timetable, surrounded by everything that he so dearly loved. I had never loved Drew and Cindy more than on that morning. Together we made the most difficult decision there is to make, and we walked away knowing that we made it equally together.

That conversation was never mentioned again. The decision was made and there was no turning back. I know a little piece of Drew died then and there, right next to the barn. Maybe he felt like he had failed his duty as a father to keep his son safe but, then again, maybe he recognized the act of letting his son go was the bravest thing he'll probably ever do in his life.

"Great deeds are usually wrought at great risks."

—Herodotus (484 BC – 430 BC)

VISITORS

The Online Guestbook

The following day, many letters were posted on Marley's website in response to Uncle Jay's alert. The first entries were written by our best friend Jay, and by Marley's Uncle Jay. Whenever time permitted, we would jump on Drew and Cindy's computer to read the new entries. Sometimes we would read them aloud, laughing or crying together.

As the online visitors were increasing, so were the the phone calls. Relatives from far away wanted to visit using the only personal means available. As the news of Marley's impending death spread, visitors started driving all the way out to the Colestin to bring food, flowers, and to say farewell in person.

Thursday, June 26, 2003
Guestbook entry by Jay

This is Marley's friend Jay from Ashland. (Not his Uncle Jay.) I just wanted to say thanks to the Marley Man for being such a great friend and teacher. You've taught me how to live in the present, stay strong in the face of pain, and get in touch with my inner badass. We've had so many great adventures together! I especially enjoyed peeling out in my Nova in your neighbor's driveway. Or trying to hang on to the back of the Mule while you were racing it up and over the bunny hills. Or swinging on the rope you hadn't tied off! Too much fun. Anyway, I love you and Jennifer and Catie very much. Thank you all so much for letting me be a part of your life for the last five years. You will always be a huge part of who I am, and I'm the better for it.

-Jay-
Ashland, OR

Thursday, June 26, 2003
Guestbook entry by Uncle Jay, Mill Valley, CA

Early on, I met a guy who embodies all the qualities and characteristics that are necessary for becoming a world-class explorer or discoverer.

If he were born around 1000 B.C., he probably would have been a Phoenician trader. He would be flying on the wind with a cargo of Greek wine and olive oil bound for North Africa, taking uncharted short and long cuts as he ran from coastal pirates destined for profits in Egypt.

If he were born in 1000 A.D., he probably would be barking orders from the deck of a Viking longboat headed for Constantinople soon to be a leader of the Varagian Guard. "Pull those oars! Do I have to do it all myself?" His name? Something like Gunnbjorn Vmarleyson.

Born around 1450, his name would have been Vasco Da Marsa Bara. He would be finding better routes to South Africa, making large sweeps across the Atlantic and then, just for the heck of it, finding a way to India to start a new trade route.

If it were the 21st century, he would be a cowboy heading west somewhere near the Oregon trail on a horse or ATV, finding an ocean of friends, busting new trails, and leading others by strong example. His qualities of courage, compassion, enthusiasm, fearlessness to admit fear, boundless energy, inventiveness even under pressure, camaraderie, an unimaginable capacity to endure and keep going, faith that the journey always continues, wildness, a love for stories, a need to be outside, a good snort of soda, and a never-ending hunger for pushing through the outer limits. His name, of course, is Marley Pratt.

The Journal

While folks were visiting with Marley, the girls were busy creating a spot down by the river. It was a beautiful little hidden sanctuary, close to the barn, with a mowed path that opened up to a small, hidden meadow next to a gentle flow of clean water running over smooth river rocks. There were boulders to sit on at the water's edge and wild iris growing in the surrounding thicket.

The girls lined the entrance with stones and brought down a chair for older folk. They used a mound of earth as an altar for pictures, flowers, and other tokens of love. They asked CJ to purchase a beautiful journal and fancy pens to be left at the altar for family and visitors to write in. As family and new arrivals waited their turn to be with Marley, they too decorated the space with stonepiles of all sizes and other creative works of art. We all really enjoyed sneaking off alone for a few minutes to enjoy the evolution of the river spot and to read what others had written as we cooled our feet in the water.

Written by Marley's stepsister Vanessa

Marley, my love,

You are an amazing human being. You have shown me strength, courage, and love. Together we have accomplished so much. So many great experiences and treasured memories. You've taught so many people how to endure in hard times and really, fully appreciate life and all that it is.

REMEMBER: BE FREE!

Love, your ever so loving sister,
—Vanessa
(or better known as, "Yo Sis!")

ya baby ya!!!
Am and always will be.

Thursday, June 26, 2003
Subject: "NEWMAN REPORTS"

• A personal e-mail which included many in Marley's Network
From: Jay

Hi to Mom and Dad, the rest of my family, West coast family, new friends, and old friends.

My friend Marley Pratt is living out his last days. He may go this weekend or push on for a few more weeks—it all depends on how long he wants to stick around and fight. As some of you know, Marley (who's 18 now) has waged an epic battle against cancer for the last three and a half years. He's deteriorating fast and his quality of life is pretty low. It's been a rough two weeks. Up until then, he'd still been able to maintain a relatively fun and active life (except for the half dozen operations, chemo, radiation treatments, and living in constant pain). But now he's only in pain, he can't walk, and he can't even get on his four-wheeler to forget about it all. He can barely even talk. It's pretty sad, and he's really mad right now...but at the same time, he is so full of love and affection. He's always had a unique sense of clarity and purpose, but now that has intensified into feeling his emotions—whatever they are—to the fullest. I'm so honored to know him. He's such a great life teacher. Although he's on a lot of pain meds, he can still acknowledge me and flick me the bird when I call him "one-lung." (I joke that he'll be okay unless the doctors amputate his middle fingers—then he'll have no way to communicate.)

It has sort of become my unofficial job to transport friends to and from Ashland to Marley's dad's house in the Colestin Valley, about 45 minutes south of here. In addition, I'm notifying all of the Ashland friends and giving them the news. It's a tough job, but it helps me to deal with it by explaining it to others. Yesterday, I was talking to one of Marley's friends, who is developmentally disabled. He wasn't getting why they can't just fix Marley like they have in the past. In trying to explain it in the most simple way I could, I helped explain it to myself. There has been a war raging inside Marley for years. Sometimes the cancer wins a battle—and something has to be taken away or radiated by the doctors—and sometimes Marley wins a battle by defying the odds and finding some other part of himself to take up the slack. But the war has been going on for so long now that there isn't much left inside Marley to fight it. And the final battle seems to be under way.

I realize that I've been pretty sheltered from having to deal with death in my life, except for the sudden death of my high school friend and my three grandparents. I haven't lost anyone really close to me for more than ten years. And with Marley, I've been preparing for this time since I first heard the word "cancer" attributed to him. So at this point, I feel I'm ready. And I'm not sad. There's no reason to be sad while he's still alive. When he's gone, I'll grieve…hopefully in a healthy way…but I won't know until I get there.

So I just wanted to give you all a heads up. Mom, maybe you can send this to your prayer list(s) and ask for good thoughts to be sent to Marley, his mom Jennifer, and 13-year-old sister Catie, who's also been a trouper throughout this whole ordeal. As well as Marley's father Drew, stepmother Cindy, and stepsisters Laura and Vanessa. And cousin Selene, who recently lost her father and is on her way up here to be with Marley.

Other than this whole drama, I'm doing okay. But now I have to try and get some work done here at the office…which hasn't been easy. But hey, someone has got to bring the world better bathroom reading. You'd think I'd find it easier to focus without Marley here smacking the back of my head telling me he's bored. You'd think.

I love you all.
-Jay-

GRAND CENTRAL

Party-time

As the Hospice team arrived the morning after Marley returned to the Colestin Valley, a stream of cars came down the long driveway. There were eight of us staying there, with more family on the way. It's a good thing Drew and Cindy had a big yard and plenty of parking. It was also a good thing they had two refrigerators and a giant freezer in the carport, because food was arriving with each guest.

Wednesday, just after Uncle Jay's announcement letter went out, mainly just close friends visited. Everything was relatively calm. Marley was alert and talkative and enjoyed the company as he lounged on the double bed surrounded by those he loved. Drew was busy clearing a spot in the mud room, just down the hall from Marley's room, for the oxygen machine. We fed the tubing to Marley's bedside. Cindy and I did our best to make sure that while Mr. Social was entertained, he was comfortable and always had something to drink. We were most thankful that Cindy's parents Dick and Pauline were arriving later that night. Something told us we were going to need help.

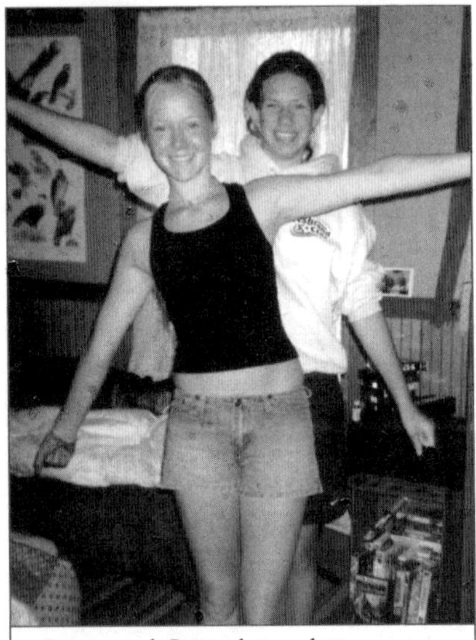

Laura and Catie doing their routine

By Thursday morning, the news had traveled, and the ranch became known as "Grand Central." The phone rang off the hook. Pauline took up position in the kitchen, making sure food was always on the table for us to nibble on as we rushed by. Dick took post in the living room to oversee the action and to keep everything calm. The girls rotated between being in Marley's room, jumping on the trampoline, or playing in the swimming pool. Amidst all this action, Cindy and I were doing our best to coordinate trips to the airport.

The Real World

That afternoon, Catie and I drove to the airport in Dreadford to pick up my sister Julia. I had no idea when I got behind the wheel of the Suburban that it was a dumb idea. I had been doing a brilliant job of keeping our little protected world together but, when I left the Colestin Valley and joined thousands of other people on the highway who had no clue that my son was dying, I felt completely lost. It was like I was experiencing a sensory overload, and I could barely pay attention to road signs and turn signals.

Everyone was minding their own business, worrying about paying the bills or upset at how slow the traffic was moving. I was shocked, remembering how completely shallow and petty we all can be. I wanted to scream, "Wake up, folks! Remember to pay attention to the people in your lives. Smell the roses while you have the chance!" Instead, Catie and I chose to talk about how beautiful everything was, how vibrant the colors were, and how glad we were that everyone was gathering around Marley.

I felt safe again only when I was pulling down Drew's long driveway and heard the dogs barking from their pens. We arrived to see about fifteen cars parked by the barn and scores of people standing in the yard and sitting on the front porch looking through the photo albums. I knew there was little time to relax after my harrowing adventure into the "real world." At least I was surrounded by loving and caring people who had dared to venture into the *real* real world. It was a world of truth, honoring a hero who was making his passage to another realm.

"There's no place like home."

—Dorothy (Judy Garland)
***The Wizard of Oz* (1939)**

BRIANNA

Marley's Best Girl

Marley was just seven months old when he met our neighbor Brianna. It was love at first sight when this little blond four-year-old girl wandered down our driveway. Even then, he knew what he liked. Brianna was his "golden girl." During her daily visits, I would take off her pretty little dress and put her in grubby clothes so she could play in the mud with "Mars Bar." It was a match made in heaven.

Brianna was in college. Her life was now full of traveling, school, and boyfriends, but she was never too far away, even though she had moved four hours north. At the beginning of the summer, she had announced that she was scrapping her current plans in order to help care for Marley. Catie and Marley were thrilled to have a playmate that could drive.

Brianna came down to the ranch every day—she wanted to be close. If she wasn't cuddled on the bed next to Marley, she was out on the front porch looking through the photo albums and talking with visitors.

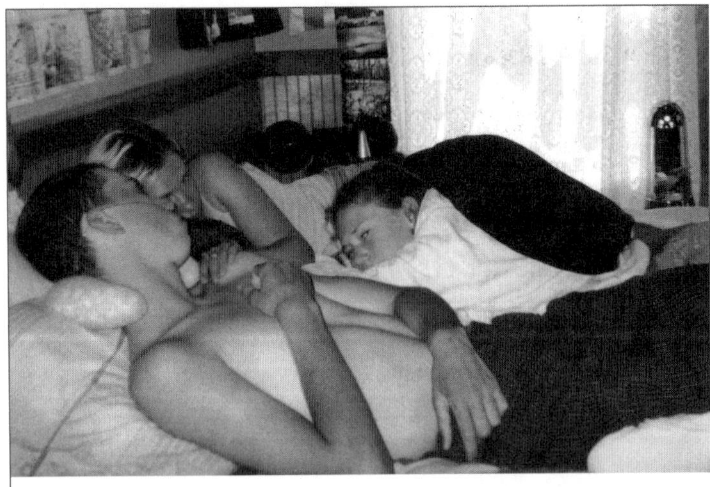

While Marley rested, Brianna and Catie stayed close

COYOTE'S CALL

The Lukes

Like Brianna, Luke and Lucas never asked for our permission to hang out down at the ranch; they were just there. They spent a lot of time lounging on the front porch with the girls. When Marley was resting, they would take off on their dirt bikes and scare up some trouble, making sure they left enormous plumes of road dust in their wake.

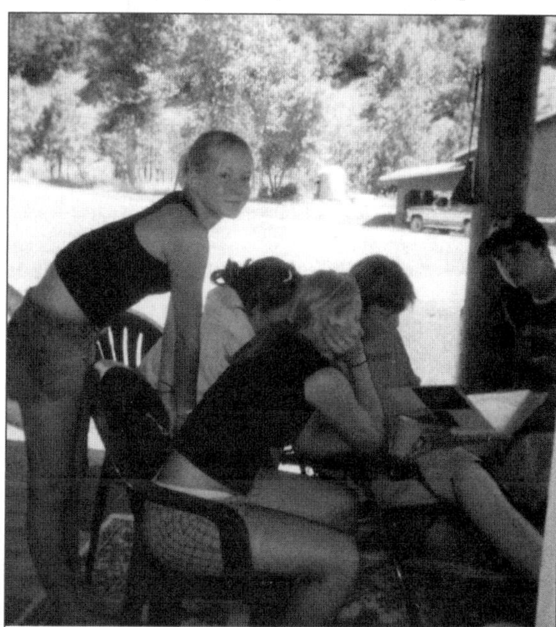

The kids on the porch looking through photo albums

Written by the Coyotes

Dear Marley

You have been the best friend anyone could ask for. The Coyotes will go on no matter where you go (because you will always be there in our hearts).

We love you bud,
Luke and Lucas

HONORING THE FIGHTER

Above and Beyond

On Thursday evening, the Colestin Valley Volunteer Fire Department Chief, his crew, and a representative from Fire District Five came to honor Marley. Thirty of us stood by as two state vehicles came down the long drive. They were dressed in their formal uniforms as they entered Marley's room. Visitors squeezed into the room with them, and the rest of us went outside and watched through the open windows. Cameras were clicking away as Marley was presented with a certificate from the College of the Siskiyous. He had passed his First Responder Medical Training and received two college credits for enduring the grueling course required in order to become an official firefighter.

The Fire Chief proudly presented Marley his firefighter's badge, officially marking his graduation from junior volunteer firefighter to the big league. He was also given an honorary plaque which read:

> "The Colestin Rural Fire District Firefighter of the Year Award 2003 Presented to Marley Pratt for Dedication Above and Beyond the Call of Duty."

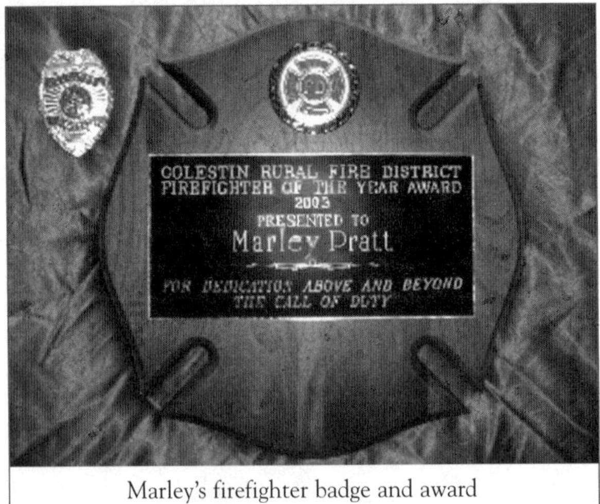

Marley's firefighter badge and award

AXEY'S GOOD-BYE

Like Peas and Carrots

After an action-packed day, it turned out to be a horrible night. Marley's pain dramatically increased and breathing was difficult. We started him on the oxygen, which helped, but he was slipping further away from us as the new day began. We all groaned when the first car came down the driveway, but we all nodded in approval when Axey and his mother Agathia walked towards the house.

Axey and Marley met when they were ten years old. Marley didn't talk very well, and Axey couldn't see at all—he was blind. Marley took the role of guiding and protecting Axey whenever they were together. They bonded like wood and glue and communicated like they knew each other from lifetimes past. Throughout the years, Axey trusted Marley to lead him at school, to go bike riding on dirt roads, horseback riding in the woods, and jumping off cliffs into the lake. It was pretty phenomenal. They always remained friends, treating each other with a sweetness most young men are terrified to show each other.

Marley's love of hugging and holding hands was key to their relationship. It simply didn't occur to Marley that loving others like this wasn't cool. With Axey, the ability to touch was required. Axey had no trouble with how weird Marley was or the way he talked. They were quite a pair.

The Blind Can See

I ushered mother and son into Marley's room. Axey sat next to the bed at Marley's right elbow, Agathia sat at the foot of the bed, and I was on the other side of Marley. Agathia was trying to keep the mood upbeat and positive. I knew it was time to talk straight to Axey. I started by describing everything—painting a picture of Marley's position, the equipment, the lava lamps, etc.. Marley was not responsive—all of his energy seemed to be focused on taking very shallow breaths. Axey could hear his rapid breath and wanted to touch his friend. Agathia got nervous, not wanting Axey to hurt Marley, but to her relief, I encouraged it. Axey gently let me guide his hands to Marley's chest. Together we explored the oxygen tubes in his nostrils. He curiously explored Marley's face and his thin shoulders and arms. He found Marley's long-fingered hand and just held it while he asked scores of questions. The last one was the toughest. "Will he get better?" I had to respond with, "No, Axey, I think this is the last time you'll 'see' Marley. You have had a really good time together but now, it's time to say good-bye." The tears were welling in my eyes as I looked at Agathia. Streams of tears were running down her face as she tried desperately to accept what I had just said.

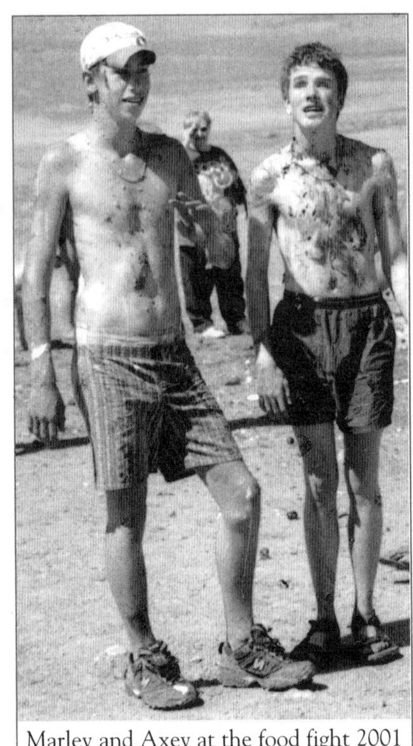

Marley and Axey at the food fight 2001

Axey seemed to know exactly what was happening and took it in stride. He said his good-byes to his dear friend lying peacefully before him. He thanked Marley for never judging him and always loving him and then he turned to me and asked if he could give Marley a kiss. I said, "Of course" and helped to guide his face to Marley's. Just as Axey bent close, Marley's long right arm rose and flopped across Axey's back. Then the left arm slowly lifted and joined the other arm. Without opening his eyes, Marley quietly said, "I love you, bud." Then his arms slid back to their place, crossed over his belly. Agathia and I cried. We knew we were privileged to witness perhaps the sweetest farewell between two dear friends possible.

BENNY BOY

The Long Good-bye

Ben and Marley had been dear friends for most of their lives, but after Marley was diagnosed with cancer, he had drifted away from spending time with Ben. Marley needed to go fast and ride hard, and that was not Ben's strong suit. The Coyotes better satisfied Marley's need for speed.

Ben visited me at the office regularly to see how Marley was. He always wanted connection, and never feared to show his love and concern for Marley. As with Marley, Ben wasn't like other boys their age. Ben had some health problems that weren't easy to identify. I'm not sure if Ben ever really understood what was happening to Marley. Sometimes I thought he did and then he'd ask, "So when's Marley going to get better?" When Mars first got sick, Ben was hospitalized for having seizures. Over the years, Ben's confusion increased as his ailment was managed with medication, while Marley just got sicker and sicker.

Three Peas in a Pod

Ben, Axey, and Marley were great friends, even though they were very different with very different issues. (It seemed that this wasn't the first lifetime spent together.) Although it was unplanned, on the final day of receiving visitors, Ben and his father Kevin arrived right after Axey and his mother Agathia. I knew we must be close to saying good-bye to Marley.

Ben and Kevin waited on the front porch while Axey said good-bye to Marley. Afterward, Ben and Kevin sat beside Marley. They told some very funny stories of times spent together over the years. When Ben told the one about Marley crashing into a tree in Ben's go-kart, we all laughed. I knew when I saw a corner of Marley's mouth curl that he could hear us even though he was floating somewhere between the worlds.

When Ben said good-bye, I wasn't sure if he knew that it was the last time. But I'm sure someday they will meet again.

REALITY CHECK

Calling a Spade a Spade

After Ben and Kevin left the ranch, Drew and I knew we had to take a few minutes alone with Marley. He had begun to stir, needing more pain medication and to be readjusted in bed. We stood by our son to let him know what this new day would look like. We had to make sure Marley knew what was happening.

We started by asking Marley if he knew why all these people had been visiting him over the last four days. He shrugged his shoulders. Our response was, "They're coming to say good-bye." It was like some energy field started crackling around the three of us. "Marley, this is the last time you're probably going to be seeing these people. They love you very much, and this is difficult for everyone. Do your best to help them let go."

I just *had* to make sure Marley understood what we were saying and I didn't know how to put it gently. I leaned forward and asked, "Honey, do you realize that you're dying?"

He looked up, his eyes opened wide and he focused on Drew with shocked, puppy dog eyes and whined, "But I don't want to die." Drew's shoulders visibly sagged with the pain. Actually voicing those words somehow violated the possibility that Marley would make a miracle comeback—even though we all rationally knew this just wasn't in the cards anymore.

"The real hero is always a hero by mistake; he dreams of being an honest coward like everybody else."

—Umberto Eco, *Travels in Hyperreality*

We huddled close and told him everything was going to be okay. "Soon you won't have to feel any more pain. You get to go Home and visit with Uncle Steven. You also get to meet your grandparents, Marley. They'll all be right there waiting for you. All you have to do is relax."

A new light washed over his face. I could hear him thinking. "All right, maybe this isn't so bad after all." My sister Julia came in to tell us Lucas' mother was here to visit with Mars. We asked him if he was okay with having more company, and he nodded.

Elizabeth, the mother of Marley's best friend and co-Coyote, had arrived with her two other children, Andrea and Mark. Andrea had been training to be a volunteer firefighter along with Lucas, Marley, Catie, and Luke. She was a competent, quiet, loving, and reserved teenager. Mark was doing his best to comprehend what was happening. He was the little brother that was usually left in the dust while the Coyotes powered up their engines and rode off into the sunset. Mark loved Marley, who probably paid him more attention than his older brother Lucas did. Mark always seemed to express awe and respect when he was around Marley.

Elizabeth walked up the front porch smiling and holding her arms open. I hugged her tight, drinking in her experience with grief. Her husband Rex had died in a car accident just a few years earlier. She had survived by putting one foot in front of the other and smiling through her tears. Even though she denied much of her pain, she was always available emotionally—she had done a damned good job of keeping her heart open while raising three exceptional children. As we hugged, she melted and the floodgate of her pain let loose.

No Woman, No Cry

When she pulled away from my arms, she smeared her tears from side to side, cursing, "Damn it! I swore I wouldn't cry."

I could only say, "Be serious, Girl! Why?" I took her hand and Drew and Cindy led the way to a quiet, shady spot at the side of the house. We all talked. She cried. Sometimes there's no stopping the flood. We just have to let it flow until there's no more. When it was time, she gathered up Mark and Andrea and I led them into Marley's room.

With Andrea at Marley's right, Mark on his left, and Elizabeth and me standing at the foot of his bed, Marley was remarkably alert and ready for them. Elizabeth put on her best sunshiney face and greeted Marley with her twinkling, swollen red eyes. After everything we had just discussed outside, she still said, "Don't worry, Marley, you'll be up and riding around in no time." My mouth dropped open and I had no idea how to deal with this contradiction. Before I could close my mouth, Marley saved the day.

It was as if he had spent weeks, not minutes, rehearsing his final speech to these three very important people in his life. "No, Elizabeth, I'm dying, but it's all right. I love you. You gotta take care of Lucas and these two for me (he nodded toward the two children at either side of him)." At this point, rivers of tears were streaming down the faces of the four of us. Marley was perfectly calm and sure of himself. He turned to Andrea and spoke directly to her, then turned to Mark and did the same. He told them how good they were and he told them exactly what to do. It was stunning to watch my son who had, just minutes before, learned he was dying, turn into the wise guru. He deeply touched the souls of those struggling to let him go. I was in awe.

While Marley was attending to her children, Elizabeth changed her position as fast as Marley had. She acknowledged his courage and reminded him that her late husband would be right there to help Marley as soon as he crossed over.

She said, "Oh Marley, I'm so glad you finally get to meet Rex. You two will get along so well. You'll be just fine."

I think Marley had had enough of emotional talk, so he said, "Did you all see the award I got last night?" They nodded, replacing their tears with genuine smiles and laughter as Marley joked about being the only Coyote to receive that award. After the smiling subsided, everyone hugged him one last time and walked out the door laughing. My whole soul was filled with an intense pride. I was proud that I *might* have had something to do with how great that young man was. I aspire to be just like him when it's my turn to be on my deathbed.

"The real voyage of discovery consists
not in seeking new landscapes,
but in having new eyes."

—Marcel Proust

SELENE BEANIE

Broken Hearts

Selene had been such an instrumental player in Marley's life. She had been called to be close for the first two years of Marley's illness—a gift I will forever be thankful for—but the real world had swept her away. Ashland is a small town, and she needed to spread her wings. I'm sure it was also really hard for her to watch Marley slowly deteriorate, especially in light of the fact that her father was on the same road. When she had chosen to move to Oakland to go to art school, I knew she was taking care of herself. I greatly respected the courage it took for her to call her limit.

It was hard not having her there at the end to share this remarkable experience, but she was already dancing on the razor's edge. Steven's recent death was incredibly painful for her. She was still raw from grief's grip and didn't think she had the strength to witness yet another of her beloveds die. Nevertheless, Selene drove six hours to visit Marley on his deathbed. Seeing Marley broke her heart, and she just couldn't bear to stay any longer than a few hours, so she turned around and drove back to the Bay Area that same day. As difficult as it was, I'm really glad she completed with Marley before he left, and was held by those who love her.

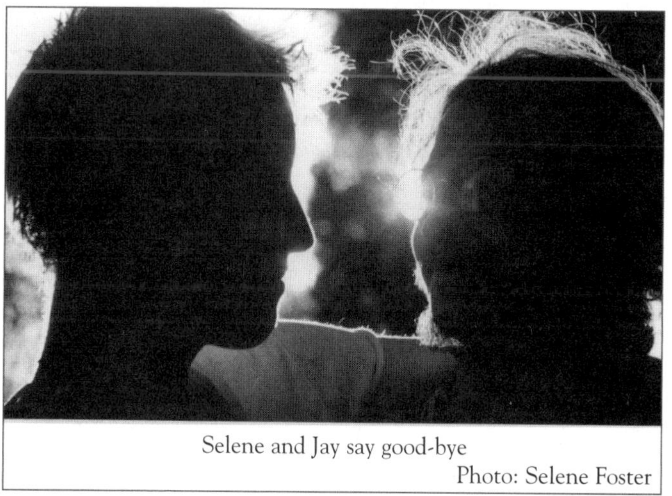

Selene and Jay say good-bye

Photo: Selene Foster

Friday, June 27, 2003
Written by Cousin Selene

Marley, Mars Bar, friend, brother, crazy-ass,

There will be very few things I do in my life without your voice in my ear telling me not to be a pansy, telling me nothing that is safe is worth doing, that I am capable of more than I think I am.

I will miss you madly, desperately, always.

I don't know that I will ever find another whose hugs I look forward to as much as I have yours. How many times have you enveloped me with your love? And I realize now, you are the only man in my life who I could sit next to and feel as though there is nowhere else in the world I would rather be. I can only hope there were a few moments you felt as comforted by my presence as I have felt by yours.

Thank you for giving me purpose in my life, Marley—for reminding me on a daily basis that we are here to be alive, to play, and to take care of each other. Now you will be taken care of by all the creatures of this earth. And I will look forward to seeing you again. My death will be easier knowing you will be there. It's more than everything, all of it, forever.

May the force be with you,
Selene
(A.K.A. "Blondie")

"When your parent dies you have lost your past. When your child dies you have lost your future."

—Dr. Elliot Luby

HOME ALONE

Shutting the Gates

The love surrounding Marley was beyond belief, but the sheer number of people that came to deliver that love was overwhelming. All of us ended up in the position of playing host to a never-ending party. Marley was exhausted by the time the last car left a trail of dust down the valley. He was trying to leave us, and the life force that came with those who loved him was keeping him here, attached to life. It was an incredibly difficult decision, but we had to create a protected, quiet space so he could leave us in peace.

"Life is pleasant. Death is peaceful. It's the transition that's troublesome."

—Isaac Asimov

We had a family meeting on Friday night. We shared stories of the day's events and even though we were all amazed by the sweet interactions, we concluded that Marley wasn't getting the amount of care that he needed. Some of the issues were practical, like not having enough toilet paper or having to guard the oxygen tubing from being stepped on or pinched by the door. Too many people meant more work and more stress.

We decided to close and lock the gates. We had to discuss what this really meant. We knew Marley's teachers, Tim, Pat, Kate, Katie, and Jim were scheduled to arrive on Saturday morning. These were some of the most important people to Marley's life since he was seven years old but.... Jay, Brianna, Luke, Lucas, Andrea, Sherry, and CJ wanted to be close to Marley until the moment of his death but.... We had to draw a line. It had to be clean—all or nothing—or we were going to start arguing amongst ourselves as to who was more important to Marley's life. After much discussion we agreed: family only, with one exception; the Nortons.

The Nortons were in Hawaii when they were called about Marley's condition. They had to change their flight plans and were to arrive the next night. They were Colestin neighbors and were considered non-kin family. Even I had to consider the impact not saying good-bye to Marley would have on their two little girls, Hannah and Nakita. The Nortons were Drew and Cindy's closest support, and they would have given the world for us. As it was, they had supplied the housing for all of the relatives that had already arrived.

Biting the Tube that Feeds You

Friday night was a stressful night. The intensity of the day was too much for Marley, and his pain levels rose to an all-time high. We increased the pain medication and hoped he would get some well deserved sleep. But Marley was agitated all night. The oxygen tubing was bothering his nostrils and the tops of his ears. We had cut the nose pieces short and filed them smooth. We had added padding and adjusted the tubing to alleviate the rubbing on his ears. But nothing satisfied him.

I slept with one eye open all night, making sure he was as comfortable as humanly possible. Every time he pulled off the oxygen, I would quietly wait for him to drift off and I would slip it back on again. At one point, I heard an odd chewing sound. I thought there was a mouse in the floorboards, until I heard Marley spit and something hard hit the wood floor and slid a few feet. I crawled on the floor, finding that he'd spat out the nose piece to the oxygen tube. *That* was a very effective way to thwart my efforts to help him breathe easier.

"Shit!" I thought, "Now what am I supposed to do?" His breathing became labored almost immediately. I held the single strand of tubing just under his nose while I tried to clear my head to think straight. Drew and Cindy were asleep upstairs. They would never hear me unless I screamed. I held my breath, dropped the tube, and ran into the kitchen where the medical supplies were. I dug around, found another nose piece, skidded around the corner to hook it up, and put it back on Marley's face. Being without the oxygen for a few minutes made him a little more willing to accept my solution.

Saturday Cartoons

The next morning was quiet and peaceful. The girls had made a really beautiful sign to post on the gate that explained why we had locked it. Phone calls were made to those we knew were planning to visit. Our sense of relief was so strong that we knew we had made the right decision. We finally had time to process the last few days.

The girls spent the morning lying in bed with Marley. They watched home videos and action movies. Marley slipped in and out of consciousness and seemed very satisfied to have Catie and Laura endlessly practice their impromptu dance routines in his room. When one of us would kick them out so we could have our turn to quietly be with him, they would scuttle off to the swimming pool to practice their water ballet routine. I loved the way the two youngest dealt with watching their brother die. They would have their times of riding waves of tearful grief, and then a few minutes later they were laughing and playing. It all seemed so natural.

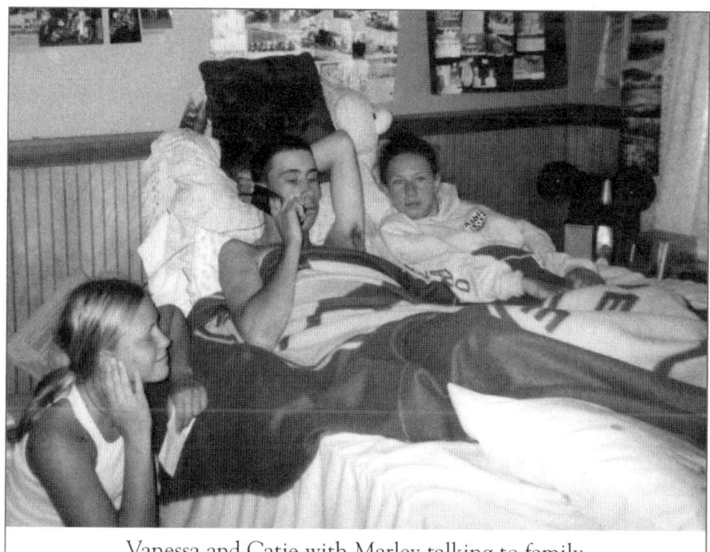

Vanessa and Catie with Marley talking to family

I spent a lot of time talking on the phone to my siblings. It was comforting to know they were all there, at least in spirit. I'll never forget when my brother Ric called from Minnesota to verbally hug me and to tell me "he knew." He knew how it felt to watch a child die—he had done it exactly eighteen years earlier with his son Sean. We both cried. We cried for ourselves and we cried for each other. I don't think I had ever felt so understood as during that phone call.

Throughout the day, we had to survive the pangs of guilt as people would arrive at the gate, stop to read the sign, leave whatever they brought next to the fence post, and depart. Midday, Cindy walked into Marley's room to find Brianna snuggled close to Marley's side. Brianna had decided to take matters into her own hands and had jumped the fence behind the house and snuck into Marley's room. We let her have a few minutes more and she left, satisfied with her final farewell. Luke and Lucas tore down the road on their ATVs and spun donuts in front of the gate sending giant plumes of dust high in the air that slowly drifted over the hay fields. They later told us that they figured the sound of the engines would help Marley feel better. They were probably right.

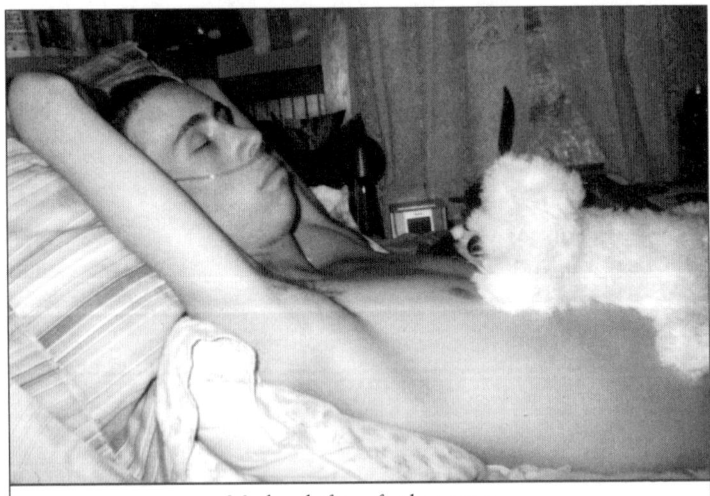

Marley drifting further away

Saturday, June 28, 2003
Subject: "A BRIEF HELLO AND GOOD-BYE"

Dear Marley Fans,

I wanted to touch bases briefly to let you know Marley is leaving us with honors. I cannot spend the time to write, but will as soon as I am able.

On Wednesday, Marley was moved from my home to Drew and Cindy's. He was born at home and he will die at home. The time has been sweet. Tuesday through Friday, a constant stream of folks came to say good-bye to Marley. Family members have had enough time to drive and fly to be close if they felt called to come. The support is unlimited. The love has flowed through all unconditionally.

As Marley has slipped further into the space between the worlds, we felt the need to have just family around. There were many who did not get a chance to physically complete with Marley, and for this we are sorry, but all of you are deeply felt. Know that he knows he is totally loved by you, and now he is being cared for with amazing skill and intuition.

As we were fluffing his pillows, trying to make him more comfortable today, he came briefly to consciousness for one of his "visits" with us. He looked me in the eye and said, "Mom? I'm bored. When can I go home?" With all the love in my heart, I replied, "Honey, you're on your way. All you have to do is relax and you'll find your way there. I can't come with you, but your Uncle Steven is there. Just think, you finally get to meet my parents. They'll be waiting for you too!" As he closed his eyes he said, "Oh, that's good."

Hug yourselves as you help release this most amazing human.

As always, with love,
Jennifer

SUNDAY, SUNDAY, SUNDAY!

Double Dosing

Cindy and I had become an amazing nursing team. No one administered the drugs except for the two of us. It had become increasingly difficult, because Marley was starting to refuse the liquid morphine and was unable (or unwilling) to swallow the little slow-acting morphine tab. By midmorning on Sunday, he was no longer drinking anything either. Cindy and I knew we might be in trouble with our patient.

Up until that point, we had been able to get Marley to let us squirt the liquid morphine in his mouth by having a lime popsicle ready to pop in his mouth afterward. But he started shaking his head no and pinching his lips together. Our biggest scare came when we were giving Marley an Oxycontin pill. The coating on this little pill allows the morphine to slowly release. We were warned not to cut the pills because it would give him a full dose very quickly. It had become a two-person job, trying to get the pill down his throat. That morning, we thought we were successful, until that little shit spit the damned pill across the room! We tried giving him another, and after nearly biting Cindy's finger off, he bit the pill in two. We panicked and tried desperately to swipe both halves out of his mouth.

We just stood there and looked at each other. We whispered, "Oh my God, did we just give him an overdose? Drew will never forgive us if we just killed him." We decided to remain calm and wait. In the meantime, we called Hospice for advice. They told us not to worry and said we could use morphine patches instead, and that they would order them for us. They reminded us that refusing food, then liquids, and even pain medications were all normal signs that the time may be very close. They also suggested it was time to be aware of other signs that death may be hours or minutes away, like half-opened or glazed eyes, restlessness or a surge of energy, a request for a favorite meal, and wetting or soiling the bed. Regardless, this was Marley's time, and we should follow his lead.

"There are two major events in life. Birth is one. Dying is the other."

—Stanley Keleman

Irrigation Day

All the ranchers in the Colestin shared water rights. They were all on a schedule, each having a different day to use the water to drench their fields. Sunday was Drew and Cindy's day so, no matter what was going on, work had to be done. I called Rhys to see if he would come help move the irrigation pipes and also bring the prescription of pain patches. He jumped at the invitation to cross the gate into our sacred territory.

The pipes ran the length of the hay fields and had to be moved at least twice so the width of the field could get sprayed with the giant sprinklers. With enough people, the task was almost fun. A team of two disconnected each twenty-foot section and moved it, forming a new straight line. It became a game to see which team could reconnect the pipes not only faster but accurately. The object was to avoid a hydrant-force spray once the water was turned back on. Julia and the grandparents stayed in the house with Marley, as the rest of the gang went into the field. I didn't feel comfortable being so far from Mars, so I decided to go weed Cindy's neglected garden. Just as the pipe movers were piling into the Mule to return, Julia yelled at me from the front porch.

The Last Supper

As I raced towards the house, I signaled to the Mule team to hurry home. When I rounded the corner to Marley's room, his grandmother Pauline was sitting next to him supporting him. When I tried to imagine what Marley might request for his last meal, I expected it to be something like his favorite Mexican meat sandwich or a big slab of juicy beef and potato wedges. I had no idea it was going to be a Mountain Dew. Yes, indeedy, Marley had sat up in bed, fully conscious for the first time in about thirty hours. Julia had found a Mountain Dew and was delivering it to him with a straw poking out the hole.

One of his giant hands wrapped around the can and he started sucking on the straw like he intended to drink the entire can in one gulp. I sat down on the other side of him and said, "Whoa now." He paid no attention to me. His sucking reminded me of the way he used to nurse...like there was no tomorrow! I tried to be sneaky and pinched the straw to extract it. Boy, what a dumb move that was! Never interfere with a dying person's final meal; even if you think it may kill them. Live and learn. He started to squeeze the can. Julia, Pauline, and I were gaping at him as he proceeded to crush the can like it was a sponge. After that, he seemed satisfied and lay back down.

Cindy had entered the room and was helping to straighten the sheets. I went to put his oxygen tube over his head and he started to put the tubing on like it was a T-shirt. The tubing was now looped around his chest. I had to convince Marley that we had to take the "invisible shirt" back off. It was pretty funny trying to "undress him" from the clear tubing without laughing too hard. Just when I got it in place, he reached up and pulled the tubing off and threw it on the floor. Once we stopped laughing, we decided to just let him relax before we tried again.

The Final Hours

We gathered around the table in the kitchen—none of us wanted to be far away. Just before dinner we put his first pain patch on, but Marley was restless. It didn't seem to be the pain that was agitating him. He just wanted to move. We took turns keeping a close watch on him. I loved my private times with him. I massaged his feet and legs and talked about how cool I thought heaven might be. He wasn't conscious but I knew he could hear me.

I kept saying things like, "Just remember to breathe and relax. Everything's just perfect. If you see a light, go towards it, and don't be afraid. There are people there waiting for you. It'll be okay. Just think how much fun you'll have when there's no more pain and nothing to stop you from doing anything. Catie will be fine. Drew and Cindy and the girls love you and want you to be free. I will make sure that everybody is taken care of. Don't worry about us. It won't be long until we get to be together again. Just breathe and relax, my boy. I love you."

The grandparents and Steve drove to their cottages half a mile away at 10 P.M. Just after their departure, Marley wanted to sit up in Steven's green folding recliner. While Drew and Rhys moved him to the chair, Cindy and I changed his sheets. In Boston, I had learned a great technique of putting a half folded top sheet on top of the fitted sheet. It meant that two people could easily shift Marley, it helped prevent bed sores, and it made for quick changes if any accidents occurred.

It was nice to see Marley semi-coherent. The girls came in and knelt beside Marley's chair to socialize. Rhys and Julia stood with their arms around each other by the open door, framed by the hall light. Marley seemed really peaceful, and yet at the same time he was anxious. He couldn't seem to get comfortable. We put him back in bed and left him to rest. I lay down next to him and was quiet, just listening to him breathe. The fluids had filled the space around his lungs so that quick shallow breathing was his only option. He stopped breathing for a few seconds and I heard a rush of fluids. I slipped my hand near his hip and realized he had just urinated.

I called for Cindy and said we needed to do a quick bed change. Drew came in with her to help. We had just changed the sheets and had a liner under the half sheet, so it didn't take much effort. We got him to the sitting position, and Drew lifted him to stand. Cindy slipped off his PJs while I changed the half sheet and the pad beneath it. All three of us had moved to flank Marley on all sides, preparing to sit him back down on the bed and dress him.

Marley's arms were slung around Drew's shoulders. Drew was nose to nose with Marley and in the calmest, sweetest voice Drew said, "It's okay buddy. It's all right. I know this hurts but it's almost over."

Then, in a voice that startled us, Marley loudly said, "Dad!"

Drew responded with, "I'm here."

Marley's body went limp. As if he had no muscles in his neck, his head fell back and I caught it in my hand. I knew he was gone.

THE LAST BREATH

And Then He Was Gone

Halfway between the standing and sitting position, Marley left us. The last breath came and went—nothing new replaced the old. Gone was the rhythm of the rise and fall, the in and out. As Cindy, Drew, and I laid Marley's body down on the bed with the realization he had just taken his last breath, Drew's fingers went to the side of Marley's throat to find the possibility of a pulse. My fear, that Drew's instinct was to breathe life back into his son, made me hold my breath. I waited for Drew's next move. My face was just inches away from both Marley's chest and Drew's face. I witnessed the miniscule muscles on Drew's forehead and around his mouth, revealing the inner process as fast as if it were my own. I knew the instant his instinct turned to release as he realized he had to let his boy go Home in peace. I inhaled once again, relieved I wasn't going to be put in the position of trying to stop Drew from reviving Marley. It was a selfless thing for Drew to do, and I'm proud of him for his courage to let Death take our son away.

Washing over the three of us was the shock of how final death is. For just a few seconds, it felt as though we were caught in between the two worlds—time stood still—none of us could move. We just held him with our faces inches from each other. Our boy's true being slipped out of my arms and deeper into the darker, calmer, simpler world of the dead. I realized I could not help my child any longer. I could not follow him. He was, for the very first time, on his own. I didn't even dare call his name, in fear that I would draw him back to the world he had just left—a world full of pain. As quickly as the wave washed in, it swept us back into the world of the living. There wasn't even time for tears. They would come later.

Rising Above

I noticed that just behind us was Julia. She stood as if frozen with her hand held over her mouth. As the three of us rose to rotate

Marley's lifeless, naked body, she came to help us by lifting his feet from the floor and lifting his head toward the pillows like we had done scores of times during the last week. But this time Marley wasn't there to help. We knew the others were gathered around the kitchen table in the next room and that they should know the end had come, as quickly as possible. So we just covered him with his favorite John Deere blanket and Drew turned to face the living. All eyes were on Drew as he said, "Everybody's gotta go in there." They all paused in a vacuum as they awaited the reason. Then he said, "Marley just died." Catie leapt toward Drew. I was powerless to move for those first few seconds, but when I rounded the corner, I saw that Drew had drawn Catie as close to him as a father and daughter can be. He stood there holding her until the next wave of chaos began to swirl.

Laura was kneeling on the bed beside Marley's body—her own body heaving with sobs of grief. She finally let go and the flood of her emotions filled the room with honesty. That little girl looked as though she had been abandoned by the only thing she knew. It was harsh to watch the rawness of her sorrow. My heart was breaking. When Catie and Vanessa came close, joining Laura and me on the bed, I felt for a moment that I was lost in a swirling darkness, caught in the riptide of a pureness of feeling I had never experienced before. These young women wept tears that were not connected to other pains of their past. This was the moment that was to create their future memory of disconnection to the world as they knew it. It is likely that all of the pain in their adult lives could be traced right back to this minute I was witnessing.

Confusion

Cindy left the room. I had to follow her. Rhys followed me. She was rushing around the house, flicking all the light switches on and telling us to do the same with such an urgency Rhys and I looked at each other in complete confusion.

"Turn them on! Turn all the lights on!" She ordered.

We thought she was following some ancient custom and that

if we didn't obey her command, maybe the souls she thought were coming to take Marley's spirit away wouldn't be able to find him. Then I thought maybe she was doing this so that her parents and brother could find their way back to the house in the dark, as they had been called to join us. But that didn't make sense… they knew where the house was, and they had a car with headlights.

Cindy was an electrician and there were light switches everywhere! After a half a minute of this madness, Rhys and I stopped and again looked at each other and shrugged our shoulders. Had Cindy popped her cork? Just then, Cindy stopped dead in her tracks and looked around as if she suddenly woke up. She flicked off the light switch that her shaking hand was on and shook her head and said, "I don't know what I was thinking. I'm sorry." Then the three of us turned most of the lights back off.

It only took a few minutes for Steve, Dick, and Pauline to arrive, and we all gathered around Marley. The room was left dark except for several lit candles and a pathway of yellow light that spilled into the room from the hallway. All nine of us found spots to nestle together and just be, letting the cells in our souls settle into a new way of living life without Marley. I half sat, half curled in a ball to the left of Marley's head as the stories began to roll, one after another for the next two hours, along with tears and laughter and an intense love for one another. We all recognized that we were sharing a moment that could never be re-created.

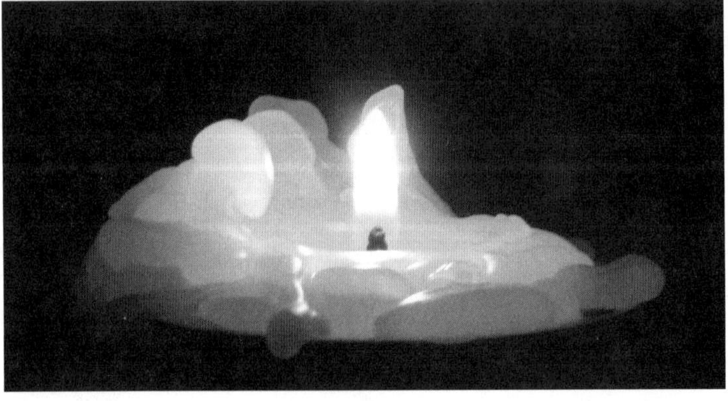

Chapter Seventeen:

Marley Rides

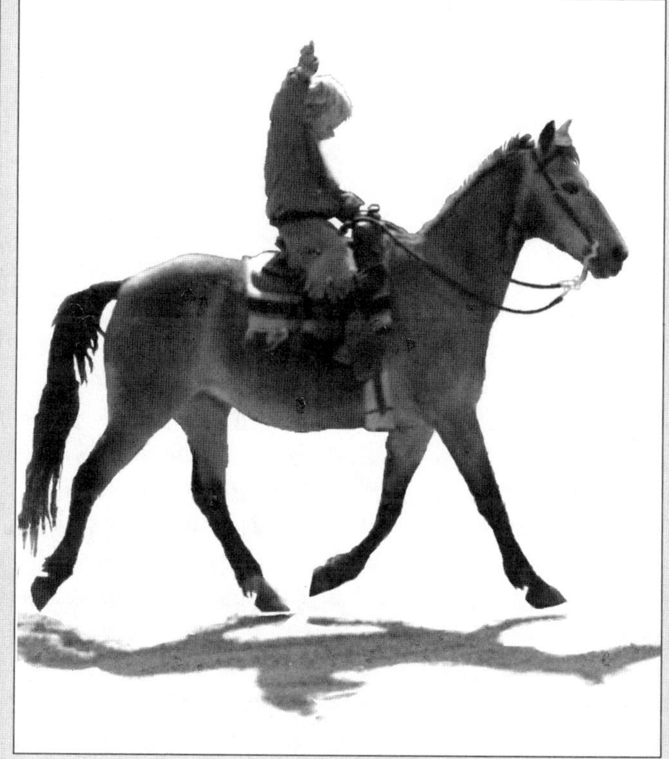

Marley, age 5, on his horse Nike
Photo: Jennifer

A NEW CHAPTER

Rest in Peace

To have the courage to keep living meant we needed to let go of the past. We realized that we could not all stay gathered around Marley telling stories the entire night. Cindy's parents said they had to leave to get some sleep. None of us wanted to leave, because unconsciously I think we knew that a new chapter in our lives had begun. We were all in shock, and no one wanted to turn the page.

We all got up and stretched. We proceeded to bump into each other, fumbling for our next steps. Julia reminded us to drink water, which gave me a temporary goal in life. And then Cindy asked me where I wanted to sleep. Once again, confusion stirred in my soul like a San Francisco fog. I had been sleeping on a cot at the foot of Marley's bed every night since we'd arrived at Drew and Cindy's. But now I was no longer needed to assist Marley in the wee hours. He didn't need me for anything anymore and never would again. Ever.

Cindy had offered to set up a tent nearby in the woods, but it felt as though an umbilical cord was still connected to Marley and it wouldn't stretch that far. If I went too far from his body, I felt sick to my stomach. All I could do was shake my head and mutter, "No. Not yet." Rhys came to my rescue and put his arm around my shoulder and suggested we sleep in the Suburban, which was parked a mere forty feet away. I relaxed. That seemed to be the limit of this strange invisible cord coming from just above my navel. Rhys didn't mind. I think he would have held me standing in a closet if that's what I needed.

The fabric of my reality had ripped apart. The hole in my heart ached. I wanted to deny the truth—to sleep near and protect Marley "just one more time." But I knew I had to honor his passage by stepping across a threshold myself. Just as Marley had courageously lived during the last three and a half years, we were the ones that now had to be brave. His role was over. The story was no longer about Marley, it was about us.

Rhys and I made a soft, comfy bed for the two of us in the back of my Suburban. It felt treasonous to fall into Rhys' arms and be held my first night. I had to keep shaking the vision of Marley's head falling back into my palm as he died. All I could hear was Marley calling out to Drew. I was scared. It felt like my chest had been punched hard. My heart hurt. My best friend had left me.

Just as I prepared to climb up onto the bed, a wash of absolute terror came over me as I met my new companion…Pain. Pain held my heart out before me, still pumping. I panicked. I grabbed my heart, shoved it back in my chest and ran fast back to Marley's room. My excuse to Rhys was that I had to get my down comforter from the cot in Marley's room. I ran into his room and grabbed the blanket, and then I stood near his still body. I felt calm clutching the comforter. There was no room for Pain near Marley. I could breathe again, but I knew I couldn't stay long.

Turning my back on Marley and walking toward Pain was one of the most courageous things I've ever done. Fortunately, Rhys was there to dull the grip of Pain. I felt safe in his arms as I fell into a coma-like slumber. My dreams of neon blue grass and balls of pure light were surreal and incredibly vivid.

The Mourning After

At first light, my eyes shot open. I sat bolt upright and looked out the tinted windows toward the house. There was a kind of a panic that flooded through me. I looked down at Rhys, who was sound asleep. Quietly, I scrambled out of our cocoon of blankets and made a beeline to Marley. As I tiptoed through the house, I was aware of the silence—it was dead quiet. The oxygen tank had been turned off, and no other bodies were stirring. I entered Marley's room, halfway expecting a miracle. His body was still there, but he wasn't. My secret disappointment made my shoulders slump.

I had told Drew I wanted to draw Marley before we did anything beyond what we had done the night before. He rolled his eyes in semi-disgust that I would want to do such a thing, but he agreed. He thought it was morbid, but I knew from experience the process was magically transformative. When I was sixteen, I had drawn my father just after he died, and again, when I was 22 years old, I had done this within hours of my mother's last breath. I knew it wasn't gruesome or unhealthy—it was healing.

During those precious minutes, alone with my son's face, I was in a state of grace. No lie. It was a simple drawing, but it captured that amazing Being in a way no photograph could. I finished, knowing deep within that I had gotten what I came for. Never again would I be able to notice every line on his face. Time stood still while I watched Death take my boy away.

***"There is no death.
Only a change of worlds."***

—Chief Seattle

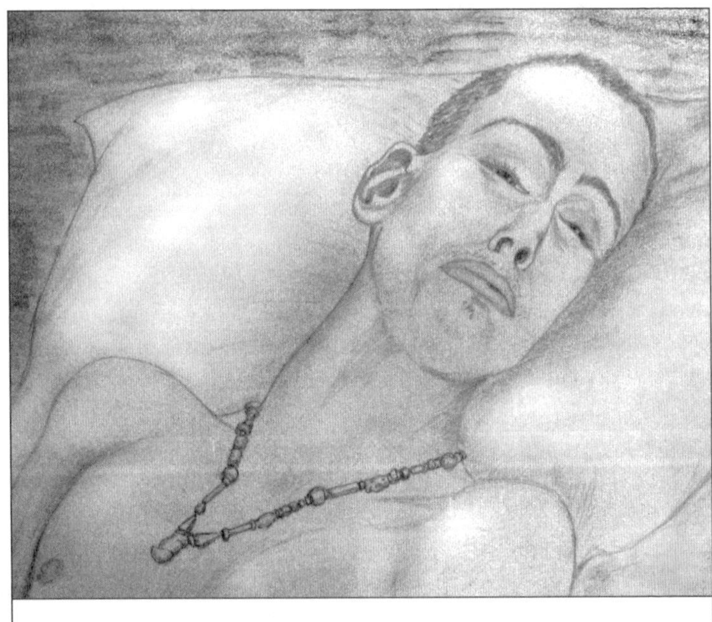

Post-death sketch of Marley

Monday, June 30, 2003
Subject: "THE MARLEY MAN RIDES"

Beloveds,

The Marley Man is free! He died last night (Sunday) at 11 P.M. Right through to the end, he led us on an amazing journey. I thought I had a handle on what a "good" death was like but, in true Marley fashion, he directed a most phenomenal final act.

The dying process took seven days (Sunday to Sunday). At the time of death, he was being moved. This was not an easy operation—it required several of us. At the end, Drew, Cindy, and I were all holding him, laying him back down on the bed, as he took one last breath. That was it. He was gone. No more pain.

It was so quick that the three of us could hardly believe that it was the end. After we laid his body on the bed, the rest of the family gathered 'round. We lit candles in his room. We cried and we laughed as we told Marley stories. After the initial shock wore off and emotional exhaustion set in, we could finally go to bed knowing our lives would never be the same.

For the next few days, the family will be tending to Marley's body in preparation for cremation. We have to take each step in this process slowly, deciding whether we can handle visitors or not. I will be updating my home voicemail daily. For right now, we are holding each other close and being quiet.

I have a feeling this is just the beginning of Marley's lessons, so stay tuned as this next chapter unfolds. Thank you so much for being a part of Marley's life. The boy certainly knew how to love in a very special way. We are blown away by how many people's lives he deeply touched.

With love,
Jennifer

DOWN BY THE RIVER

Lost in Silence

The first day without Marley was a calm, sunny, summer day. There was not a breath of wind and everything felt surreal. No one wanted to talk very loudly, like we were somehow afraid we would wake the dead or disturb some sort of otherworldly ritual. We walked around literally bumping into each other as we aimlessly moved about. I would walk outside and down the front porch steps as if I were on my way to do something, and then I would stop and realize I had no idea why I had gone outside. I wasn't the only one—everyone felt lost.

Going down to the river to Marley's altar seemed to be one thing we all could do. It was a good place to go to have intimate conversations and to check in with each other or simply be alone. Marley wasn't with us any more, so this was the day most of the family continued talking to him on paper—privately writing letters to him in the Guestbook.

Written by Cindy

My sweet child—

I am so happy that you are free at last. I am so proud of you. I tried to teach you things and you tried to teach me. We learned from each other and it wasn't always easy! But we loved each other since the day we first met, and that made it all be okay.

You fought a losing battle and yet you won the war. Your courage and spirit were an inspiration to so many people. You are a true warrior. My heart goes with you, and I pray that the wind is blowing in your face.

Cindy

June 30, 2003
Guestbook entry by Cindy's parents

Dear Marley,

You are a tree,
Our tree of life
Your roots grounding us
In the realities of life.
Your branches reaching out,
Shading us in our sorrow but
Offering us the beauty of your life
Shimmering in the dappled sunlight
of our futures.

Love,
Dick and Pauline

Containment Difficulties

Rhys took it upon himself to be my shadow, making sure I didn't walk into walls or do anything stupid. He would show up at my elbow with a glass of water to replace the one I had inevitably misplaced. It was comforting to have his body there whenever I just needed a hug or to lean against something stable.

When it was time to talk about what the next steps were, Rhys was right there. The first thing was to call Hospice, but I was scared. I told Drew and Cindy about my fear that someone was going to take Marley away from me. I burst out crying and said I couldn't handle that.

When my father died at home, we barely had an hour before the funeral home ghouls came to take my dad's body away. As a sixteen-year-old, I watched my father be carried away in a black plastic bag, and it was awful. When my mother died, we knew enough to wait for several hours before calling the coroner. We had enough time to say our good-byes, wash her body, and dress her in the beautiful gown she called her shroud. Even so, they still came and carted her off to store her in a refrigerator until cremation. When Steven died, I learned that we could see the body again before cremation...but that wasn't enough. I just couldn't handle having my baby taken away from me. I just couldn't.

Cindy talked to Kris at Hospice, and she assured us that because Marley had died from a terminal disease, an autopsy was not required. We could tend to his body until cremation. Kris told us we needed to keep Marley's room cold and to get dry ice to pack around his body. She also said she would be arriving shortly to give us Hospice's death kit and would help us create a ceremony while preparing his body.

The next step was to talk about the container he was going to be cremated in. I knew the cardboard boxes funeral homes carry were legal and cheap. Cindy said her parents had offered to cover the cost of a casket if we wanted one. It was then I told Drew and Cindy I had investigated funeral parlors and had an insurance policy that should cover the funeral costs. Rhys told us the story of how our friend Joska had made the casket for his little girl when she died. He said the process of working the wood and having a focus helped Joska deal with his pain. Drew liked that idea, but was overwhelmed on how to do that. Rhys had heard that do-it-yourself kits were available, and suggested we talk to the funeral home.

It was decided that Rhys would drive Drew to the funeral home that afternoon to make the cremation arrangements and to make the container decisions. Rhys also volunteered to pick up a supply of dry ice in Dreadford before Hospice arrived. Cindy called some of their neighbors to see if anyone had an air conditioner. Within a few minutes, one was being installed in the window of Marley's room. Once again, our lives had a focus.

The Death Kit

The kit Kris brought to us was a beautiful purple box that contained four white cotton cloths, a baggie for a lock of hair, a bottle of rose water, and another of lavender oil. The box had a place to put a picture of Marley and enough room to put a few keep-sakes.

Kris was very gentle with us. She talked about everything we might experience, the rituals that are commonly done and their origins, and the mechanics of how the body works postmortem.

Because of having had those hours with my mother, I had already warned the family that the blood starts to settle to the lowest parts of the body as rigor mortis sets in. I told them about dressing my mother—when we rolled her onto her side, I was so shocked by seeing her back a dark, purplish red that I dropped her! This time I knew what to expect and could warn the others too.

Kris explained that often, when a person dies, all of their muscles relax and the contents of their stomachs and bowels spill forth. Thus the washing ceremony was required. Fortunately, in our case, it was simply a symbolic ritual of cleansing and letting go. In the days before air conditioning, especially in the summer, bodies would decompose quickly, and the scented water and oils would help cover any smells. She also told us, that's the whole idea behind sending flowers when someone dies. Lilies have always been a favorite because they emit such a strong, sweet scent.

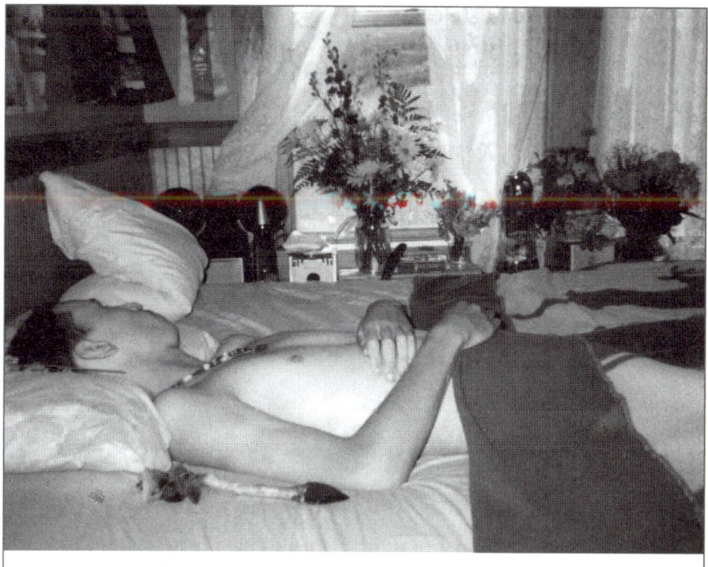

Marley's body just before the cleansing ceremony

> ***"It should be a sacred day for you when one of your people dies... A sacred day when a soul is released and returns to its home."***
>
> **—Black Elk**

After Marley was washed and dressed, Kris warned us not to be alarmed by the effects of the dry ice. She laid a layer of towels on top of Marley and placed a slab of dry ice, wrapped in a paper bag, on both his chest and his belly. Another two slabs were stored in an ice chest for when we needed replacements. Dry ice is used because it evaporates instead of melting and doesn't get everything all wet. It freezes anything it comes in contact with, so she said not to be scared if we saw ice crystals forming on his skin. The last step was to cover him with several layers of blankets as insulation.

Simply Pine

As evening approached, Drew and Rhys returned from their journey to the outside world to get a container for Marley's departure day. They opened the back doors of the Suburban and unloaded a very beautiful, simple pine casket with wood handles that ran the length of the coffin. Drew said he couldn't help himself; the cardboard box wasn't good enough for his boy, and they didn't have any kits. Rhys and Drew decided that instead of focusing his energy on making a box, Drew could instead decorate one during the next two days.

It was a very good day, designing ways to honor Marley's life by tending to his body. I was incredibly relieved that the kind people at the funeral home had agreed to work with us. No one was going to stop me from caring for my boy until his body was no longer. I had three days to lie next to him, memorize every line, and let him go.

> ***"One doesn't discover new lands without consenting to lose sight of the shore."***
>
> **—Andre Gide**

Tuesday, July 1, 2003
Subject: "DAY TWO – POST DEPARTURE"

Dear Network,

Another day passes since Marley went HOME. It's hard, really hard. The tears keep falling and our hearts hurt, and yet there is much joy. Our family unit is safely tucked away in what seems like a very sacred space. We have decided this first stage will be with just the immediate family—three private days with Marley's body before cremation. This was a very hard decision because Marley has a lot of very important people in his life that could easily be considered family. I cannot say thank you enough for loving Marley and having the courage to be loved by him. I hope he rocked your world enough so that loving will never be same.

Yesterday, with the help of Kris, our beautiful Hospice nurse, we set a bowl of rose water to warm in the sun in preparation for bathing Marley's body. Kris gave us each a clean, white cotton cloth as we gathered around his bed. Moving through their fear of touching a dead body, the girls began the bathing process as Kris held the bowl of flower water for them. The rest of us gathered around them as they gently cleaned Marley's face and neck. Then they went outside and ran together, waving the cloths in the sunshine. Through the lace-covered curtains, we watched those three beautiful creatures leaping with joy as we finished bathing his whole body. We then rubbed him with lavender oil and dressed him in his formal firefighter's shirt and badge, blue jeans, and cowboy boots. He looks so official and handsome. We are so proud of him. Today he lies fully dressed and ready for action.

Drew and my partner Rhys went to get a simple pine casket. We ripped out all the fluffy lace and satin lining—we all agreed that was not Marley's style. The denim quilt his grandmother

Pauline made for him will become the new lining. Rhys and I are sleeping in the back of my Suburban, and this morning, at first light, I woke up and looked toward the house. Drew was in the carport carving Marley's initials on the top of the casket. He had already fired up his forge and had repeatedly burned Marley's cattle brand to form a border around the outside of the coffin. The girls will be decorating the inside of the box this afternoon.

Each day is a new day spent breathing and letting go. The importance of having Marley's body remain at home with us has been incredible. It has helped us all with the shock of disbelief that he is gone. All of us have come to appreciate the old ways of caring for the dead. It seems so natural and so simple.

Soon we will make decisions about gathering for a memorial to honor Marley's life and death by dancing, crying, laughing, and screaming and shouting. But for now, this process needs to be for family as we prepare for Marley's cremation tomorrow evening.

We love you all. Thank you,
Jennifer

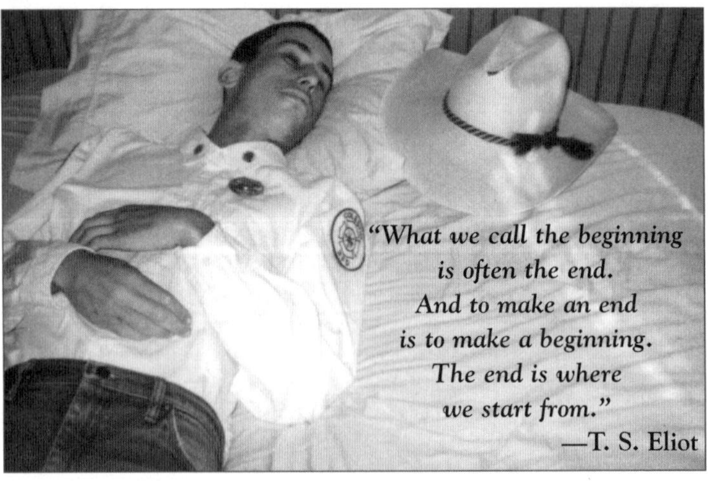

Written by my sister Constant

My beloved Marley,

You ate life up. You carved your own path straight up the steepest side of the mountain and came racing down full tilt boogy! You were my sweet boy and I loved your innocent, unabridged heart. I loved your unedited mind and voice—bold, audacious, no apology. And yet, you were so tender and kind.

I remember the day I took you to school for you to share your experience of having cancer with your classmates. You were so calm, straightforward, and courageous. Students and teachers alike were put at ease just by your manner. You opened the eyes, minds, and hearts of so many by sharing your experience and telling your story.

I am humbled by your ability to love, your determination, never growing up, and surrendering so simply and swiftly. That was such wisdom for your family. You took care of us all by that. You took care of you in that.

You touched my life with one lesson after another. Lessons of love and care, boldness, the power of communication (with or without words), growling, and free falling. You are the master of letting go.

I utterly love you,
Constant

"Nothing in his life
Became him like the leaving it."

—Shakespeare

Monday, July 7, 2003
Subject: "MARLEY DONATION UPDATE"

Dearest friends,

I am trying to find computer time to continue this amazing story. Until then…here are some answers to questions most asked.

Thank you all for your support and love.
Jennifer

Celebrating Marley's Life

Mark your calendar. We have scheduled Marley's memorial on July 21st. (Details to come.)

Three ways you can honor Marley

There are two special organizations that you can send funds to in Marley's name.

1) The Colestin Rural Fire Department (Marley lived to serve the Colestin Fire Dept.)

2) Ronald McDonald House
229 10th St., Brookline, MA 02446
(These folks were very kind when Marley had his lung removed.)

3) Frequent flyer miles – The man who prints our books at Banta asked if he could donate his frequent flyer miles to help get family to Marley's memorial service. Thank you, Paul. I cannot tell you how grateful we are to accept the 2,500 miles you have granted us. Once again, you have shown me that every once in a while, I will find real, honest-to-goodness humans hiding in the jungles of corporate land!

DECORATIONS

Great Minds

Drew had done an amazing job of personalizing the outside of Marley's coffin, and the girls had gone to town decorating the inside. There were no rules, no guidelines for what it was supposed to look like. Marley's name was written on the inside lid using strips of duct tape. I heard much laughter coming from the carport as the girls worked with each other. Using acrylics and markers, they painted vines and flowers and wrote poetry for Marley. They brought color and warmth to the pine canvas.

Aside from the florist and the Hospice nurses, no one else had entered our little private world. As the afternoon approached, we were all feeling like we were missing something…or someone. I went to talk to Drew and Cindy about including the Coyotes in this process. Drew and Cindy looked at each other and said, "We were just talking about inviting Luke and Lucas down to help the girls!" We went to check with the girls, and apparently they had come to the same conclusion—the art project needed their talent.

Within minutes the sound of engines could be heard, and a cloud of dust appeared. The boys were a bit timid as they approached the open coffin in the carport. I asked them if they wanted to visit with Marley's body. They looked at each other with expressions of both fear and excitement. I felt honored to be their guide as I led them through the hall and into Marley's very cold, air conditioned room. When Luke entered, he took a step back and said, "Oh God." The more I talked and told them about the details of what happens to bodies after death, the more both boys felt comfortable. They moved in closer, touched his face, looked under the covers at Marley fully dressed with his badge on. We all laughed when Luke knocked on Marley's very frozen chest and when I described how hard it was to get cowboy boots on a dead person.

A Work of Art

The boys spent hours on the interior of the coffin. They drew a speedometer, ranging from 0 to 3,000 mph, at the foot of the box "so Marley could see how fast he was going." Two guesses at what speed Lucas drew the needle at! A steering wheel was drawn on the inside of the lid and a hand brake on either side. Lucas just couldn't resist drawing headlights on the outside of the coffin, while Luke drew horizontal yellow, orange, and red flames on both sides. Marley's vehicle to the land beyond life was ready to go!

Constant Rides

My sister Constant had flown in from San Diego and decided she wanted to try out Marley's electric wheelchair. While the kids were busy in the carport, Rhys and I were standing next to the Suburban by the barn. Rhys' pickup was parked about 20 feet away. When we heard Constant's giddy shrieks of laughter, we looked towards the house to see her coming at us at eight miles an hour down the bumpy gravel driveway. Watching her expression as her breasts were bouncing uncontrollably had us doubled over until we realized she was going too fast to make the turn between the two rigs. In seconds flat, she slammed right into the rear tire of Rhys' truck.

The impact bounced the chair back three feet. Rhys and I ran to Constant, thinking this couldn't be good. Her ankle had taken the impact as it was between the chair's footrest and the tire. Constant couldn't stop laughing even though I could see she was hurt. She was looking up talking to Marley, saying things like, "God! Now I know how you must have felt…that was so much fun!" She looked down at her foot and started to laugh again. "It's hurts so bad, but that was *so much fun*!"

Her skin wasn't broken, but there was a serious dent in the back of her ankle. It was going to be a very nasty bruise. I worried that she had broken a few of the bones on the top of her foot. As I placed her foot back onto the footrest (which was now bent to the side) we joked that at least she was already in a wheelchair, and it was going to be easy to get her back to the house. It was a miracle: No bones were broken; she didn't sprain her ankle or cut the artery or tendon. The next day she had a minor limp, and two days later she was as good as new!

Tuesday, July 8, 2003
Subject: "DAY THREE – POST DEPARTURE"

Dear Friends,

What a long strange trip it's been. The story since Marley has died is every bit as amazing as the three and a half years he dealt with cancer and the fifteen years before that. What a tale I have to tell!

The third day of our post-death vigil was the most organized, for it was the day we all had to say good-bye to Marley's beautiful body. Drew's parents, Cindy's sister, and my nephew Winston had flown in to join us. We had gathered the night before to discuss the plan for cremation day so we all knew what to expect and what to do.

As we woke up, we barely talked. Everything seemed ultra quiet. It was as though a peaceful blanket covered all. Even the horses, dogs, and birds seemed especially quiet. Vanessa was dressed in a bright yellow sarong and black tank top. She looked so beautiful as she headed for the river with her violin to where an altar for Marley had been set up. I gathered cleaning supplies and headed for my Suburban, which was to become the hearse for the 5 P.M. appointment at the crematorium. As I cleaned, Vanessa practiced the tune she was going to play for Marley later that afternoon. The sounds that serenaded me as I polished the Suburban sent me to another world.

Midmorning, Drew approached from the carport, as Cindy came from the barn, while I was walking towards the house. We met in the middle of their circular yard. We spoke of how weird the morning felt. Just then, a blue heron flew toward us and slowly circled, gently touching each treetop around us. This graceful bird's motion seemed so filled with purpose. As it departed, all three of us burst into tears and hugged.

Catie came out dressed in a maroon tank top and a black skirt as Laura came out dressed in a black tank top and maroon skirt. Seeing the three girls together, so color coordinated, was breathtaking. They simply radiated wisdom and beauty. They joined me as I decorated the Suburban using window paint and streamers of orange bailing twine and rope.

Later, everyone gathered around Marley in the bedroom. We pulled back the covers, packed up the dry ice, and each took our turn honoring him. Some sang songs or played instruments. Others read poems or spoke from their hearts. Julia read the letters sent from those who could not be there. Catie played Marley's favorite country western song on the CD player REALLY loud, which sent us into peals of laughter and rivers of tears. It was Aaron Tippin's *Big Boys' Toys*. I highly recommend finding a way to listen to this song…it's sooooo Marley!

At 2 P.M. we moved the casket from the carport into the living room. Drew, Cindy, Rhys, Winston, and I placed Marley on his denim quilt and used it to carry Marley to his fully decorated coffin. As solemn as this event was, moving a long, dead body through narrow halls and door frames was no easy trick. All it took was Rhys speaking aloud his fear of accidentally ramming Marley's head into the wall, and we almost dropped him while laughing as the nervous tension released. After gently placing Marley in the casket, we lifted it onto a rolling stand and placed all of the flowers around it.

There in the living room, we had created a space much like what happens in a funeral parlor. Every family member had a chance to visit with Marley's body one last time and to place something special in with him to be burned. His John Deere blanket was with him, along with his horse's bridle, his lariat, chaps, knife, *Cabela's* catalog, necklaces that had been made for him, many notes, pictures, Uncle Steven's arrow point, a beautiful cross with gems inlaid, and, of course, a roll of duct tape. (Unfortunately, his saddle didn't fit!) The casket was closed and was carried to my decorated Suburban by the men.

Before leaving, Drew fired off six rounds from his .30–30 rifle. The spirit world definitely knew Marley was coming! The procession to town consisted of two Suburbans: the first driven by Rhys containing Marley, Drew, Cindy, and me, the second with Marley's grandparents, sisters, cousin, and three aunts. We all laughed and feared for our lives as we entered Highway 5, when no less than 20 semis surrounded us as we climbed the mountain pass. Even in our Suburban convoy, we felt puny and in danger of being squished. All of us thought this was Marley's way of letting us know he was still in control of things!

Drew, Cindy, Catie, Vanessa, Laura, and I went with the casket into the bowels of the crematorium oven room, leaving the others just outside. Together we all kissed his sweet face one last time, closed the casket, pushed the button to open the oven door, pushed the casket in, and finally, together we pushed the button that closed the door that separated our bodies forever. We then joined the others, drove home, and commenced to dance, tell Marley stories, and play Marley style. It was a tremendous release and a great close to one of the most intense days of our lives.

Live well,
Jennifer

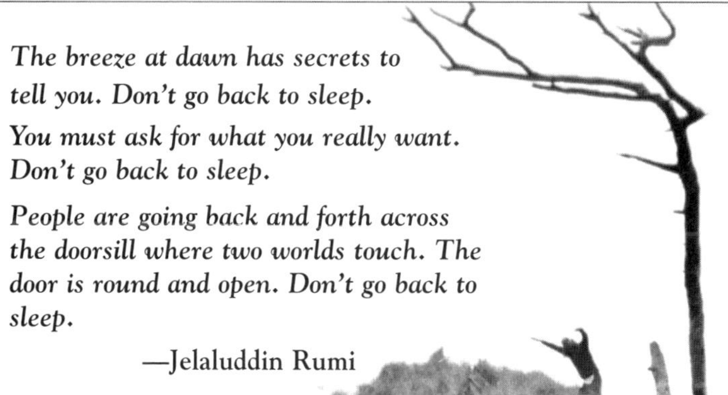

The breeze at dawn has secrets to tell you. Don't go back to sleep.

You must ask for what you really want. Don't go back to sleep.

People are going back and forth across the doorsill where two worlds touch. The door is round and open. Don't go back to sleep.

—Jelaluddin Rumi

CELEBRATING LOSS

Refocusing

Before driving back from the crematorium, we gathered in the parking lot next to the two Suburbans, feeling kind of lost. We looked at each other silently saying, "So, now what?" One of the kids asked if we could go get some ice cream. Drew, Cindy, and I groaned, realizing we were not ready to face the real world yet. Fortunately, grandparents and aunties exist. They took the lead and decided that one vehicle would go back to the ranch and the other would venture out into the world to buy ice cream. It was a perfect plan.

In retrospect, I realized the three surviving sisters had different needs and reactions to Marley's death than the three of us parents. At that moment, in the funeral home parking lot, for the first time in a long time, the focus could be aimed somewhere other than Marley. They needed some attention too! The support of family and friends was imperative for Marley's siblings to be able to lean on, yet nothing can replace the focus of parents.

I was physically, mentally, and emotionally in one piece, yet my whole being felt as though some odd hallucinogenic drug was in my system. Nothing seemed real, I had trouble focusing, and the ground seemed to be moving as though very mild earthquakes were rolling below me. I lost my balance every once in a while, for no apparent reason. I knew Catie existed and was close, yet I was in a bubble that made me feel incapable of parenting.

As soon as we arrived back in the safety zone of Drew and Cindy's ranch, like bees to a fragrant flower, we headed for the carport where there was a stash of cold beers and an enormous bottle of tequila (thanks to the folks at the Hilt store). Even Constant and Julia, who normally don't drink and certainly not tequila, held out their little hands for a shot glass. We were standing in a small circle, savoring the melting warmth of the drink while debriefing about the recent events. When the others returned, they joined us in the carport, expanding the circle.

We were all standing there together feeling a little lost

because no one had any particular task to perform. The pressure no longer existed, so we finally found ourselves relaxing. Because each of us had different focuses over the past few days, we shared the little things that had made big differences. Most of the stories were funny, and the tension was draining away. Some of the tales had us slapping our thighs and gagging for air through tears of joy and laughter.

Cindy told us about this weird noise she heard just before Marley died; it was like nothing she'd ever heard before. It came in waves, at odd times, with no apparent rhyme or reason. She heard it in the middle of the night and again the next morning. At first, she thought it was coming from far off and that it must have been a neighbor down the road. Then she realized that the sound's location wasn't moving or changing from its consistent yet varying pattern. Days later, while wandering behind the house, she finally located the source buried in the hillside. It was one of Marley's large toy trucks—an emergency vehicle with a siren and an engine that revved in three speeds. For some reason, after a year of being lost under dirt and overgrown weeds, having survived two summers and the heavy snows of one winter, the damned thing went off on its own. She reached up on the shelves behind where we were standing and showed it to us, pushing the buttons so we could hear the sounds of the mud-crusted toy. Can dead people, with a sense of humor, control the physical plane? How were the buttons activated? Was it just coincidence? All we *did* know was that the story was funny and deserved to be honored with another shot of tequila.

Let the Party Begin!

Vanessa brought out the stereo and played "Let the Good Times Roll." Still wearing our finest clothing from the day's ceremony, we all started dancing in the late afternoon sunshine. It felt so good to be outside, to dance, and to laugh. Everyone looked so incredibly beautiful, especially the three girls. I cannot describe the overwhelming joy, freedom, and love that we all felt for each other that evening. It was remarkable. If any of us had been religious, I'm sure it would have felt sinful to feel so good.

The music kept playing and we kept dancing. At one point, Constant was twirling around with her arms outstretched, looking up at the sky. Three of us saw that she was drifting dangerously close to a two-foot high drop-off, and we yelled at her to stop. She laughed and said, "I see it! I see it!" And then she proceeded to dance right off the edge anyway! She crumpled to the grass below, rolled over, and started to laugh. Instinctively we all jumped off the wall at the same time and piled on top of her. That's when the fun began!

One by one we changed into comfortable clothing and the music kept us all dancing, that is, until all hell broke loose. I was on the phone with Joseph in North Carolina, to include him in the festivities just as the water fight began. I don't know who started it, but as an experienced water fighter, I can say it was the best water fight I've ever participated in. The ammo was abundant; there was a pool on one side of the house, a hot tub on the other, and three 5-gallon water containers on the front porch. Giant squirt guns appeared and the hose was busy filling up any other container available. At this point, both sets of grandparents elected to go inside as water was flying everywhere. No one in their right mind would have ever guessed that my son had been pushed into the cremation oven just hours earlier.

As darkness fell, the game subsided and we all calmed down. The only thing left to do was to get into the hot tub. At one point nine of us were in the tub at once. We started massaging nearby feet and laughed because no one could identify even their own feet. Slowly everyone went to get changed and to eat a little food before bed. Rhys and I stayed in the tub a little longer, thankful for the quiet. Once again, he swept me off my feet when he kissed me. After years of being the closest of friends, the time to move closer presented itself. It occurred to me that as soon as Marley was gone, really gone, something in me shifted so I could focus on loving and being loved by yet another.

Saturday, July 5, 2003
Subject: "REFLECTIONS"

• From Joseph

Hey, Phurr (one of my nicknames):

I loved all the stories I have been told about the actual events of this past week. I loved being called from sleep to hear the hoop-la and your blow-by-blow account of the celebration. It was so very hard not to be there. I was absent but only in physical form. Spiritually, psychically, emotionally, I was with you as you bathed Marley's body. I stood my vigils, helped to dress him, and watched him be consumed by fire.

I feel I need reflect so little to you about how it was for me with Marley. He was of the soul with me. A wise and wonderful young man who taught so much, even in his final days, simply by mouthing such words as, "Mom, I'm bored. Can't I go Home now?" The depth of his understanding was so profound—spoken so simply, asking so little of that human moment, just to die now. Oh, Jennifer.

I know the void is there. He is no more in the flesh. There will be great grief and great relief and a mixture of both, as well as so many other emotions. The heart connection to Marley was so great. I have wept for him—my tears became sobs that racked my body. I hurt so deeply in my loss of him. His presence meant so much to me even from so far away.

I am grateful that Rhys was there for you and you have been held. I am thankful Jules and Constant were there too, for that same reason. I am also grateful I will be there for the memorial celebration.

I love you.
Joseph

Thursday, July 10, 2003
Subject: "DAY FOUR – POST DEPARTURE"

Dearest Marley-People,

As weird as it may sound, what happened after Marley died seems to be very important. As climactic as Marley's death was, these four days afterward have been intensely rewarding. The healing process has been rich and swift, because we intuitively avoided our culture's standard post-death procedures. I know that this part of the story *needs* to be told too. So after many weeks of not being around a computer, I'll finish telling you what happened in the days following Marley's death.

On day four, post-death, Drew, Cindy, and I returned to the crematorium to retrieve Marley's remains. Drew pushed the button to open the oven door, and the three of us just stood shoulder to shoulder looking at the contents within. All we could do was say, "Wow!" We had no idea what to expect. No one that we knew, professional or friend, had seen this.

Our self-appointed task was to scrape everything remaining into a bin at the front of the 7'x 4' oven. Our boy—as well as all of the items that were put into his casket—had been transformed and were displayed before us. We took turns putting on heavy gloves (17 hours later, it was still hot) and we unceremoniously scraped the pieces forward with a long-handled wire brush, then we vacuumed out the oven to try to get every last particle (a shop vac with a long attachment was used). Then I pushed the button to close the oven door.

Large portions of Marley's skeleton had remained intact. I had learned when Marley's Uncle Steven died that generally cremation includes pulverization of the bones unless requested otherwise. Apparently this standard began when people became distressed when their urns were filled with chunks instead of fine ash that "sprinkles" easily. I requested that Marley's remains not be pulverized.

The next step was to take the contents of the bin and lay it all out on a stainless steel table. The three of us began to comb through all of it and made use of the giant magnet used to collect the metal objects. We picked out the 2-pound prosthesis that used to be Marley's right knee, some of the larger pieces of the hip, skull, and vertebra, and then we began to manually pulverize the rest with our bare hands. The action of taking his very porous bones and crushing them to ash was powerful.

The girls had refrained from joining us but, after experiencing this, we knew they too would benefit from this process and would probably think it was pretty cool. So we brought the treasures home to share with the rest of the family. We spent hours around a table marveling at Marley's cremains spread out before us, sorting and identifying everything. We found Marley's teeth, the tiny metal teeth of the zipper from his jeans, and the diamonds from the jeweled necklace (unaffected by 2000° temperatures). Once again, Marley took us on a journey we hadn't expected and would have never known about. It was amazing.

I love you all with a new and larger heart,
Jennifer

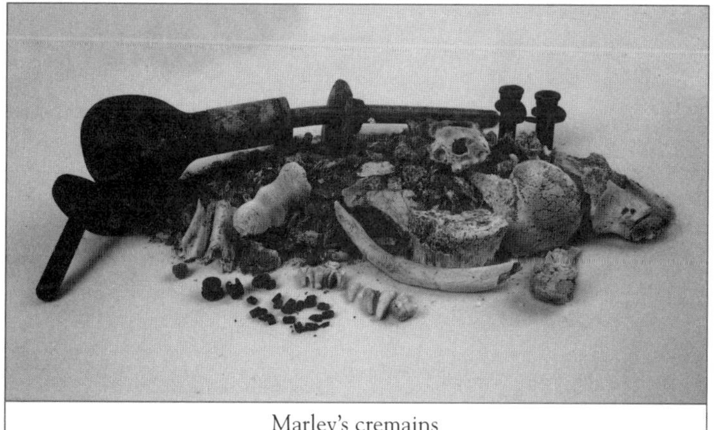

Marley's cremains

SOLO TIME

Going Home

After spending the afternoon sorting through the treasures of Marley's remains, Cindy asked me if I wanted to spend another night. As terrified as I was of leaving, I knew it was time to go home. Drew and I figured if we split custody of the kids, we should split what was left of Marley's body as well. Each pile of bone, metal, teeth, etc. was divided so we could individually decide how to disperse the "ashes." The knee prosthesis was the only problem. Each of us would keep it for a while, and then, we decided, it should go to Uncle Jay so he could work it into one of his amazing sculptures.

The two-week schedule for Catie was temporarily disregarded. She could switch back and forth as often as she wanted until life settled down again. She decided to come home with me, Rhys, Constant, Andrea, Julia, and Winston. Because no one wanted to cook, and Julia and her son were scheduled to fly back to North Carolina early the following morning, we drove to town for dinner. It was the first time I was in public since Marley's death but it seemed all right, because I was flanked on all sides by protectors.

When we arrived at my house, the first thing Winston did was to get instructions from Catie about how to drive the ATV. He roared down the road, and I realized I would never get to worry about Marley's safety again. My ears were so trained that I could hear Winston's return minutes before anyone else. When he hit the driveway, to honor Marley, Winston did a few fast donuts, spitting gravel and blowing dust into the twilight sky. I didn't know whether to laugh or cry…so I laughed.

It was a beautiful summer night, and we sat outside telling stories. I loved being home, but was scared about how I was going to handle being reminded of Marley's absence every time I looked anywhere. His Legos were right next to the outside couch, just where he had left them on the last night we were home. I knew I would be okay when Julia made Andrea and Rhys promise one of them would be with me during the first month until the shock wore off. And life goes on….

Chapter Eighteen:

The Fine Art of Grieving

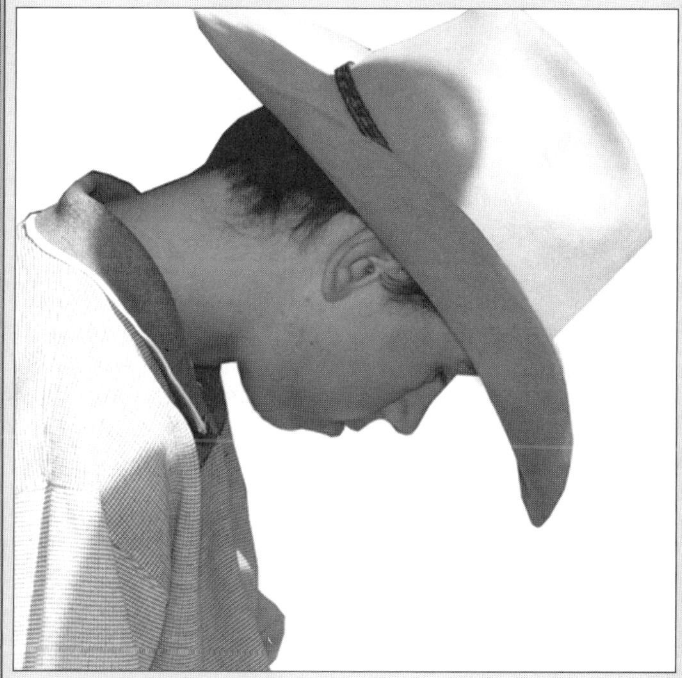

Marley

Photo: Debbie Thornton

The Butterfly Effect

My Angel
by Vanessa Blount, age 16

One breath apart from all others.
Parents sigh at the first sight of their newborn baby.
A boy, welcomed into this world, one not like any other.

One tear, encompassing all of my pain, helpless despair, heartache, and love.
A tear not for myself, but for someone close to me,
someone I love.

One laugh that shall ring in my heart forever true of one voice, that of my angel.
One smile, one smile that shall forever remain imprinted in my thoughts.

One knot that shall forever remain a knot. So worthy of what it has become, the endless tangle of rope will never willingly go back.

A lone cowboy, never afraid.
Tall tales that echo in my heart, always repeating, but softly fading away.

One family, like so many others, but with one exception: We were blessed with an angel.
Have you ever seen an angel?

They don't wear halos, have wings, or possess robes fit for kings.
Angels bring you strength and courage disguised in the form of sorrow.

Angels show you how to forgive, celebrate life, and run with your dreams. They show you what ambition is all about.

They bring you on a journey through every emotion imaginable.
Tears, loneliness, help, fire, passion, inspiration, simplicity, change, appreciation, admiration, and hope.

They gift you with their presence, but it is for you to realize on your own that it is not limitless.

This is the story of one angel, my angel.

My angel was the only person I ever knew to be a hippie, cowboy, and a crazy redneck all in one.

The only person who I ever knew to try and bring a snowball to school, in the car, in his hands, on a 30-minute car ride, and to his dismay all that remained was a puddle of water in his lap.

The only person to save a drowning frog that I was so convinced was in danger for its life.

Endless horseback adventures, accompanied with the realization that it's a lot quicker to escape a swinging punch with four legs instead of two.

When a discussion about graveyards arose while gazing out the car window, my mother explained to us that graveyards are the places where people's bodies are buried after they die. My angel asked, "What about the heads?"

Never fearing the unknown.

Rope swings, sunburns, star thistle, yellow jackets, naked bodies, and no shoes.

Baths in a fire-heated outdoor clawfoot tub, with umbrellas, in the rain.

Mud (no further explanation).

Firefighter of the year.

Stopping a moving vehicle so he could jump out and pick some flowers on the side of the road for his little lady friend at school.

Countless forts, teepees, club houses, and ideas.

The location of a long-past dead cow forever remained our treasured archeological digging site. Our bone garden.

We had room to roam; we were free, but not free enough for my angel.

Our little technician. He could take anything and everything apart, but when it came to putting things back together....

My cow wrestling companion.

The only person besides myself to have the title "the big kids" over our two little sisters "the little girls."

My partner in crime, my right-hand man, my big brother, my angel.

One day.

The day I cried until my eyes almost shut,
The day I screamed at the top of my lungs,
The day I hurt like I've never hurt before—the day my angel left me for his freedom.

They say the word "cancer" is an explanation for what stole him away from us, but really it's just a word to pin the blame on, almost like God.

As time went on, my perspective of the situation changed. Instead of thinking he was stolen from us, I began to realize that his greatness exceeded that of any other.

He wasn't just meant for me and my family (which wasn't easy to come to terms with), but he was so special that he was meant for the whole world to have a piece of him. Drifting from place to place and person to person, my angel lives on.

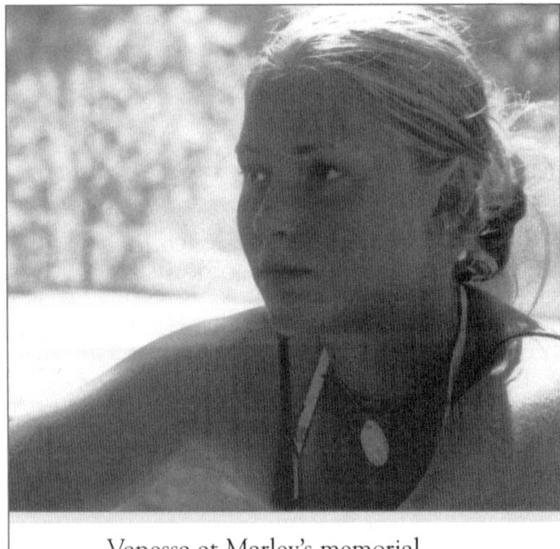

Vanessa at Marley's memorial
Photo: Reagan Burrell

18 years old.

One breath apart from all others. I watch my parents try to collect themselves as they struggle for air, watching our beloved son and brother leave this world.

A boy—one not like any other.

THE FENSTEMMERS – PART II

Mystery Solved

During the first two years of Marley's illness, we had received two incredible mystery gifts from two different people with the same odd last name, both with bogus return addresses. After that, we didn't hear from our anonymous friends until just before Marley's memorial.

When Catie and I saw the box from "The Fenstemmers" we both knew we were in for some loving. We sat on the couch out on the front porch, with a mixture of anticipation and sadness that Marley wasn't with us.

In the past, there were two gift containers in each package, one for Marley and one for Catie; but this box contained gift boxes for Catie and *me*. They were special and tender little gifts like stone hearts and gold angel pins packed in beautiful little silver heart-shaped boxes lined with velvet. Embroidered handkerchiefs were the wrapping for delicate crystal pendants designed to hang in a window to reflect the sun's light in rainbow patterns. Catie and I sat quietly, slowly unveiling each piece of intentional love as our hearts melted. Once again we were awestruck at the care and timing of the Fenstemmers' gifts. We both felt truly cared for.

Never before had any correspondence been included in the packages, only name tags. But there at the bottom of my box was a letter. It explained why we had been blessed by the Fenstemmers and why we hadn't heard from them for so long.

We had lost the Fenstemmer connection in 2001 when Franco no longer had the time to volunteer his services as our website manager. With the help of Debbie, we created a new website, but because the Fenstemmers weren't on the master list, they were never notified. Nevertheless, the Fenstemmers were back in our lives and it felt good, like having a fairy godmother return after an extended vacation.

July 2003

Dear Jennifer and Catie,

We Fenstemmers are a far-flung family, but we enjoy working together as a team to do good works in the world. We particularly enjoy small anonymous endowments to underprivileged people as well as surprise gift packages to deserving people—especially those who are hoeing a hard row and doing it with grit, determination, and faith. We found Marley's story on the Internet and unanimously agreed to support him in his struggle.

We were saddened by his death, especially because we didn't know it was coming up so soon, and we missed our last chance to serve him. The Internet was our only connection, and when the website went down, we had no information until finding the online obituary in your local paper.

Thank you for taking such good care of the soul that was Marley and for being so generous with your love. Here is a token of our appreciation for the hard work and heartache you undertook on his behalf.

Hurray for Marley in his wonderful new life!
Hurray for Catie and Jennifer for their abundant love!

Sincerely,
The Fenstemmer Family

We Are One

Support comes in all shapes and sizes, and I'm learning to accept it in all forms. I am surprised by how gifts can be so impactful long after they've been given, so I try to stay open to receiving no matter how I feel.

Friday, July 9, 2003
Subject: "LESSONS OF GRIEF"

• From: Glen

My friend Jennifer,

Recently, I lost both my wife and my mother within a few weeks. Initially, I found myself walking around kind of mumbling to myself, at times crying uncontrollably, and at times just feeling frozen, like all I wanted to do was to curl up into a ball.

I've learned there is a big difference between grief and mourning. Grief is the pain and anguish I have inside. Mourning is my external expression of that pain and anguish (or anger, pity, or a million other feelings.) Grief is NOT something I get over; it is something I go through. And the way to go through it is to allow myself to mourn. Men in particular don't do a very good job of expressing feelings other than anger.

The word "bereavement" comes from a middle English word meaning "to rob"—which expresses how many people who have lost loved ones feel. It's vital for me to remember:

First: Whatever negative or painful feelings come up—or even if feelings of relief come up—after the death of a loved one, it is all a part of a natural process of healing.

Second: It can take 18 to 24 months just to stabilize during this mourning period.

Third: It is vital that I let others know how I feel, and that I make a commitment to find ways to express the pain I feel.

Fourth: All negative feelings I express, including sadness, anger and self-pity, are appropriate and self-therapeutic.

Their death has been an opportunity for me to look at my own mortality and my faith, or in some cases lack of it. I remain committed to feel the pain I need to feel, and express it in the best way I know how.

Peace shall come,
Glen

LIFE WITH A PURPOSE

Focal Point

Planning the memorial celebration to honor Marley's life was something I thankfully had to focus on during the first three weeks of living without Marley. With the help of Debbie and Jay, a really nice tri-fold invitation was created. I spent days sitting in my outdoor living room addressing envelopes and planning the event. It still felt like I was in a state of shock, but at least I had a focus.

Condolence letters arrived daily, and many were still writing to Marley on the website Guestbook. Constant, Julia, and Andrea had all left during the second week, and Catie had gone back to Drew's. Rhys took a month off from work to be by my side and act as chauffeur if I needed to go to town. Being in public scared me to death after the first time I tried to go to the grocery store. Having to face getting hugs, making decisions, and realizing I had to relearn how to shop and cook was awful. Eating at restaurants was even worse: I was a sitting duck for well-wishers. So I avoided town as much as possible. Staring off into space, crying, writing in my journal, and being close to Rhys were the only things I could deal with.

"Grief teaches the steadiest minds to waver."

—Sophocles

Losing a child is a truly terrible thing, and comfort in any form was good. Jay and Brianna came up to my place to design a special space in the woods so we could have a place to put Marley's ashes and his favorite things. The sacred spot they created was a circle of stones overlooking a steep ravine. They placed a chair in the center and put his favorite keepsakes around the circle. It really helped to have a place that I could go sit.

Trying to stay as close to Marley as possible meant I spent many hours sitting at his altar. Each day I spent less time visiting Marley's spot and more time focusing on making plans for the memorial celebration.

Saturday, July 10, 2003
Subject: "MEMORIAL INVITATION"

MARLEY'S MEMORIAL GATHERING

Marley Jacob Pratt died Sunday, June 29th at 11:00 P.M. This vibrant, courageous young man touched the hearts and souls of so many. We invite you to gather to celebrate the 18 years he generously shared with us.

When asked what he wanted his memorial service to be like, two weeks before he died, he requested that each of us share our favorite Marley-story around a campfire in a wilderness setting. He knew the power of flickering light in the darkness allows for a greater level of caring and honesty. He wanted us to get to know each other. He wanted us to get to know him. He wanted us to get to know ourselves.

Marley's life was never easy. He required us to stretch beyond our comfort zone. He asks, even now, for us to take a Monday off from the "normal" world to join his family in the "real" world. He would always ask, "What's *really* important? What you're doing now or playing with me?" Hmmm. He tried so hard to teach us to "be here now," to forget the rules, and to work hard at playing. Let's honor his life by gathering Marley-style!

• We'll start the day with Marley-play: floating down the river, hiking, fishing, throwing horseshoes, and playing volleyball. • At 5 P.M. a BBQ/POTLUCK will commence. • At 7 P.M. the evening ceremonies begin with a bagpipe salute by the fire department honor guard. • Then we'll gather 'round the fire and each of us will share our best Marley-story.

Camp with us that night and howl at the moon. Bring fishing gear, bathing suits, towels, toys, warm clothes, lawn chairs, musical instruments, a tent, food, and drink. Be prepared!

THE MEMORIAL

Gifts of Heaven

Family started arriving from all over the country the day before the memorial. It was Sunday, and once again it was irrigation day at Drew and Cindy's. So we all gathered at the ranch for pipe moving fun, a big dinner, and the "give-away." We displayed Marley's things for family to go through and take what they wanted. Luke and Lucas were the first to take what they wanted. It turned out to be a very funny fashion show with lots of laughter.

The memorial was at the Tree of Heaven campground. We spent three days playing by the river, being surrounded by almost everyone who knew Marley. A newspaper reporter came and spent the second day with us, interviewing people and getting a taste of who Marley was. Tents were set up everywhere, banners were hung, a memorial altar was created around the fountain that had been made for Marley's Monster Bash. Jay painstakingly dismantled it from its spot at the office and re-mantled it at Tree of Heaven. As much joy as was there, the altar was a place for people to go to cry, place their gifts, or to just sit in silence.

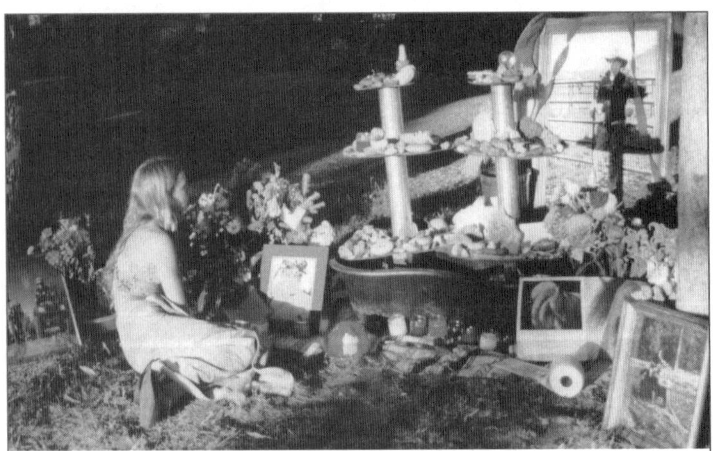

A guest at Marley's memorial altar
(Note the shadow cross on the picture of Marley)
Photo: Selene Foster

Let the Grieving Begin!

A heat wave hit Southern Oregon on the second day of the memorial celebration. The temperature peaked at a blistering 118° that afternoon. It was impossibly hot, but the Tree of Heaven campground was in a deep ravine, fully shaded, and with a river ready for massive water play. Plans had to change: It was simply too hot for a fire ceremony to be the focal point of the evening. We couldn't bear to grill or eat hot salmon, chicken, or even the home-grown beef that Drew and Cindy brought. Munching cold-cuts and clutching cold beers was all most of us could handle. Some folks even dragged their folding chairs and put them right in the river.

The fire department's honor guard was scheduled to start the evening's ceremony with a bagpipe procession, but sadly they had to cancel. Due to the heat wave, they were busy fighting scores of brush fires. That afternoon, we had to shake our heads in amazement when a grass fire started in the same ravine as the campground and the fire department was called to put it out. Rhys, wearing Marley's fire jacket, joined Drew and a few other thrill-seekers in helping the firemen who came to the rescue.

"Victory often changes her side."

—Homer

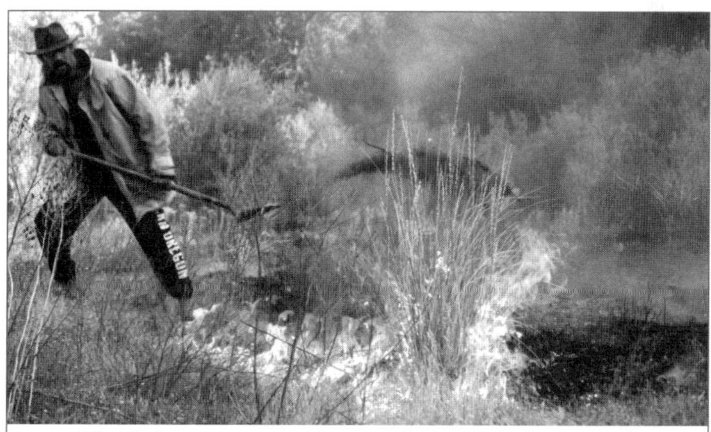

Rhys helping to put out the grass fire at Marley's memorial
Photo: Jay Newman

Several of the firefighters were members of the honor guard, and after the fire was controlled, they joined us, laughing at the circumstances. They said that they would have brought their bagpipes if they had known they'd end up coming to the memorial anyway! Marley didn't get his official tribute, but he did get the crew there and some hot entertainment.

Still wet from swimming, hundreds joined in a circle for the evening event. Annie, Jeff, and another dear friend began by singing the songs Annie had sung at my house the night Marley started his dying process. Then one by one, people of all ages and backgrounds stood in front of the altar to tell their Marley-story. Some had us laughing to the point of tears and others made us cry.

I heard things about my son I never knew, told by people I had never met. A police officer told us about the last time he saw Marley; he was speeding through a cemetery on his electric wheelchair. He said because it was Marley, there was nothing to do but shake his head, return Marley's big smile, and wave back at him. Several young women had the same theme to their stories; they said they weren't sure if they would ever find a man who would love them the way Marley did—unconditionally and so fully. So many voices, so much heart. After two hours with no end in sight of people wanting to share their tales, as darkness fell, I suggested we move over to the small fire that Jay had started.

Although it was hot, the glow of the fire pit was exactly what Marley wanted. Musicians gathered as folks milled around and collected in small pockets of connection. The party continued into the wee hours. As guests fell into their tents to sleep, slowly the sound of the river overpowered us all. Jay, Jeff, and I stayed up all night sitting inches away from an enormous portrait of Marley that had been given to us for the event. I was incredibly thankful to have friends close by. I knew as people left the next morning that it was up to me to start a new life—one that would honor Marley's death.

"Death is more universal than life;
everyone dies but not everyone lives."

—A. Sachs

Thursday, July 31, 2003
Subject: "IN RETROSPECT"

Dearest Clan,

One month has passed since Marley left. I have trouble understanding that he's truly gone. I'm sure this will take time. My mind is just beginning to focus, and it's a little easier to be around people. Every time I encounter people, I hear new Marley-stories. It's like a continuation of his memorial.

I know he understood more at 18 years old than most of us might learn in a lifetime. I ponder who Marley was, why he had such a profound effect on people of all ages and backgrounds, and what he ended up teaching us. All I do seem to know is that Marley was an unusual kid. I will start to investigate if there are others like him, really like him. Are there other kids teaching the same things? Lessons like how to love unconditionally no matter who you are or what your story is, how to have the courage to continue walking when there are no bones beneath, the strength to resist what doesn't make any sense, and the wisdom to know who you are and what you stand for all the time. I want to start paying attention!

I'm not sure what happens next. I'll take it one step at a time.

Catie, Laura, and Vanessa are at Cindy's family home in Wisconsin. I fly there tomorrow to pick Catie up, and then together we'll drive to Minnesota to return to where I was born. Family…yum!

Thank you,
Jennifer

P.S. Nike, Marley's beloved horse of fifteen years, lay down in the pasture and refused to continue. After everyone said goodbye to this remarkable horse, Drew put him down. Now Marley has his horse and together they can RIDE!

Monday, August 04, 2003
Written by non-kin family Jeff

Hey all in Marley-land,

I'm honored to be a part of this network of people. The memorial a few weeks ago reminded me of just what an incredible, amazing, soulful group surrounded Mars. By the time I gathered the nerve to speak at the memorial, we dispersed and I didn't get a chance to honor Mars verbally.

This is something close to what I might have said: Mars, I miss you more than I expected. I hear your voice in the strangest of places and swear I see you out of the corner of my eye every now and again. Lanky teenagers, motorized wheelchairs, some kid yelling "mah-ah-m!" These things bring you back for a split second, and I'm left with this peculiar feeling of fleeting recognition. Like a haunting, I guess, but in the best way possible.

It's hard to choose a Marley-moment to single out. Often they were little moments, like the sweet hugs you'd give at odd, unexpected moments, or the times you'd cajole me into playing or mock me for working rather than playing. I remember five or six years ago when we used to wrestle. One evening outside the office, you just up and sacked me out of the blue. I remember hitting the ground and hearing (and feeling) several loud pops. When I stood up I felt better than I had all day. You'd just adjusted me. Best chiro work I've ever had done—you should have charged me.

A couple of weeks before your death, you appeared in one of my dreams. I'll never forget it. We were at the BRI office, which in the dream was out in the woods somewhere. I was dressed up and waiting for friends to pick me up to go out. You walked by and begged me to play with you, but I wasn't up for it and didn't want to get my clothes dirty (boring adult). You went on your merry way and I continued talking to whomever was in the office with me. After a few minutes you reappeared in the doorway with squeeze bottles of ketchup and mustard, threatening to squirt me with them. I gave you a look that said don't you dare. In real life I think you would have just threatened and backed down. But in the dream you fired. I was pissed, livid. I had just heard about your toxic calcemia, though, and knew that you might not be around much longer. I couldn't bear the thought of my last words to you being angry. So I choked down my anger and walked outside.

Annie walked up at that point, you came over and we hung out for a bit. I can't remember exactly how, but the three of us were somehow hugging. Not in the conventional sense—our bodies were connected via arms wrapped around one another, linked side-by-side. It felt more like a hug than it looked. Regardless, it was a great feeling of connection. After a bit, we separated and I, for some strange reason, jokingly hugged a tree. Then we heard Jennifer and Jay approaching. You were behind me now, kneeling over a log on the ground, and started tugging on my shirt. I groaned inwardly thinking you were going to give me some kind of grief, then turned to face the sarcasm/taunting I was expecting. Instead I turned around to see you looking up at me with the most wide-open, beautiful, heart-breakingly loving expression on your face. I melted.

Then I awoke. It was about four in the morning. And I just lay there in my bed sobbing until I fell back to sleep. I know it's not very cowboy of me to say, but that was just the beginning—I've cried more in the past month and a half than I have in my entire lifetime. For me, that's a gift. Mars, I've been honored to be a part of your life for the past six years and more so to be a part of your dying process.

Thank you so much. I love you.
Jeff, Ashland, OR

Monday, August 25, 2003
Subject: "REMEMBERING TO BREATHE"

Dearest Marley-People,

Just wanted to briefly check in with you. We're doing all right, I think we inherited Marley's courage.

It's easier to breathe (during the first month it felt like someone was holding my chest really tight). Remembering that the Marley-man is not with us is the hard part. We all have our own Marley-habits that have to be unlearned. I don't have to buy two gallons of orange juice when I shop, Catie doesn't have to scoot the car seat up as far as possible, I don't have to collect dirty dishes from Marley's room at the office before I leave, and although it's hard to remember, I don't have to count the pills he's supposed to take every night. It's getting easier every day.

Catie and I returned from our trip to Wisconsin and Minnesota safe and sound. It was great hanging out with Laura and Vanessa and playing in the lake. It was so nice to laugh. It occurred to me that I had never taken a road trip with only one child in the car. I discovered that Catie is truly a remarkable creature—it was a pleasure traveling with her. She's a wonderful mix of woman and little girl. She's incredibly strong yet so very tender. I am in awe of how well she's dealing with the loss of her brother.

Unfortunately the day before we returned, we received a call from Ashland with more bad news—our puppy was run over and died. Now Marley not only has his horse, he has his puppy too! Here's to Amazing Grace, may she romp free.

I love you all and thank you for being a part of this story.
Blessings,
Jennifer

The Butterfly Effect

COYOTES— AN ENDANGERED SPECIES?

by Lucas Rex Morgan, age 15

As I sit here, I think to myself what things have changed my life and I'm pondering why these things have happened. A few years ago, I lost my father, and every day since then I have thought of my life as more precious. Every breath I draw in is a gift. I also think how a young man I only knew for a short while changed my life in many ways. His name is Marley Pratt, and he will always have a connection with my way of living.

On the outside, Marley may have looked and sounded pretty rough, but on the inside, his views were certain and his personality was solid. He knew exactly who he was. He always dreamed of being a cowboy—growing up on the cattle drive, living a good tough life, and riding into the sunset after a hard day. I saw that dusty old cowboy in him all the time I knew him. There was one small detail he left out; his horse was made of steel. He lived a fast life but not a bad one. He did grow up on a ranch in the high plains and did live the tough lifestyle of a cowboy, that is, until he got cancer. From then on, his life would never be the same. Sometimes I wonder how he lived as long as he did. All I know is that he was the toughest, orneriest hombre I ever laid eyes on.

After a struggle with the Make-A-Wish Foundation, he got his Mule. He named her Annabelle after a girl he liked that moved away. That Mule was no sweetheart; she was slow, heavy, and handled like a lumber wagon, but we all loved her. But when we were going down a hill, with the wind behind us, and Marley hit the gas, Annabelle would give us the biggest adrenaline rush we could get.

About two years after I met Marley, he became extremely ill. The "extremely" lasted for a week before my idol, Marley Jacob Pratt, died at 11 P.M. on June 29th, 2003. With a good life behind him, two desperados stood in the distance of a dusk summer day and watched him leave the earth. He is gone now, but that doesn't make me feel constant sorrow every waking moment, for I value life every day, and I know I am lucky to be alive. (Surviving the time I knew him amazes me!)

Marley was crazy, and when I say crazy, I mean no-fear, all-out monster of a person. I've heard legends of him jumping out of 15-foot trees and jumping his bicycle off rim rocks. He also liked to test how good gravity worked while in the Mule. Once we actually got it about four feet in the air but after that stunt, the suspension didn't really work too good any more. His dad was oblivious of how many times the Mule has been rolled over (about four times).

We didn't know what the word "fast" meant until Marley got his Arctic Cat 400 for Christmas. Going 55 miles an hour with all three of us on the quad gave us a pretty good idea. Marley's "Wild Cat" stayed at his mom's place except for the one time he rode it to the Colestin about four months after he got it. In that one day Marley rolled her twice! The Wild Cat had a scary sounding muffler tone—just hearing it sent shivers through me.

When the question comes up, 'Why was Marley a good friend?' I can say that Marley was not just my best friend; he was my brother. He had something in his emotional attitude that made him different from any other person. He never feared anything, and he had a great tolerance for pain.

He never really spoke about the possibility of dying because that's not what you're supposed to think about. Not that he was afraid of dying, it's just that he wanted to live life. (Who cares about the future!) I've never gotten angry at Marley. I think it's because I come from a family that loves each other no matter how bad of a thing the other has done, and like I said, Marley was my brother. Marley has gotten pretty mad at Luke. He got mad at me for making fun of his voice once or twice. Actually, the night he broke his hip and never walked again, he was really pissed at Luke. He just felt sick of him. He was going on about how Luke had no respect for nature. He couldn't stay mad for long, though, because he only lived nine days more. I tried to be with him as much as I could.

To give him the utmost credit and to make him happy when

he died, my uncle set up a day in that week that Marley would be honored as the Colestin Rural Fire District fireman of the year for 2003. Spite the pain, spite the misery, Marley cracked the biggest smile he could. There was a tear in the eye of just about everyone in that house.

In memory, Marley will be honored as a fighter, a strong person, and a Coyote. His redwood cross looks over the sacred Colestin Valley, and the heavens open up with sunlight and speckle on the granite. The Coyotes will ride with Marley in our midst, when the blistering desert unleashes our machines from its heat waves. With pride, may his spirit live on. He will be missed.

"The Coyotes?" you ask. "Where will we go?" The remaining Coyotes are still here! We need someone to not replace Marley but to sort of take his place until my brother Mark can learn to ride and be as badass as Marley was. I don't think it's ever going to be the same without the Mule smashin' the back my quad or hearing Marley's "Yipiocyay!" just before making his descent down a steep hill in neutral, but we will keep on riding. We will keep on living with everything we have. The coyotes live…forever.

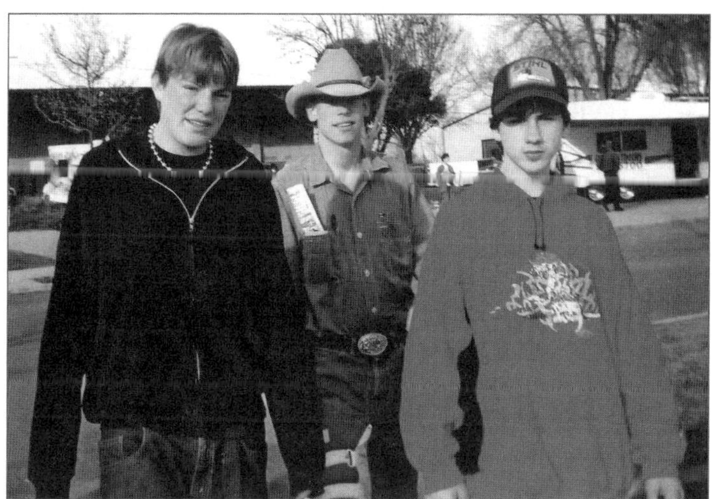

The Coyotes; Luke, Marley, and Lucas (May 2003)

Photo: Elizabeth Morgan

Sunday, November 2, 2003
Subject: "TRACKING LOSS"

Dearest Marley Network,

TRACKS

Four months ago, a perfectly square, naturally formed stone was tossed into a very deep, perfectly still pond surrounded by a chaotic world. And Marley was gone. Now, I hear reports that the ripples are still hitting the shore, which is amazing because the pond seemed very small at the time. I guess looks can be deceiving. It turns out Marley's pond is vast—the parameters have yet to be discovered. Sometimes I think I'm an island, but I am continuously reminded I am not. I know it's time to write and yet I have no clue what to say or how to say it.

SIDE TRACKED

I've done pretty well communicating the facts surrounding the events of Marley's illness and transition, but everything seems to be changing. The story has changed and so, it seems, must the reporting. The events are no longer tangible. Words are painfully inadequate.

Five months ago, when people would recount an experience they had with Marley, a "real life" explanation of the events would follow. Now people recount experiences they've had with Marley post death. Because he's not physically here, the stories are now of dreams, visitations, odd feelings, etc. and the words choke in their throats. Apparently these post-fatal experiences are no less real. In fact, it seems they can feel more impactful. The words used to describe them seem pale (black and white in a world full of color), frustrating many. The worst part is because their experience wasn't tangible, it's often not trusted.

BACK TRACK

About a month after Marley passed over, I drafted a letter to the 17,000 members of the Bathroom Readers' Institute, the group devoted to reading the books we create every year. This letter explained there had been a death at the BRI and that our standard level of communicating with them may be next to nothing. And instead, we would be focusing on doing everything within our power to meet our deadline so they would have their 2003 edition of the *Bathroom Reader* (aptly named, *Uncle John's UNSTOPPABLE Bathroom Reader*). I'm proud to say, not only did we meet the deadline, we produced possibly the best book so far! Making these books under the best of circumstances is always a challenge, but to do it while grieving...well...we did it, and we did it with grace.

The purpose of sending the letter to BRI members was to buy us some time and explain our lack of communication. Building this bridge between our work and our personal lives resulted in a much bigger network. The response to that letter was amazing. Over 100 heartfelt e-mails were sent to the BRI, and scores visited Marley's website, many telling their own story on the Guestbook. Many letters said things like, "I always knew you all must enjoy your work and each other; that's why the books are so much fun. I am very sorry for your loss."

ON TRACK

The point to this story is, the story is not yet over. Things change—everything changes—but nothing ever dies (stops, ceases to exist). This story is not just about Marley. It is not just about our family. It is about an amazing network of people who changed the life and death of a boy and who were brave enough to be changed by him. This story is never-ending, because the ripple effect of our love is now the history from which we build our futures. Thank you for your courage.

I love you very much,
Jennifer

LIFE IS BUT A DREAM

Spirit form

The night I wrote the "Tracking Loss" e-mail was the eve of Marley's four-month anniversary of being in spirit form. That night I had my first Marley dream.

We met in the doorway to my bedroom. I was with Catie and Rhys. Surprised by seeing him, I exclaimed, "Marley! You're dead!" He smiled one of his ear-to-ear grins, cocked his head, and with his long middle finger, rubbed between his eyebrows. (Marley always did have a sassy way of flipping me off!) He then flopped down on the bed, and I was able to sit with him as I laid my hand on his heart place. It was a really sweet dream.

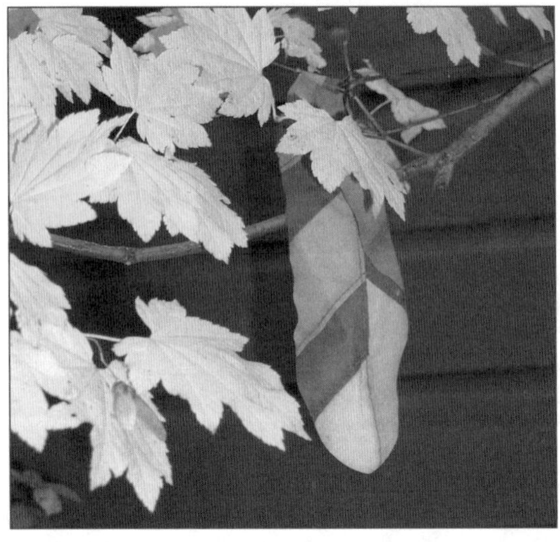

"It is wonderful that five thousand years have now elapsed since the creation of the world, and still it is undecided whether or not there has ever been an instance of the spirit of any person appearing after death. All argument is against it, but all belief is for it."

—Samuel Johnson

Friday, January 16, 2004
Subject: "NEW YEAR'S RESOLUTION"

It's a new year.

I can't even remember the last letter sent to you. I write to you all the time at home, but getting the info digitized requires staying at work late where there's a computer and electricity! Thus, many letters never quite make it to you. This one will… because I'm actually writing it on my new laptop, in my new office at home and by the natural light of the sun. [Valley girl voice] Ohh my God!

Another reason you haven't heard from me is because I've been busy training Julia to take over the management of the Bathroom Readers' Press. Yup! That's right. As of December 5th, I quit. It's a bit like jumping off a cliff in the fog, but I am following my gut instinct. There are still a few steps to take before I'm ready to land, so I hope it's a high cliff.

I've just spent a large portion of my savings adding on to my cabin in the woods. This was supposed to happen last summer to allow Marley wheelchair access and to give Catie a "real" room (she's been in the loft since she could climb the ladder). Needless to say, it didn't happen as planned. Marley didn't get a chance to see his new room, but he would have loved it. It's now being used as a place for me to write our story: *MARLEY RIDES*.

I will concentrate on writing this award-winning book in record time, assuming it will become an award-winning screenplay. I trust that a great publisher will jump at the opportunity to help produce and distribute this gem. And, of course, millions of readers are eager to buy several copies of *MARLEY RIDES*. And all this will happen before I run out of money! The world according to Jennifer—a very strange place indeed, but it's the best world I've seen…so off the cliff I jump! The next few months of diving into this story will either make or break me.

On a very personal note: Please do your best to never be a grieving parent—it so sucks, you can't possibly imagine. Nothing I've ever experienced holds a candle to this. I'm functioning fine, it all looks good on the outside, yet my heart hurts so bad, it's hard to breathe.

Catie is skiing as much as possible and has joined the Mount Ashland Racing Association. She pounds down the food, towers above me, and is very pretty (it's difficult to remember she's only 14). She has been focusing on friends this year rather than academics, which is fine given the circumstances. She continues to be a total pleasure in my life.

I love and thank you all for being a part of this story.
On a Path with Heart,
Jennifer

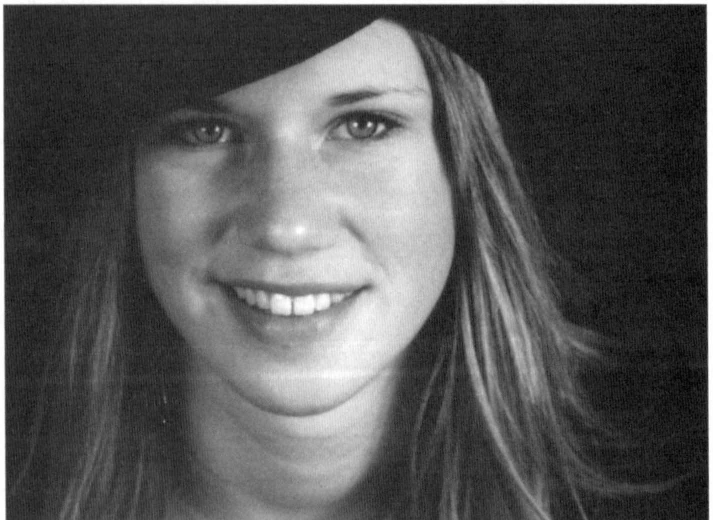

Pretty Catie

Photo: Debra Thornton

GESTATION

Weather Patterns

It took nine months for Marley to grow in my womb, and it took me the same amount of time to feel human after he died. Some days were good, some were bad, and some were all across the board. I had quit my job to write this book and to focus on me, Catie, and Rhys, but secretly I didn't want to live without Marley.

Enough time had passed that most of my friends thought I was doing fine. I didn't think they wanted to know how I *really* felt, but they would still ask anyway. Even if they were brave enough to listen, there seemed to be no way to convey how it felt inside. I felt crazy. I felt alone. I felt numb.

On my nine-month anniversary, my soul had grown cold from trying to keep it all together. I had laryngitis—a fitting disease for someone who was avoiding honest communication and feeling pain. I jumped in a hot bath with a book called *The Grieving Parent*. I was stopped dead in my tracks when I read:

> "Worst of all, far worse than lying awake all night were the mornings. There seemed to be a daily brief period shortly after I opened my eyes when I completely forgot Robby was dead. Then, like a tidal wave, remembrance would come and engulf me and make me feel as if I were drowning. I had to fight my way out of bed every day—and I mean every day. Nothing in life can be more emotionally draining than struggling to leave one's bed. If it takes all that much to get up, what energy is left for the rest of the day?"

Boy, did she hit the nail on the head! The internal storm clouds began to slowly roll in. I curled up in a ball on the couch with the the roll of pictures I took of Marley just after he died.

It had been months since I'd looked at those pictures. Within seconds the tears flooded until I was gasping for air. When I could cry no more, I could feel the warmth within once again. Mourning was the miracle that allowed me to continue living.

Sunday, February 8, 2004
Subject: "BLAST OFF!"

Never a Dull Moment!

Oh my God! Marley had a great 19th birthday party on Friday night. I took a week off of writing *MARLEY RIDES* to prepare the perfect celebration. The goal was to give Marley the memorial he requested. Marley said he wanted us to gather around a campfire after his ashes were launched in a giant firework. This was not an option during Marley's memorial, because of the blistering temperatures. His birthday seemed to be the time to fulfill his wishes.

We planned to set off the fireworks from the top of a craggy butte I live below. Beacon Hill was a favorite destination of Marley's while cruising on his ATV. All we needed was a clear night with no wind. It was beautiful all week, until Friday morning. Rhys and I sat on the front porch watching the rain. Just as we decided to cancel the event, the skies cleared.

The tiki lamps were being filled as the first brave soul arrived. It was time for Drew and our volunteer pyrotechnician to take off on the ATV to go to the launching pad to set the explosives. The first display was a 6-foot wide x 4-foot tall "set piece." This was made of plywood cut in the shape of the brand which Marley designed (his initials, scrambled, all touching: JMP). At 8 P.M. the fuse to the set piece was lit in the middle of the pasture. It worked perfectly, lighting Marley's symbol in a glorious display of color which hissed and spat sparks for about 30 seconds. As this died out, the crew on top of Beacon Hill set off the first of two perfectly executed fireworks.

The first one was for Laura (Marley's stepsister, four years his junior). Marley and Laura have always shared this same special day, so it was a great time to celebrate her first solo birthday. A four-inch shell was launched in her honor. The firework itself went 200 feet in the air, but because the launching pad was at the top of Beacon Hill, the effect had double the drama. After much cheering, we paused for the main event.

Count: One, two, three, four…BOOM! In your mind's eye see the white tail rising, then the shell exploding, igniting 100 blue stars, creating the large outer petals of the burst and 30 red to green stars exploding in the center. As the shell blew up, creating the most amazing eye candy, Marley's ashes were dispersed. Everybody whooped, howled, clapped, and cheered. Hugs all around as we walked back to the fire pit to tell tall tales.

Our beloved pyrotechnician put in many hours building a firework worthy of Marley—one big enough to represent this remarkable young man and strong enough to carry his ashes high, high in the sky. It was an eight-inch plastic shell that shot out of three-foot mortar that shot upward 300 feet. It was pretty amazing.

Around the campfire, Drew told us about the many times Marley got his Kawasaki Mule stuck in the mud. One time, the UPS driver stopped to pull him out. Then he "got stuck" again and waited for the next unsuspecting person to come along, to feel sorry for him, and to pull him out. (What a way to kill time!)

Jay related the first time he and JD met Lucas. Marley took JD and Jay for a Mule ride and passed Lucas on a 3-wheeler. Marley said, "That's Lucas, he's cool." Then he proceeded to get the Mule stuck in the middle of the mud bog so Lucas would have to pull him out.

It was a great night and Marley would have loved it. I had the distinct feeling he was there. It was one of the few days I didn't miss him. At midnight, when it stated snowing, I knew he must have had something to do with the weather clearing too!

I love you all,
Jennifer

The Butterfly Effect

This story was received a year after our last gift box had arrived from the Fenstemmers. Not only did it provide another piece to the mystery, but it made me remember the impact we have on each other's lives even if we don't know each other.

MY MARLEY MIRACLE
by "Marvin Fenstemmer"

When I was young, I had some neighbors who were very poor. One Christmas I assembled a splendid gift package for them and left it on their doorstep in the middle of the night. They never knew I was the one who did the deed. They talked about it for weeks, and it thrilled my heart every time I heard them wondering who had been so kind. From that moment on, I was addicted to playing secret Santa, or secret Valentine, or simply secret friend. As the years passed, I became better and better at it—and more and more addicted.

I feed my addiction by shopping as often as possible at garage sales, thrift shops, and flea markets. I collect tiny trinkets and interesting tokens, pretty necklaces, miniature bells, beads, lace, music boxes.... In short, toys, treats, and treasures of every type. I sort them out and store them in my basement. Then, when I cross paths with someone who, for whatever reason, needs an extra special surprise, I assemble these treasures into the nicest gifts I can possibly create and I deliver them—anonymously—to the recipient. Children are my favorite target, especially kids who are suffering some sort of hardship.

When I heard about a kid named Marley who lived in a town several hundred miles away, I knew he was going to be receiving a heavy duty dose of my mystery magic.

Marley was a special kid. He was unable to read or write, yet he could completely disassemble and reassemble a motorcycle.

Marley was 15 years old when he was diagnosed with a rare form of cancer. As he grew, the cancer grew too. Yet he displayed a courage and optimism that inspired those around him. During the three years he struggled with the illness, he received many magical packages from me without ever knowing who sent them.

Marley died in the summer of 2003.

Later that summer, I was once again hitting the garage sales, collecting items for the next recipient. I spied a deliciously pretty jewelry box, inlaid with mother-of-pearl. It was missing its hinges and the latch was broken, so it was priced at only a dollar. Inside, there was a tangle of costume jewelry. I knew I could replace the hinges and repair the latch. I offered fifty cents for the lot. The deal was done.

Later that afternoon, I sat down to see what was inside the box. I sorted through a collection of odd earrings and broken necklaces and assorted coins—nothing much of interest or value. But then, in the bottom of the box I found a pin. The pin was made of wire bent in the shape of letters. As I rubbed the dust off, I saw that the letters spelled a name…and the name was Marley.

I guess I could dismiss this as coincidence had Marley been named Bob or John or Tom. But Marley was the only person I knew who was named Marley. I could not fathom how a pin spelling out his name found its way into the bottom of a beautiful broken box that I bought for fifty cents. Truly, it seems the only reasonable explanation is that Marley put it there for me.

I consider this my thank-you gift from a young man named Marley who never had a chance to thank me while he lived. This story is my way of saying, "You're welcome."

Sometimes miracles can be very small indeed. Sometimes as small as a pretty pin inside a broken box.

June 19, 2004
Marvin Fenstemmer
123 North Southeast Ave. West
Albuquerque, NM 543211/2

THE FENSTEMMERS – PART III

The Mystery Continues

I don't know if the "Fenstemmer family" is a one-person show or not; it really doesn't matter. For simplicity's sake, if "they" exist, I'll just call "them" Marvin. I hope Marvin knows how much his gift-giving has given to my family. I hope someday I can actually hand him the gift that Marley and Catie made for him that was returned. It is among the few special things of Marley's that I've saved. These items surround me in his room, which is now the place where I write every day.

The Fenstemmers gave the gift of unconditional giving—a rare and very special thing, especially these days. Marvin's story reminds me of a wonderful movie I watched with Marley just before he died, called, *Pay It Forward.* It's based on a book by Catherine Ryan Hyde, who created an action plan within a work of fiction. It was about the efforts of one boy who is caught up by an intriguing assignment from his new social studies teacher. The assignment was to think of something to change the world and put it into action. Young Trevor conjures the notion of paying a favor not back, but forward—repaying a good deed done to three new people, who in turn must pay it forward to three new people, and so on.

Since the book's release in 2000, a real-life social movement has emerged, not just in the U.S., but worldwide. What began as a work of fiction has already become much more.

Like Catherine Ryan Hyde's idea and Marvin Fenstemmer's actions, I sincerely hope this story about Marley's Network—the ideas, actions, and prayers—will impact the lives of many. I hope the gift of Marley's courage and his desire to bring people together rubs off on millions of people. If their lives are beneficially changed by his life and my re-telling of it, and they want to give thanks, I ask they pay it forward with their own courage and desire for unity. It is in this way I will send my thanks to all of those who were a part of Marley's Network.

"And we should consider every day lost
in which we have not danced at least once.
And we should call every truth false
which was not accompanied
by at least one laugh."

—Friedrich Nietzsche

RESOURCES

Making Sense of Living and Dying:

We Who Have Gone Before by Steven Foster with illustrations by Selene Foster © 2002, Lost Borders Press

The Roaring of the Sacred River by Steven Foster and Meredith Little © 1989, Prentice Hall Press

Last Letter to the Pebble People: Aldie Soars by Virginia Hine © 1977, Unity Press

Networking by Jessica Lipnack and Jeffrey Stamps © 1982, Doubleday

The Denial of Death by Ernest Becker © 1973, The Free Press

Living Your Dying by Stanley Keleman © 1974, Random House

The Caregiver Helpbook by Schmall, Cleland, & Sturdevant © 2000, Legacy Health System

The Home Care Companion's Quick Tips for Caregivers by Marion Karpinski © 2000 Healing Arts Communications

Caring for Your Own Dead: A Complete Guide for Those Who Wish to Handle Funeral Arrangements Themselves by Lisa Carlson © 1987, Upper Access Publishers

The School of Lost Borders <www.schooloflostborders.com>

Hospice <www.HospiceFoundation.com> (800) 854-3402

Pay It Forward Foundation <www.PayitForwardFoundation.org>

Make-A-Wish Foundation <www.wish.org>

Ronald McDonald Houses <www.rmhc.org> (630) 623-7048

Natural Burial Company <www.NaturalBurialCompany.com> (503) 442-1430

Green Burials <www.GreenBurials.org>

Grieving:

The Bereaved Parent by Harriet Sarnoff Schiff © 1977, Penguin Books

Healing a Parent's Grieving Heart: 100 Practical Ideas by Alan D. Wolfelt © 2002 Companion Press

The Courage to Grieve by Judy Tatelbaum © 1980, Lippincott & Crowell

Medical Stuff:

The Complete Cancer Survival Guide by Peter Teeley & Philip Bashe © 2000, Doubleday

Fundamentals of Anatomy and Physiology by Frederic H. Martini © 1995, Prentice Hall

The Encyclopedia of Medicinal Plants by Andrew Chevallier © 1996, DK Publishing

The World Book Medical Encyclopedia © 1989, World Book, Inc.

Wall Chart of Human Anatomy © 2001, Anatographica, LLC

Encyclopedia Anatomica © 1999, Taschen (This is the one that grossed even Marley out!)

Ulman Cancer Fund for Young Adults <www.ulmanfund.org>

National Children's Cancer Society <www.children-cancer.com>

Special Love for Children with Cancer <www.speciallove.org>

Sibling Support Project <www.chmc.org/departmt/sibsupp/default.htm>

Family Resource Library Project <www.interlog.com/fcc/library.html>

Candlelighter Childhood Cancer Foundation <www.candlelighters.ca>

CancerNet <http://cancernet.nci.nih.gov>

Families of Children with Cancer Resource links <www.interlog.com>

Quotations:

One Makes the Difference by Julia Butterfly Hill © 2002, Harper San Francisco

Where Two Worlds Touch: Spiritual Rites of Passage by Gloria D. Karpinski © 1990, Ballantine Books

The Medicine Wheel: Earth Astrology by Sun Bear and Wabun © 1980, Prentice-Hall

Uncle John's Colossal Collection of Quotable Quotes by the Bathroom Readers' Institute © 2004, Bathroom Readers' Press

Uncle John's Quintessential Collection of Notable Quotables by the BRI © 2006, Bathroom Readers' Press

Sacred Journey of the Peaceful Warrior by Dan Millman © 1991, KJ Kramer

ORDERING INFORMATION

To order copies of *Marley Rides*, contact:

Hart2Heart Innovations
PO Box 580
Ashland, OR 97520

www.MarleyRides.com
jennifer@hart2heart.com

Cost:
Each copy of ***Marley Rides*** cost $20.
Wholesale discounts available for resale.

Shipping & Handling:
Book rate (7 – 10 days) $4. per book
Priority (3 – 5 days) $7. per book

Payment:
Send a check (please include the shipping address), or go to the website (*www.MarleyRides.com*) to pay with a credit card.

Continued Networking:

It's always a wonder to learn how folks hear about *Marley Rides*. If you are so inclined, please write about your journey to Marley's world and how it has effected you.

Word of mouth is a powerful marketing tool. This book was created on a shoe-string budget, and was self-published. If there's anything you can do to help *Marley Rides* touch the hearts of more people, please let me know!

Jennifer